Traditional Herbal Medicine in Northern Thailand

Comparative Studies of Health Systems and Medical Care

For a list of titles in the series Comparative Studies of Health Systems and Medical Care, see back of book.

VIGGO BRUN & TROND SCHUMACHER

Traditional Herbal Medicine in Northern Thailand

with a list of medicinal plants by Terje Bjørnland and Trond Schumacher

UNIVERSITY OF CALIFORNIA PRESS
Berkeley / Los Angeles / London

University of California Press
Berkeley and Los Angeles, California

University of California Press, Ltd.
London, England

Library of Congress Cataloging in Publication Data

Brun, Viggo, 1943–
Traditional herbal medicine in northern Thailand.

(Comparative studies of health systems and medical care)

Bibliography: p.
Includes index.
1. Medicine—Thailand. 2. Folk medicine—Thailand.
3. Herbs—Therapeutic use. I. Schumacher, Trond,
1949– II. Title. III. Series.
R611.T45B78 1986 610'.9593 84-28026
ISBN 0-520-05271-4

Printed in the United States of America

1 2 3 4 5 6 7 8 9

Dedicated to our main informants

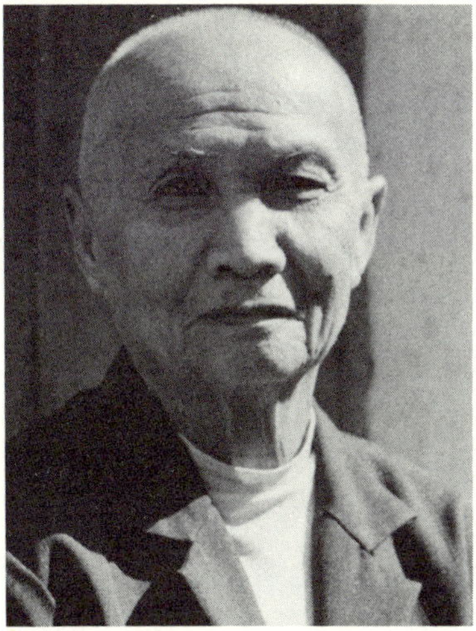

PO LIANG TAN THAMMAKHRONG
Myang Nga Village, Lamphun
(1900–1979)
(*Photo: Terje Bjørnland*)

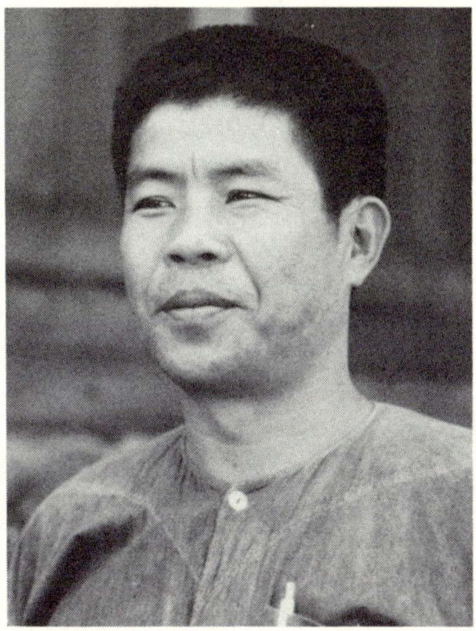

PRADIT NANTHAWI
Pong Noi Village, Chiangmai
(*Photo: Viggo Brun*)

Contents

Preface

This book presents the results of an interdisciplinary study aiming at a description and analysis of the herbal medical tradition of Northern Thailand. Field studies were carried out from June 1978 to February 1979 in the provinces of Chiangmai and Lamphun in Northern Thailand by a team consisting of Viggo Brun, lecturer in Thai at the University of Copenhagen, Trond Schumacher, medical doctor and botanist, University of Oslo, and Terje Bjørnland, chemist and botanist, University of Oslo. Interviews and discussions with informants were carried out in the local dialect, partly by Mr. Brun, and partly through bilingual (Northern/Central Thai–English) assistants assigned to Dr. Schumacher and Mr. Bjørnland. The processing of the data has, parallel with other duties, continued for four years at our respective universities in Oslo and Copenhagen after our return.

The study naturally falls into three parts: an ethnomedical, a botanical, and a chemical one; however, only the ethnomedical results are published in this volume. The botanical and chemical data will be published separately.

A list of the collected medicinal plants together with their uses is presented in the Appendix. The aim of the ethnomedical part was to study the local disease system, that is, to arrive at an understanding of the local disease terms, their classification, and the underlying theories behind this classification. As far as possible we also wanted to identify the local disease terms with cosmopolitan concepts. The collection of medical data turned out to require much more time than expected, and thus became the most extensive part of our studies. Our approach was intensive rather than extensive, in that we chose in-depth interviews with a few herbalists within a limited area, rather than superficial interviews with many herbalists in a larger area. We hoped in that way to secure a representative amount of data of high quality. These in-depth interviews were supplemented with sporadic interviews with other herbalists, with nonherbalists (patients and villagers), and also—in order to make sure we had not overlooked any disease terms or basic medical vocabulary—with a study of local medical manuscripts.

Our relationship with the herbalists was a personal one based on mutual interest. We did not enter into any formal teacher-pupil relationship with any of them, nor did we make any promises or formal arrangements regarding economic compensation for the information they provided. We did help them in various ways, however, when natural occasions arose—with transportation, buying things they needed, contributing cash to specific purposes, and so forth. But there were no direct obligations involved on either side. The herbalists talked freely about the diseases, and we experienced no obstacles in getting data of this type. A general problem was the lack of standardization of the medical vocabulary. It also proved difficult to separate sporadic knowledge acquired from the urban traditional medical schools from the knowledge of the rural medical tradition proper. And, finally, it was sometimes difficult to know when the herbalists were inventing answers to questions they did not know anything about—a problem familiar to all ethnographers.

Our idea was to let an herbalist describe the pertinent disease concepts in his own way, making sure, though, that questions concerning the cause, the symptoms, the possible progressions, the treatment, and so on, were raised, as well as questions like "Are there other types of . . . ?" and "What is the difference between . . . ?" in order to elicit possible subcategories and borders with other concepts. The information thus obtained was written down with phonemic transcription to keep the local expressions intact. When this cognitive part of the interview was over, the physician of the team asked some additional questions pertinent to diagnoses and to a possible delimitation and elucidation of the concepts.

Obviously, a meaningful interpretation of the relationship between the diseases in the two medical systems—the Northern Thai and the cosmopolitan—could not rest on a verbal description only, but had to be supplemented with direct observations of diseased persons, which we made together with the herbalists. This latter requirement proved difficult to fulfill in practice. Patients arrive erratically and infrequently to consult the herbalists, who normally have only a few consultations each day. Also the herbalists do not keep records of their patients' names and addresses, so it was impossible to trace them, unless we accidentally stumbled into one of them during our interviews. The result is that in many cases the biomedical diagnoses rest on oral information only, and must therefore be regarded as preliminary suggestions. The instances when a diagnosis is based on direct observations as well have been marked with an asterisk in the text.

We have made a particularly detailed study of skin diseases because skin diseases are rather common among the villagers, and quite a few of the patients consulting the local herbalists were dermatological cases. Furthermore, with the kind assistance of the Dermatological Section of the Chiangmai Clinic, we were also able to arrange an artificial clinical situation in which one of the traditional healers together with the physician of our team—Dr. Schumacher—had the chance to make their diagnoses and observations on patients at the clinic simultaneously without, however, Dr. Schumacher making any attempt to offer treatment. About one hundred patients were observed in this manner.

Our study is limited to the medical practices of the herbalists. We made no study of mental diseases, nor of other practices related to diseases and their treatment, such as shamanism, divination, and other rituals, although on occasion they will be briefly referred to. We did not study the local health-care system, and we made no systematic investigations into the sociological aspects of the tradition.

We have, however, found it natural to present a description of the urban variant of Thai traditional medicine—here called the "Royal Tradition of Wat Pho"—as a contrast to the rural variant of Northern Thailand. This we feel is rather important, first because we want to emphasize the differences between the two traditions and, second, because it is the urban school that has received the attention of most scholars up to now, and which is generally regarded as *the* medical tradition in Thailand. Still, we want to emphasize that our study of the urban variant is not a complete one. We have only included information from the written sources of this tradition, and from only one out of several textbooks, namely, the one on traditional pharmacy.

We have been able to locate quite a few sources related to the ethnomedical and historical aspects of the tradition. As there exist no extensive bibliographies on this subject elsewhere, we have decided to include all references we have come across, even if we have not been in a position to consult all of them.

The outline of the book is as follows: we first describe briefly the historical and cultural setting of which the tradition is a part (chapter 1: Introduction), followed by a description and analysis of the royal medical tradition based on printed data (chapter 2). Then follows a description of the medical tradition in rural Northern Thailand based on our own data. In chapter 3 we record briefly the position of herbalism in relation to other traditional methods of cure, the knowledge of the tradition and the way it is transferred, the basic medical vocabulary and concepts, and the general outline of the disease panorama. In chapter 4 each of the local disease concepts is described in detail, and classified into a larger unit. In chapter 5, we discuss the confused relationship between drugs and diseases in Northern Thailand and suggest a way to solve the confusion and, lastly, chapter 6 gives an overview of the general position of traditional medicine in present-day Thai society.

Due to the abundance of data and the nature of the subject, it has proved impossible to incorporate all the information on one particular topic in one and the same place. Instead of having numerous cross-references in the text, we decided to assemble the references in indexes at the end of the book. These indexes are vital for an effective use of the book.

Northern Thai words are rendered according to a standard phonemic transcription, as used by Søren Egerod in "Studies in Thai Dialectology," *Acta Orientalia* 26 (1961).

Translation of disease terms is, generally speaking, problematic, and not always possible or relevant. We have chosen to give—as far as we can—a literal translation of the disease terms when they appear as headings to a section; in the text block we have normally left them untranslated.

The outline of the book and the description and analysis of the Northern Thai medical tradition and concepts in chapters 3 and 4 are the result of a truly cooperative effort. The collection of data, and the writing of the first draft of the remaining chapters were, however, the fruit of individual efforts. Chapters 1, 2, and 6, plus sections 5.2, 5.3, 5.5, and 5.6, are Viggo Brun's; Trond Schumacher is the author of sections 4.1, 5.1, and 5.4.* In spite of this natural and necessary division of labor due to our different academic backgrounds and knowledge, we have both profited from each other's comments and criticisms. The book as it stands is thus a product of an interdisciplinary cooperation—and at times compromise—between the humanities and the natural sciences.

*The collection and identification of the botanical material in the Appendix is a result of joint efforts by T. Bjørnland and T. Schumacher.

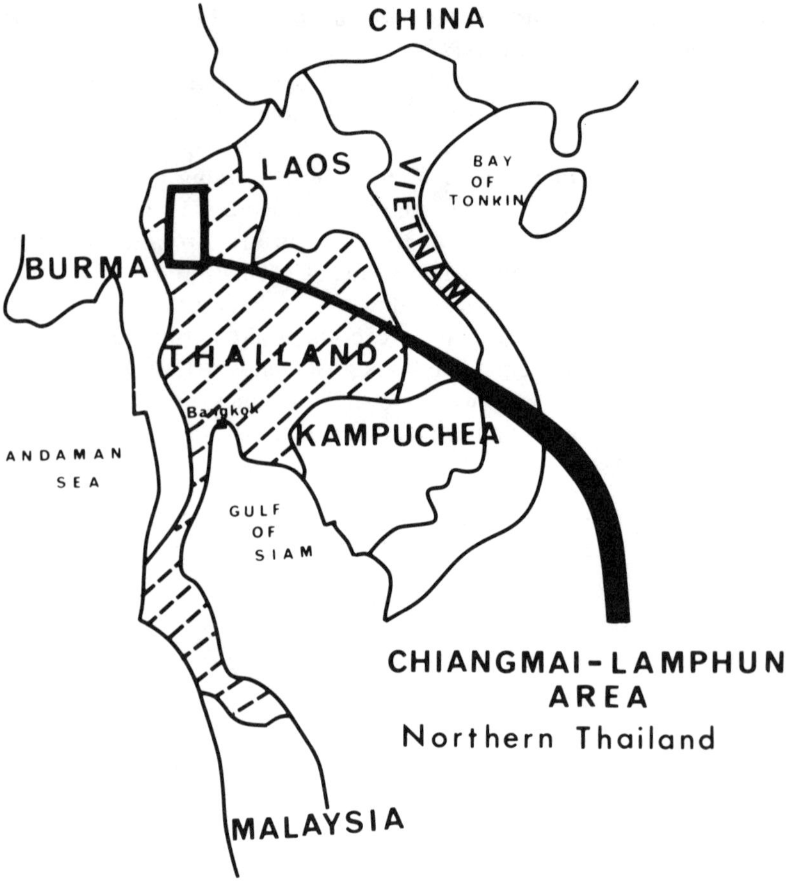

Research area in Southeast Asian Context

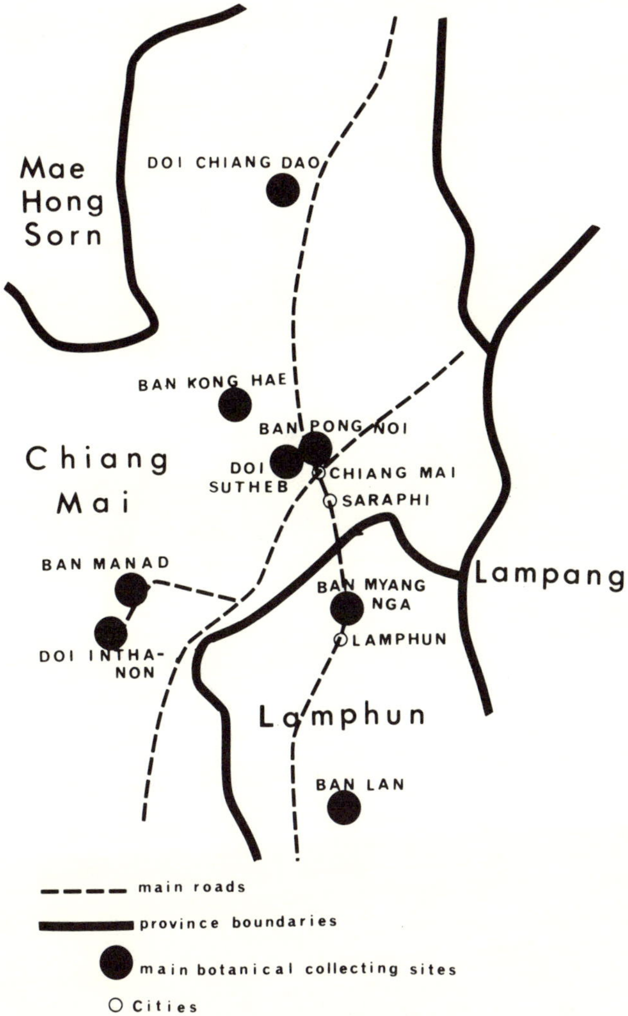

Research areas of Chiang Mai and Lamphun provinces, Northern Thailand

Acknowledgments

This book has been made possible by the assistance and support of the following institutions and individuals:

The Norwegian Agency for Development (NORAD) supplied all the necessary funds for the project, and the National Research Council (NRC) in Bangkok secured the research permit in Thailand. We extend our deepest thanks and appreciation to both institutions for their generosity and cooperation.

Terje Bjørnland, the chemist-botanist of our team, has, with discussions and suggestions, influenced the general outline in the ethnomedical part of our study.

The data were supplied by local informants. We are particularly indebted to Po Liang Tan Thammakhrong (Myang Nga, Lamphun), Mo Camnong Tonkid (Saraphi, Chiangmai), and Po Liang Nan Mi Wannaphrom (Lamphun), but a host of other informants supplied data as well. On the botanical side we have been lucky to share the enormous knowledge of our botanical guide, Pradit Nanthawi (Pong Noi, Chiangmai).

We had several part-time assistants working for us during various periods: Det Yainthorn, Vicharn Horprayoon, Nuntawut Juncaroen, Ugrit Xuto, and Prakhong Piamsiri.

We also thank the following people who copied medical manuscripts for us: Maha Chom Thebmongkhon (Sanpajangnom, Lamphun), Po Liang Nan Mi Wannaphrom (Lamphun), Khru Anan Wisaj (Pa Daet, Saraphi, Chiangmai), and Nan Di Munninta (Pong Noi, Chiangmai).

Dr. Trevor Smith at the Chiangmai Clinic graciously allowed us access to an office in the clinic and also to his patients and his files, which made possible an intensive comparative study of skin diseases.

We had several inspiring discussions with Thai scholars and experts and received many suggestions from them. We especially want to thank Bencha Yoddumnern and Awrathaj Caroensilapa, both from Social Science and Humanities, Mahidol University, and Panida Karnchanapi and staff at the Department of Medical Science, Ministry of Public Health.

Dr. Eric Grinstead helped us with the language at one stage of the writing process. Dr. Charles Leslie's positive evaluation of the manuscript and his valuable advice helped us through the final editing phase. We particularly want to thank Joan P. Leemhorst, our copy editor, for her thorough and intelligent corrections and suggestions. We remain, though, solely responsible for any errors that may occur in the book.

The people who helped us in one way or another with the botanical and chemical part of our study will be mentioned in forthcoming articles.

We appreciate the typing assistance of the secretaries at the East Asian Institute, University of Copenhagen—Marianne Klem and Kirsten Landorph—and of Charlotte Winther.

We especially want to thank the villagers in Myang Nga, Lamphun, for their overwhelming hospitality, and our wives and children who came to stay with us in Thailand, and who, then and later, tolerated our changing moods and irregular working hours.

1

Introduction

1.1. THAILAND— HISTORICAL AND CULTURAL SETTING

Traditional medicine as it exists in Northern Thailand today is the result of a long historical and cultural development, and although our study is basically a synchronic one we feel it is indispensable to trace the most important historical lines and cultural influences that have molded this tradition into what it is today. This background knowledge will—at least partly—explain the considerable regional, local, and even individual variations that exist within the Thai medical tradition, and especially the development of the urban and rural variants.

The Thais—like the Burmese and Vietnamese—are not among the original inhabitants of mainland Southeast Asia. These three ethnic groups migrated southward into the region, the Thais being the last to arrive. When the first Thai-dominated kingdoms appeared in what is present-day Northern Thailand in the thirteenth century, the Thais had already been infiltrating the area from Yunnan and other parts of southern China for centuries. The Thais continued their southward expansion, and new Thai-dominated kingdoms appeared farther and farther south: in Sukhhothai (1250–1350), in

Ayuthaya (1350–1767) and, finally, in Thonburi and Bangkok (1767–). These kingdoms were ruled by Thais, but the majority of the inhabitants were—at least originally—not necessarily Thais.

The Thai kings have, up to the last century, looked to the emperor of China for official recognition, and tributary missions were regularly sent to the Chinese court. These ties with the Chinese empire, which were mostly a matter of formality, were a prerequisite for the lively seaborne trade that developed with ports in southern China. This trade brought Chinese immigrants to Thailand, and the Chinese have come to play an important role in the social and economic development of the country.

Thai culture, however, came to be heavily influenced by India, indirectly through the Mon-Khmer civilization that dominated the lowlands of Southeast Asia at the time the Thais first arrived. These local civilizations had been for centuries strongly influenced by Indian culture. The Thai court followed the pattern of adopting (and adapting) the indianized culture of the people they conquered. During the Ayuthaya period Indian influence thus became firmly established in many domains: the concept of divine kingship replaced the original Thai version of feudalism; Indian law—the Code of Manu—became the model for Thai law; the astrologers surrounding the king were Hindus; the alphabet was modeled after Indian (and Khmer) alphabets; Indian literary genres and metrics were introduced and, of course, Buddhism became the national religion.

But besides the continual influence from the two "superpowers," India and China, Thailand had continual and reciprocal cultural exchanges with neighboring local powers, like the kingdoms of Malaysia and Indonesia, Cambodia, Laos, and particularly Burma, which was Thailand's main rival for centuries. Southeast Asia was until recently comparatively underpopulated, and the many wars fought during the centuries were fought mainly to obtain manpower. When one army conquered another, its main booty was thus prisoners of war who were brought back to be resettled in the country of the victors. This moving back and forth of sizable portions of the populations in this area contributed—together with the migrations—to an extensive mixture of the populations and their cultures. But Thailand has also had contact with cultures farther away. In Ayuthaya town there was an Arabian quarter, and at one time a king of

Ayuthaya had a royal bodyguard consisting entirely of Japanese soldiers.

And, finally, the European presence has also been felt. The first Europeans to arrive were the Portuguese in the first decade of the sixteenth century, but the Dutch, British, and French were particularly active from about 1600 to 1690. The European attempt to dominate Thailand failed, though, and was followed by a long period when Thailand was almost closed to Western influence. In the first half of the nineteenth century the Europeans were back on the Asian scene in full force, but the impact of this presence was not felt directly in Thailand until the Bowring Treaty of 1855, which had a profound economic impact. Western influence has since then been steadily growing and is today strong indeed, in both the economic and cultural domains.

This brief historical and cultural summary serves as a background against which we must evaluate the development of what we are concerned with in this study, namely Thai traditional medicine. The medical tradition in Thailand is part of a cultural tradition that has received impacts from many quarters over the centuries.

But before we go on to discuss this tradition in detail, we have to remind the reader of another important characteristic of Thai society and culture: the difference between town and countryside—between the court and the peasantry. Thai society was traditionally an intensely hierarchical and centralized society aimed at controlling the labor of the vast majority of peasants, slaves, and prisoners of war. The king and his court of royal family members, concubines, and nobles were the center of all power, administrative and economic. Culturally the external influences—especially the Indian—first pervaded the court, where they were accepted and remained, but were only partially disseminated in the countryside. In many respects, the court was a cultural enclave: Buddhism, as practiced at the court, was accompanied by Hinduistic rites and practices unknown to the peasants; court literature and drama were different indeed from the literary expressions of the peasants, and, as we shall elaborate on later, there developed at the court a medical tradition heavily influenced by Āyurvedic medicine, which in many respects was quite different from the medical tradition as practiced in the rural areas.

1.2. TRADITIONAL THAI MEDICINE

1.2.1. General characteristics

Traditional Thai medicine has until the present century been transmitted individually from teacher to pupil—partly orally and partly by means of handwritten manuscripts—and is practiced by males only. The materia medica is taken mainly from the botanical kingdom, but with ingredients also coming from the animal and mineral kingdoms. The prescriptions often contain many ingredients, and the principles of preparing and administering the medicines are common to the tradition. Magical practices and incantations are an integral part of traditional Thai medicine. Traditional herbalists do not perform any kind of surgery on or dissection of the human body,[1] and their views of anatomy and the functioning of the body are thus quite different from those of the West. Traditional medicine is the ancient art of healing indigenous to Thailand, but it has, over the centuries, received influences with various degrees of impact from surrounding medical traditions so that today it does not appear as one unified tradition. In addition to the outside influences, the aura of secrecy that surrounds the tradition has hindered communication among the practicing herbalists, a fact that has further enhanced local and individual diversity.

From a *historical* point of view there existed up to the last century two types of traditional curers: those practicing inside the court ("royal doctors") and those outside ("common doctors"), the adjectives referring to the social status of their patients.

From a *contemporary* point of view we still have to reckon with basically two types of traditional medicine:

The urban variant, which is the direct heir of the royal tradition, and which is taught at the various traditional medical schools.

---

1. Some traditional doctors now perform minor surgery, like lancing abscesses. In certain situations the fetus is removed from the womb of a woman dead in childbirth. This operation, performed at night at the cemetery, is not done by traditional doctors, though, but by people practicing black magic, who use the magically potent fetus in their occult practices. People in Northern Thailand generally have an aversion to the idea of being operated on.

It is standardized in the form of printed textbooks, it contains explicit theories, and it is the only form of traditional medicine that is officially recognized.

The rural, or village, variant is the traditional medicine as it is practiced in the countryside. This variant, which has hardly been studied up to now, consists of several regional subvariants. The characteristics of the Northern subvariant will be found in chapter 3. Needless to say, the distinction between the urban and the rural traditions is not a clear-cut one. They certainly have influenced each other and, on a practical level, they have many things in common. But in order to find out how and in what way they differ, we have to keep them apart for the time being.

From a *legal* point of view there is only one type of traditional doctor in Thailand today, namely, the doctor with a license. This license is issued by the Ministry of Public Health and can only be obtained by passing certain examinations based on the textbooks of the urban schools, which again are reprints of textbooks with roots in the medical tradition of the court.

We will use the terms *royal* and *common* in historical contexts, and *urban* and *rural*, or *village,* in contemporary contexts, but basically *royal* and *urban* are synonymous, and so are the terms *common, rural,* and *village.*

We also employ the term *herbalist* in order to distinguish this type of curer from other categories of traditional curers in Thailand.

1.2.2. History

Little is known about the history of traditional medicine in Thailand up to the mid-nineteenth century.[2] At that time there was a division of traditional practitioners into the so-called royal doctors and the common doctors.[3] The royal doctors (mɔ̌ɔlǔaŋ) were men who practiced at the royal court or at the courts of princes and nobles in the major provincial towns. They were officers of the

2. We have unfortunately not been able to consult a thesis on the history of traditional medicine in Thailand by Yuwadi Tapaniyakorn (1979).

3. phɛ̂ɛdsàad I 1964, Yoddumnern 1974, Bradley 1865.

crown, receiving salaries according to ranks given to them by the king. They were normally recruited from the relatives of practicing physicians, and so the position of royal physician was inherited. There were no rules prohibiting commoners outside the palace from being elevated to the position of royal physician, and a few cases have been reported.[4] The knowledge of the tradition was transferred individually and in an unstructured manner through an apprenticeship with a practicing physician—normally one's father or uncle.[5] In 1865 Dan B. Bradley reported that there were between sixty and one hundred royal doctors at the court.

In the reign of Rama III (1824–1852) a body of medical knowledge was for the first time made public, with stone inscriptions on the walls of Wat Chetuphon[6] near the royal palace in Bangkok, and at Wat Raja-Orasaram (wád râadchá?oorásǎaraam) in Thonburi.[7]

It has been suggested that much of what was inscribed at Wat Pho was simple and general knowledge that most people already knew. This was so because the royal doctors were reluctant to make their manuals public.[8]

During the reign of Chulalongkorn (1867–1910) a committee of royal physicians was appointed to collect and edit old medical manuals. The result of the work of this committee, referred to as *tamra luang,* was kept in the library of the palace, and was available to the court physicians only.

The first Western-trained physicians (and missionaries) in Thailand appeared in the 1820s, and during the last half of the nineteenth century an increasing number arrived, several of whom became close friends of the king.

Dan Bradley stayed in Thailand from 1835 until his death in 1873. He introduced smallpox vaccination, started a program of prevention against cholera, was the first to perform an amputation,

4. Bradley 1865:113.

5. Yoddumnern (1974) maintains, though, that there existed a Royal School of Medicine at the court, with examinations.

6. Dhani Niwat 1933, tamraa pheesàd 1977, Riley et al. 1979.

7. sǎmraan 1952.

8. saŋàd n.d.:120.

brought the first printing press to Thailand, and became a teacher of English and science to King Mongkut (Rama IV).[9]

Later, during the reign of Chulalongkorn (Rama V), Samuel Reynolds House, Peter Caven, Dr. H. Heyes, and Dr. G. B. McFarland were among the other physicians to practice in Thailand. The latter three all practiced at Siriraj Hospital and taught at Siriraj Medical School. These doctors were called on to treat patients in the palace, especially when traditional methods had failed. The traditional doctors at the court were thus regularly confronted with a medical practice which, in many cases, proved far more effective than their own. When Siriraj Hospital was established in 1887, the curriculum at the Siriraj Medical School (1889) included Western and traditional Thai options, so that the patients could choose either a Western or a traditional Thai treatment.

There exist some vivid, and revealing, descriptions from students who participated in the courses in traditional Thai medicine in the period 1889–1906.[10] They record that the traditional doctors at the school quarreled about the use of drugs, and practiced in different ways.

There was apparently no fixed curriculum, and during the first few years the four or five teachers in traditional medicine each used his own manuscripts in class. About 1895 the *tamra luang* mentioned earlier was in use at the school, but it was not printed until 1907, edited by Phraja Phitsanuprasadwed, and entitled *Phaedsad Songkhro Chababluang.* A year later a revised and abridged edition was printed under the title *Tamra Phaedsad Chababsangkheb,* now known as *Wedchasygsa.* Although several other medical manuals were printed for use in the school before 1907, the 1907 and 1908 editions are certainly the most important ones because at present the traditional medical schools in Thailand still use them as textbooks.[11]

---

9. waarásǎan sǎŋkhomsàad kaanphɛ̂ɛd 1978, 1.2:10–18.

10. waarásǎan sǎŋkhomsàad kaanphɛ̂ɛd 1978, 1.2:20–28, citing: wêedchánídsasìd phimnaj ŋaanchalɔ̌ɔŋ 50 pii sìrírâad 1939.

11. Conflicting accounts of the printing history of the early textbooks are found in the foreword of phɛ̂ɛdsàad sǒŋkhrɔ́ʔ (1964) and in sùd sɛ̀ɛŋwíchian 1978:22–26.

The method used to teach traditional medicine at the school was the "parrot" method: the teacher read aloud from his original copy, the students noted down every word, and then memorized the text. There were no explanations whatsoever. This way of teaching just wearied and bored the students, many gave up, and very few actually passed the exams. The few who did had not obtained any real understanding of what they had learned.[12]

The confrontation between traditional and modern medicine which took place at the Medical School at Siriraj Hospital from 1899 to 1906 exposed the basic weakness of traditional medicine: namely, the lack of standardization. One important explanation of this lack of standardization was the secrecy with which each herbalist surrounded his wisdom. This secrecy hindered frank exchange of knowledge and experience, and resulted inevitably in lack of standardization, fragmentation, and stagnation of the tradition as a whole. Furthermore, the Ministry of Public Health could not, of course, recognize a secret tradition, nor a tradition that was not a whole but consisted of many incoherent fragments.

These problems were overcome by simply adopting the textbook of the royal court as *the* standard textbook. This arbitrary choice glossed over the internal disagreements, inconsistences, lacunaes, and so on, within the tradition. The problems were, in other words, simply swept under the rug. But this apparent exposure of their secrets was not enough to get official approbation—other changes were also imposed, such as allowing women into the tradition, suppressing magic and incantations, at least on the surface, and introducing a necessary minimum of Western medical concepts and practices.

At any rate, there is no record of teaching or of examinations in traditional medicine at Siriraj after 1906.[13]

During the following fifty years there apparently did not exist any schools for traditional medicine, and the official medical scene was totally dominated by Western medicine. In the period between the two world wars Western medicine saw a popular breakthrough,

---

12. sùd sɛ̌ɛŋwíchian 1978:20–27.

13. sùd sɛ̌ɛŋwíchian 1978:25; see also Riley et al. 1979:141, referring to McFarland 1958:141.

especially with the arrival of antibiotics.[14] During this period the Rockefeller Foundation also began a significant subvention to the Medical School at Siriraj Hospital.[15] Still, the Ministry of Public Health did not suppress traditional medicine outright, but continued in fact to issue licenses to traditional doctors. Although up to the Second World War licenses could be acquired without passing any examinations, after the war applicants had to pass examinations arranged by the ministry in order to become officially registered.[16]

In 1957 an Association of the School of Traditional Medicine was established at Wat Pho (Wat Chetuphon) in Bangkok. Since then the association has branched out—and split—and there now exist several rival traditional medical schools in Bangkok and in some major provincial towns. As we pointed out earlier, the textbooks used at these schools are reprints, or slightly revised versions, of the 1907 and 1908 editions.[17]

The teaching at these schools is organized as follows: The students can choose either a one-year course in traditional pharmacy (pheesàd) or a course in midwifery (phádungkhan). Having completed the pharmacy course, they can go on to a two-year course in medicine. Before being allowed to practice legally, however, the students have to pass examinations organized by the Ministry of Public Health.

14. waarásǎan sǎŋkhomsàad kaanphɛ̂ɛd 1978, 1.2:10–18.

15. waarásǎan sǎŋkhomsàad kaanphɛ̂ɛd 1978, 1.2:43 ff.

16. Examples of this are found in section 3.4. The Herbalists—Personal Histories.

17. With the exception of the Āyurvedic Association at Wat Sam Phaya.

2

The Royal Tradition of Wat Pho, Bangkok

2.1. INTRODUCTION

It is the royal medical tradition that has, up to now, received the bulk of attention from those studying traditional Thai medicine, presumably because information on the royal tradition is readily available in printed textbooks. Such studies tend to ignore the medical tradition in the countryside, though, and thus promote the royal tradition as *the* Thai medical tradition. This is both erroneous and unfortunate because the royal tradition is in several respects not representative of Thai traditional medicine. In order to give an impression of the contrasts between the two traditions, we will first briefly describe the royal tradition, and then go on to discuss the Northern Thai tradition in detail.

The royal tradition is outlined in (a) the printed textbooks used at the Association of the School of Traditional Medicine at Wat

Pho dating back to about 1900,[1] (b) the stone inscriptions at Wat Pho,[2] and (c) the stone inscriptions at Wat Raja-Orasaram,[3] both dating back to the 1830s.[4] The Wat Pho manuals leave the impression of a strong Indian influence, although influences from other sources have also been detected.[5]

We want to stress that the following exposition of the royal medical tradition is based on a detailed study of only one of the volumes used at the Wat Pho school; namely, the manual of pharmacy.[6]

The logic of the sequence of material presented in this manual is not clear. We have therefore found it necessary to rearrange the contents of the manual, without, we hope, violating the inner logic of the tradition. We believe, on the contrary, that our exposition makes the system much clearer.[7] In fact, the editors of the Wat Mahathat edition of this manual[8] saw the basic weaknesses of the original edition and, while keeping the contents identical to the original, started the process of rearranging the sequence, thus making this edition much easier to study. They began to walk along a path which we will try to follow to its logical conclusion. We would recommend that future students of the royal school use the Wat Mahathat edition, and therefore we also include page references to that edition in parentheses in the footnotes.

---

1. (a) phɛ̂ɛdsàad sǒŋkhrɔ́ʔ 1964–1976, vols. 1–3. (b) khûumyykaansỳgsǎa wíchaawêedchákɔɔnthaj 1960. (c) khûumyykaansỳgsǎa wíchaawêedchákam 1970. (d) tamraa pràmuan làg pheesàd 1978. (e) pràmuan sàbphákhun jaathaj wâadûaj phrýgsàchâad 1963–1969, vols. 1–3.

2. tamraa pheesàd 1977.

3. sǎmraan 1952.

4. We did not have the chance to compare these three sources and do not know to what extent they contain identical information.

5. Riley et al. (1979) point out certain similarities between Thai and Chinese massage theory.

6. *khûumyy kaansỳgsǎa wíchaapheesàdchákɔɔnthaj* (*A Manual for Studies in Thai Pharmacy* [Wat Pho, Bangkok, 1969], referred to as Wat Pho 1969).

7. Another scholar, Jane Mulholland, has also described the Wat Pho manual. See Mulholland 1979*a*.

8. *tamraa pheesàdchákamthaj phɛ̌ɛnbooraan* (*A Textbook in Traditional Thai Pharmacy* [Wat Mahathat, Bangkok, 1973], referred to as Mahathat 1973; in footnotes as MT).

We have chosen to classify the information in the pharmacy manual into three categories: basic theories, connecting statements, and enumerations.

2.2. BASIC THEORIES (BT)

BT-1. *The theory of elements* (thâad) states that everything—including the human body—is made up of elements. In everyday speech one counts four elements: earth, water, wind, and fire, but in many theoretical contexts a fifth element is added, namely, ether.[9] When in a normal state the elements rest in balance, but in defective states the elements will generate an imbalance that results in ailments in the body. The defective states of the elements cause the elements to intensify (kamrə̂əb), to slacken (jɔ̀ɔn), or to become abnormal (phíkaan). The curing process aims at restoring the elements to their normal state, thus bringing harmony back to the body.

In the manual,[10] one finds a sequence of relationships in which the elements are related to other concepts in what is seemingly a causative chain:

> The *body* (râaŋkaaj) is the location of (pen thîitâŋ hɛ̀ɛŋ) the causative factors (samúdtàthǎan).
>
> The *causative factors* are the location of the elements (thâad).
>
> The *elements* are the location of the diseases (rôog).
>
> The *diseases* are the location of *food* (ʔaahǎan).

9. In one place defined as "wind in empty cavities" (lomnajchɔ̂ɔŋwâaŋ), Wat Pho 1969:330.

10. Wat Pho 1969:274 (MT 242).

The presentation of this chain starts with the last link and then unravels the other more fundamental causative links. If we read it from the bottom, starting with the fundamental cause, we get: Food creates diseases that disturb the elements that in turn influence the causative factors that result in ailments in the body. The important thing, we feel, is not the causative chain itself, but the fact that food is brought in as an important causative factor. This is in fact one of the very few places in the manual where a close connection between food and diseases is explicitly established.

BT-2. *The theory of tridosa* (triithôod) states that there are three humors of the body to which the cause of a disease can be immediately traced: the bile, the wind, and the mucus, collectively named tridosa. The state of the tridosa is intimately linked to the state of the elements and the seasons, although the exact relationship between the elements and the tridosa is not made explicit in the manual.

The concept of samúdtàthǎan (causative factor) is not defined in the manual but, in the causative chain outlined above, it is mentioned as something different from the elements and something less fundamental—causatively speaking—than the elements; thus we presume that samúdtàthǎan basically refers to the tridosa.

We also note that there is an overlapping between the elements and the tridosa, in that the concept "wind" is common to both. We have found no indication in the pharmacy manual that this concept should be understood to have different meanings in an element and a tridosa context, so we have taken it to be one and the same concept.

BT-3. *The taste theory* (ród) enumerates the number of tastes: Drug mixtures may have one of the three principal tastes: hot, cool, or mild (sukhǔm), while single ingredients in drugs have one (or more) of nine tastes: astringent, sweet, poisonous (mawbŷa), bitter, hot and spicy, oily, cool and fragrant, salt, and sour. Sometimes a tenth taste, bland (cŷyd), is added.

The taste theory postulates that each of the tastes has a different curative property, and thus establishes a direct link between the plants and the diseases on a theoretical level.

2.3. CONNECTIVE STATEMENTS

The textbook links the basic theories to one another and to other concepts in what can be termed *connective statements (CS), or rules.* We have arranged these statements into three groups: a group of nine plants (CS-1), the tastes (CS-2), and the parts of the plants (CS-3).

CS-1. The statements in this group have in common that they relate some or all of nine common plants to the elements, tridosa, seasons, state of the elements, and weight. In order to make the presentation of these statements as clear and brief as possible, we will symbolize each of the plants with capital letters.

CS-1.1. This group of statements links each of the elements with five specific plants, collectively called "the family of five" (bencakuun)[11] in the following way:

The individual plant of the element earth is diiplii (A).[a]

The individual plant of the element water is cháaphluu (B).[b]

The individual plant of the element wind is sàkháan (C).[c]

The individual plant of the element fire is cèedtàmuunphləəŋ (D).[d]

The individual plant of the element ether is khĭŋ hɛ̂ɛŋ (E).[e]

CS-1.1.1. Together with the dimension "weight" these five plants are used as a standard medicine to cure diseases in the "ten openings of women":[12]

10 units of A, B, C, D, and E, respectively.

11. Wat Pho 1969:183, 255, 276–277, 329–330 (MT 187 and 245). [a]Piper sylvaticum (McF 1944:330); [b]Piper sp. (McF 1944:286); [c]Piper sp. (McF 1944:835); [d]Plumbago zeylanica (McF 1944:256); [e]Zingiber officinale (McF 1944:157).

12. Wat Pho 1969:282 (MT 248).

CS-1.1.2. If the elements are defective—either intensifying, slackening, or becoming abnormal—use a prescription containing:[13]

4 units of D

6 units of C

10 units of E

12 units of B

20 units of A

CS-1.1.3. A variant of this combination occurs with the addition of the concept "part of plant," linking the prescription to discolored stools: "When the elements are defective, and cause discolored stools—like black, red, white, or green—use "the family of five" in the following way:[14]

4 units of leaf, flower, and root of D, respectively

6 units of leaf, flower, and root of C, respectively

10 units of leaf, flower, and root of E, respectively

12 units of leaf, flower, and root of B, respectively

20 units of leaf, flower, and root of A, respectively

CS-1.1.4. When the elements are defective and cause stools with one of four abnormal smells, use the "family of five" in the following way:[15]

The table should be read as follows: If it is a defective earth element that is the cause of the smelly stools, take 5 units of A, 4 units of D, 3 units of C, 2 units of B, 1 unit of E, and so forth.

13. Wat Pho 1969:282 (MT 198, 245).

14. Wat Pho 1969:280–281 (MT 245).

15. Wat Pho 1969:282–283 (MT 249–250).

	axis of symmetry ↘	Elements Earth	Fire	Wind	Water	Ether
Units of weight	5	A	D	C	B	E
	4	D	C	B	E	A
	3	C	B	E	A	D
	2	B	E	A	D	C
	1	E	A	D	C	B

↖

Fig. 1. Relationship among elements, plants, and weight in cases when stools have abnormal smell.

	axis of symmetry ↘	Elements Earth	Water	Wind	Fire	Ether
Units of weight	16	A	B	C	D	E
	8	B	C	D	E	A
	6	C	D	E	A	B
	4	D	E	A	B	C
	2	E	A	B	C	D

↖

Fig. 2. Relationship among elements, plants, and weight when the elements are defective.

CS-1.1.5. Another standard medicine for defective elements[16] is shown in figure 2.

CS-1.1.6. These statements link the "family of five" plants to tridosa and other ailments:[17]

---

16. Wat Pho 1969:281–282 (MT 246–248).

17. Wat Pho 1969:276–277. The myth behind the discovery of the relationship between these five plants, the elements, and the tridosa is retold in Mulholland 1979*a*:105.

A relieves incurable diseases (ʔachinnárôog).[18]

B relieves muscular aches and pains (mŷaj khòb).

C relieves mucus and wind diseases (sĕemaháʔ, waajoo).

D relieves diseases arising from the bile (dii).

E relieves diseases arising from the tridosa.

CS-1.2. In another part of the manual, however, there is a statement linking each of the tridosa with three other common plants:[19]

The individual plant of the wind is *Terminalia chebula*[20] (G) (sàmɔ̌ɔ thaj)

The individual plant of the bile is *Terminalia belerica*[21] (H) (sàmɔ̌ɔ phíphêeg)

The individual plant of the mucus is *Phyllanthus emblica*[22] (I) (mákhăampɔ̂ɔm)

All or some of these three plants plus the "family of five" plants plus pepper (phrígthaj) (F)—altogether nine plants—occur in elaborate arrangements, linking the concepts season, tridosa, elements, state of elements, and weight.

CS-1.2.1. A common arrangement of these nine plants into three groups gives us a three-to-one relationship between plants and seasons as shown in figure 3:[23]

18. The translation of this word is taken from phódcanaanúkrom . . . 1964:355.

19. Wat Pho 1969:330.

20. McFarland 1944:818.

21. McFarland 1944:819.

22. McFarland 1944:632. Alternative identification: Emblica officinalis (Euphorbiaceae).

23. Wat Pho 1969:248 and 277–278 (MT 197–199, 204, 208, 243).

The combination G, H, and I is called phíkàdtriiphalǎa, and is the standard medicine in the hot season.

The combination F, E, and A is called phíkàdtriikatùg, and is the standard medicine in the rainy season.

The combination D, C, and B is called phíkàdtriisǎan, and is the standard medicine in the cold season.

CS-1.2.2. A rearrangement of these plants gives us a three-to-one relationship between plants and tridosa:[24]

H, E, and D is the standard medicine to restore the bile.

G, F, and C is the standard medicine to restore the wind.

I, B, and A is the standard medicine to restore the mucus.[25]

CS-1.2.3. Statements here link the plants with seasons, tridosa, and weight units.

CS-1.2.3.1. If a disease occurs in the *hot season,* to restore the tridosa, take as shown in figure 3:[26]

CS-1.2.3.2. If a disease occurs in the *rainy season,* to restore the tridosa, take as shown in figure 4:

CS-1.2.3.3. If a disease occurs in the *cold season,* to restore the tridosa, take as shown in figure 5:[27]

---

24. Wat Pho 1969:274–275 (MT 244 also includes references to the seasons.)

25. CS-1.2.1. and CS-1.2.2. can be combined into one chart:

	Mucus	Bile	Wind
Hot season	I	H	G
Rainy season	A	E	F
Cold season	B	D	C

26. Wat Pho 1969:279 (MT 243).

27. In the Wat Mahathat manual three charts identical with those in CS-1.2.3. appear on p. 243 (MT 243 and 197–198), but an additional concept—"age span"—

	axis of symmetry ↘	bile	Tridosa wind	mucus
Units of weight	12	H	G	I
	8	G	I	H
	4	I	H	G

↖

Fig. 3. Relationship among tridosa, plants, and weight in hot season.

	axis of symmetry ↘	wind	Tridosa mucus	bile
Units of weight	12	F	A	E
	8	A	E	F
	4	E	F	A

↖

Fig. 4. Relationship among tridosa, plants, and weight in rainy season.

	axis of symmetry ↘	mucus	Tridosa bile	wind
Units of weight	12	B	D	C
	8	D	C	B
	4	C	B	D

↖

Fig. 5. Relationship among tridosa, plants, and weight in cold season.

---

has been added to the already existing ones. This CS is incomplete, in that several combinations are lacking; namely, for age spans 1–16 and 32 or more in the hot season; 1–16 and 16–32 in the rainy season; and 1–16 and 32 or more in the cold season.

CS-1.2.4. These statements link the nine standard plants with the elements, the state of the elements, and weight units in the following way:[28, 29]

	axis of symmetry ↘	FIRE intensify	FIRE slacken	FIRE abnormal	
Units of weight	1	C	A	B	
	2	A	B	C	
	3	B	C	A	↙
	4	E	H	D	↖
	8	D	E	H	
	16	H	D	E	
	1 ↗			[30]	

	WIND intensify	WIND slacken	WIND abnormal	
↘	B	D	A	
	D	A	B	
	A	B	D	↙
	F	G	C	↖
	C	F	G	
	G	C	F	
↗	E	E	E	

28. Wat Pho 1969:283–285 (MT 251–253).

29. Wat Mahathat shows the mechanics of figure 6 by arranging the concepts in a different way (p. 251).

30. Both the Wat Pho and Wat Mahathat manuals agree that this slot and the two to the left of it should be left vacant.

WATER		
intensify	slacken	abnormal
E	C	D
C	D	E
D	E	C
A	I	B
B	A	I
I	B	A
F	F	F

EARTH		
intensify	slacken	abnormal
F	E	D
E	D	F
D	F	E
C	B	A
A	C	B
B	A	C
HGI	HGI	HGI

Fig. 6. Relationship among state of elements, plants, and weight.

CS-2. The statements in this group all have in common that they relate the tastes to diseases or symptoms, elements, tridosa, age span, season, and even "the taste of blood" and "the color of skin."

CS-2.1. These statements link tastes and symptoms/diseases. There are two groups of tastes: the tastes of drug mixtures or prescriptions, and the tastes of single plants.

The tastes of drug mixtures may have one of three possible tastes: cool, hot, and mild.

> *Cool-tasting* mixtures may consist of ——— and are used to restore the fire element and to cure fever with hot poison (khâj thîi mii phíd rɔ́ɔn), and so on.
>
> *Hot-tasting* mixtures may consist of ——— and are used to restore the wind element, to cure colics and pains in the stomach, as a strengthening medicine (bamruŋ thâad), and to restore the blood of menstruating women, and so on.
>
> *Mild-tasting* mixtures may consist of ——— and are used to restore minor winds (lom kɔɔŋláˀìad) like dizziness, palpitating heart, vomiting; to cure fevers that cannot be treated with hot-tasting drugs, like "wind-fevers" (khâjphŷalom), menstruation accompanied by fever, various other winds, and "abnormal blood" (lŷad phíkaan).[31]

There are also lists with the names of prescriptions belonging to each of the three basic tastes, but without the ingredients or their curative properties.[32]

The curing properties of the ten tastes of single plants are given briefly as follows:[33]

1. Astringent — heals wounds
2. Sweet — permeates the flesh

31. Wat Pho 1969:180–182 (MT 154–185, 305–308).

32. Wat Pho 1969:350–354.

33. Wat Pho 1969:350.

3. Nauseating (mawbŷa)	cures poison (phíd)
4. Bitter	supports the blood and the bile
5. Hot	cures wind
6. Fat	cures muscles and tendons
7. Sweet and cool	makes happy and glad
8. Salt	permeates the skin
9. Sour	bites (kàd) the mucus
10. Bland (cŷyd)	cures mucus and is diuretic[34]

The relationships between the ten tastes and their curing properties are given in much more detail elsewhere in the volume. It is beyond the scope of this study to render these curing properties in full. It suffices here to give an example showing the quantity and quality of the types of information given:

Astringent-tasting plants have the property of "joining together." Used externally they heal wounds and soften the skin. Used internally they heal the intestines, cure colics (bìd) and blood in the stools, protect the elements and smooth the mucus (klɔ̀ɔm sěemáhàʔ), cure diarrhea and dysentery (ʔàtìsǎan), and so on.[35]

Then follows an enumeration of astringent-tasting plants with further details on the curing properties of each.[36]

Selective enumerations of the same kind are found in other parts of the book; for instance:

The curing properties of bitter-tasting bark.[37]

The curing properties of bitter-tasting leaves.[38]

34. Another list, said to be taken from the manual wɔɔrájookhásǎan, gives the curing properties of six tastes, namely, sweet, sour, hot, salt, bitter, and astringent. Wat Pho 1969:343 (MT 299).

35. Wat Pho 1969:181 and 186 ff.

36. Wat Pho 1969:186 ff.

37. Wat Pho 1969:324–325.

38. Wat Pho 1969:325.

The curing properties of bitter-tasting heartwood.[39]

The curing properties of sour-tasting bark.[40]

The curing properties of hot-tasting bark.[41]

Finally, relations between eight of the tastes and the parts of the body are established:[42]

Astringent	taste	permeates	the	flesh
Bitter	"	"	"	skin
Salt	"	"	"	muscles and tendons
Hot	"	"	"	bones
Sweet	"	"	"	major intestines
Sour	"	"	"	minor intestines
Sweet and cool	"	"	"	heart
Fat	"	"	"	joints

CS-2.2. Statements here link the tastes and the abnormal state of the elements:[43]

When the earth element is abnormal (phíkaan), medicines with astringent, sweet, oily, and salt tastes will restore it.

When the water element is abnormal, medicines with sour, bitter, and poisonous (mawbỳa) tastes will restore it.

39. Wat Pho 1969:326.

40. Wat Pho 1969:326–327.

41. Wat Pho 1969:327.

42. Wat Pho 1969:344 (MT 300).

43. Wat Pho 1969:183 (MT 186).

When the wind element is abnormal, medicines with mild (sukhǔm), hot, and spicy tastes will restore it.

When the fire element is abnormal, medicines with cool and bland tastes will restore it.

CS-2.3. These statements link age span, tridosa, and taste:[44]

When aged one to sixteen years, the major cause of diseases is mucus (sěemáhà?). Use sweet-, bitter-, and sour-tasting drugs.

When aged sixteen to thirty-two, the major cause of diseases is the bile and the blood. Use astringent-, bitter-, sour-, and salt-tasting drugs.

When aged thirty-two or more, the major cause of diseases is an intensifying wind, accompanied by abnormal mucus and perspiration. Use astringent-, bitter-, fragrant-, salt-, or warm-tasting drugs.

CS-2.4. These statements link seasons, elements, tridosa, and tastes:[45]

In the hot season, diseases originate in the fire element, in the bile or in an abnormal blood. Use drugs that taste cold, bitter ...

In the rainy season, diseases originate in an abnormal wind element, or an excessive or abnormal wind. Use drugs that taste hot ...

In the cold season, diseases are caused by an abnormal water element, or excessive mucus. Use drugs that taste sour, bland, mild ...

44. Wat Pho 1969:184 (MT 186–187).

45. Wat Pho 1969:184–185 (MT 186).

CS-2.5. These statements connect color of skin with taste of blood and taste of medicines:[46]

People with (color of skin)	have (taste of blood)	and should be cured with (taste of medicine)
White	sweet	hot, bitter . . .
White-yellowish	sour	salt . . .
Black-reddish	salt	any taste except salt
Black	very salt	sweet . . .

CS-3. Statements here contain collecting rules, linking part of the plant with time span of day, weekdays, and seasons.

CS-3.1. These statements link collection of part of plant with time span of the day:[47]

06–09 o'clock collect leaves, flowers, fruits, and pods.

09–12 o'clock collect branches and twigs.

12–15 o'clock collect stem, bark, and heartwood.

15–18 o'clock collect roots.

------------------------------------- (axis of symmetry)

18–21 o'clock collect roots.

21–24 o'clock collect stem, bark, and heartwood.

24–03 o'clock collect branches and twigs.

03–06 o'clock collect leaves, flowers, fruits, and pods.

CS-3.2. Statements link part of plant with time span of the day and the weekday:[48]

46. Wat Pho 1969:343 (MT 299).

47. Wat Pho 1969:178 (MT VI).

48. Wat Pho 1969:178 (MT VII).

	Morning	Late morning	Noon	Afternoon
Sunday	stem	leaf	root	bark
Monday	root	heartwood	leaf	bark
Tuesday	leaf	bark	stem	root
Wednesday	root	bark	stem	heartwood
Thursday	heartwood	leaf	root	bark
Friday	leaf	root	bark	stem
Saturday	root	stem	bark	leaf[49]

CS-3.3. Statements link part of plant with the seasons:[50]

In the hot season, collect root, heartwood . . .

In the rainy season, collect leaf, flower, fruit, or pod . . .

In the cold season, collect bark, stem, pith of bark, wood . . .

CS-3.4. Statements link weekdays with compass directions:[51, 52]

On Sundays and Tuesdays, collect plants toward the east.

On Wednesdays and Fridays, collect plants in a southern direction.

On Mondays and Saturdays, collect plants in a western direction.

On Thursdays, collect plants in a northern direction.

2.4. ENUMERATIONS

Enumerations make up the bulk of the pharmacy manual. Of the manual's 411 pages, about 250 are made up of lists and exam-

49. No apparent symmetry in the arrangement.

50. Wat Pho 1969:179 (MT VI).

51. Wat Pho 1969:179 (MT VI).

52. This collecting rule does not include part of plant.

TABLE 1

TYPES OF ENUMERATIONS IN THE PHARMACY MANUAL, WAT PHO

Type of enumeration	Entry	Information
E-1. Ingredients grouped into plants, animals, and minerals, with further subclassifications	Name	Taste, curing properties[53]
E-2. Ingredients with two names	Name	Name[54]
E-3. Ingredients that can replace one another	Name	Name[55]
E-4. Ingredients where all parts of the plant have the same taste	Name	Taste, curing properties[56]
E-5. Ingredients of which there are two or more species (cùláphíkàd)	Name	Names A, B, C . . . [57]
E-6. Groups of ingredients arranged according to number of ingredients [*sic!*]. All the ingredients have the same weight (phíkàdjaa)[58]	Number of ingredients	Name of group; name of each ingredient and its curing properties[59]
E-7. Groups of ingredients (various criteria)	Name of group	Taste, curing properties[60]
E-8. Diseases and symptoms	Disease	Name of plant(s) used as diluent (kràsǎaj) and method of preparation[61]
E-9. Groups of ingredients (various criteria)	Name of group	Name of each ingredient; taste and curing properties[62]

ples of classifications in one form or another. These lists contain a lot of detailed information—particularly about the curing properties of single plants, but they contribute nothing to the overall theoretical framework. Table 1 shows the most important enumerations, their classificatory principle (entry), and the type of information they contain.

TABLE 1 (*continued*)

Type of enumeration	Entry	Information
E-10. Prescriptions	Name of prescription	Ingredients, method of preparation, and curing properties[63]

53. Wat Pho 1969:7–163.

54. Wat Pho 1969:164–168.

55. Wat Pho 1969:168–170.

56. Wat Pho 1969:172–175.

57. Wat Pho 1969:234–242.

58. It is not clear whether these groups of plants are complete prescriptions in themselves, or whether they occur as standard subunits in prescriptions.

59. Wat Pho 1969:243–273.

60. Wat Pho 1969:307–327.

61. Wat Pho 1969:365–377.

62. Wat Pho 1969:379–393.

63. Wat Pho 1969:402–411.

2.5. ANALYSIS AND CHARACTERISTICS OF THE ROYAL TRADITION

The connective statements as they have been presented above make up a complete inventory of all the connective statements in the pharmacy manual. We will here concentrate our analysis on those statements in which the attempts to interrelate the various parts of the tradition into a coherent system are explicitly outlined.

The CS-1.1 statements postulate a relationship between the elements and five plants, and elaborate on this relationship by the introduction of weight units. The CS-1.2 statements establish a relationship between the tridosa and three specific plants. This relationship is expanded to include nine plants and the concepts of elements, state of elements, seasons, age span, and weight units. The CS-1 statements thus basically link the elements and tridosa on one hand with the plant world on the other. We note, though, that the plant world is only represented by nine plants out of a vast number of medicinal plants. The relationship must therefore be regarded as symbolic. On this symbolic level, when the statements involve more than a straightforward one-to-one relationship, they take a mechanical and symmetrical form, thus leaving us with the impression of systematic relationships.[64]

The reality is of course entirely different. If one scans the enumerations of single plants and their curative properties, one finds that it is exceedingly difficult—if not well nigh impossible—to generalize about the relationships among elements, tridosa, and plants. One will find many contradictory examples in this respect. We believe the reason for this lies in the fact that these theories were imported from India, and that, in spite of the many centuries they have been incorporated in the medical tradition, they have not been integrated into the tradition. The reason is that they *cannot* be integrated because there are no systematic links between elements, tridosa, and the plant world as a whole. The theory should not be understood to aim at such a complete systematic linkage either. It is simply an ideal model. In medical practice the explanatory power of the element and tridosa theories and the connective statements is very limited indeed. The system—if it deserves such a name—is thus a reference model to which the practicing herbalists may turn in order ultimately to legitimize their decisions and choices, but *it does not dictate their practice.* It is used for rationalizations.[65]

In spite of the fact that the CS-1 statements are merely manipulations and rearrangements of a very limited corpus of information, we note that they do not form a coherent whole, and that they should be used selectively, one by one. Any attempt to consult all the statements at once will invariably lead to contradictions and inconsistencies.

Underlying the fundamental characteristics of automatic operations, and the well-ordered symmetry of the CS-1 statements and rules, is the belief in fate and the love for aesthetics. These Indian virtues are paired with an Indian obsession; namely, that of com-

64. This is only partly true for the CS-3 group, where CS-3.1 is symmetrical along an axis (but not mechanical), while the two-dimensional CS-3.2 is neither symmetrical nor mechanical.

65. J. Filliozat arrives at a similar conclusion regarding the Āyurvedic medical system: "Thus the system of the Āyurveda is a dogmatism which interprets experience" (Filliozat 1964:30).

pleteness, which allows nothing to be outside the system. This results—in a medical context—in endless and pedantic enumerations into classes, subclasses, sub-subclasses, and so on.

The nine plants mentioned above are, besides being medical plants, also common spices used daily in the preparation of food; thus they implicitly relate the medicinal plants to nutrition.

Finally we note that the tridosa and the elements never occur together except in CS-2.4.

The imported theoretical structure involving the elements and the tridosa links the "little traditions" of Thailand with the "great medical tradition" of India, and, through the founder of the tradition, who is none other than the legendary personal physician of Lord Buddha, to Buddhism itself. These links serve to enhance the claim for authenticity and authority of the tradition.

Once we leave the statements centered around the elements and tridosa, and turn to the taste statements (CS-2), we suddenly leave the realm of mechanics and simplicity and are instead introduced to something real and complicated. Direct links are established between the plants and the full panorama of disease concepts and the parts of the body. The taste rules are never elevated to being absolute and all-encompassing, but are regarded as "rules of thumb." This makes them more useful and trustworthy than the lofty element and tridosa statements. The taste rules provide us in fact with the main links between theory and practice. But after this promising beginning, the taste theory finally ends up in enumerations of plants (arranged according to taste) and the curing properties of each of them. In other words, just a rearrangement of the information already presented in enumeration E-1.

This is not to disparage the information contained in the enumerations. On the contrary! The only part of the pharmacy manual that directly relates to practice is the enumerations, containing the names of single plants, their curing properties, and their tastes, thus establishing the all-important link between plants and diseases.

The enumerations reflect the practice of the tradition, namely, the preoccupation with the relationship between plants and diseases. A drawback is that the enumerations appear as a mass of unconnected statements, and that there is no attempt to generalize about the relationship. Generalizations would in one way or the other have to involve statistics, and the theory that would evolve from such a study would not necessarily correspond to the explicit theory as it is put forward in the official manuals. Another drawback is that in medical practice plants are seldom used alone to cure a disease, but are part of—often long—prescriptions. The relationship between the curing properties of single plants and the curing properties of a collection of plants, that is, prescriptions, is not explained in sufficient detail, and is not presented in any theoretical framework.

In figure 7 a simplified illustration of the royal medical tradition is given, showing the Indian theoretical framework being kept afloat far above the medical practice by the connective-statement balloons. The only anchorage between theory and practice is the taste theory, which links tastes to plants in a general way and thus stops the theory from drifting away and vanishing entirely. Within the square representing "practice," the only connection between plants and diseases is found in the enumerations in the manuals, in the form of countless specific relationships (represented by the vertical grid), but without—at least explicitly—any general relationship.

2.6. CONCLUSIONS

The theory of the royal medical school is imported from India, is not integrated with practice, and functions only as a frame of reference or an explanatory model. The links among each of the basic theories of the tradition—elements, tridosa, and tastes—are not firmly established, and the links they in turn ought to establish between the plants and the diseases are totally unsatisfactory. In fact, the taste theory provides the only direct—but feeble—connection between theory and practice.

It is our point of view that future studies of the royal medical tradition ought to (a) concentrate on the practice of this tradition, and not on the theory, and (b) investigate the tradition without constantly bringing in random fragments from the Āyurvedic tradi-

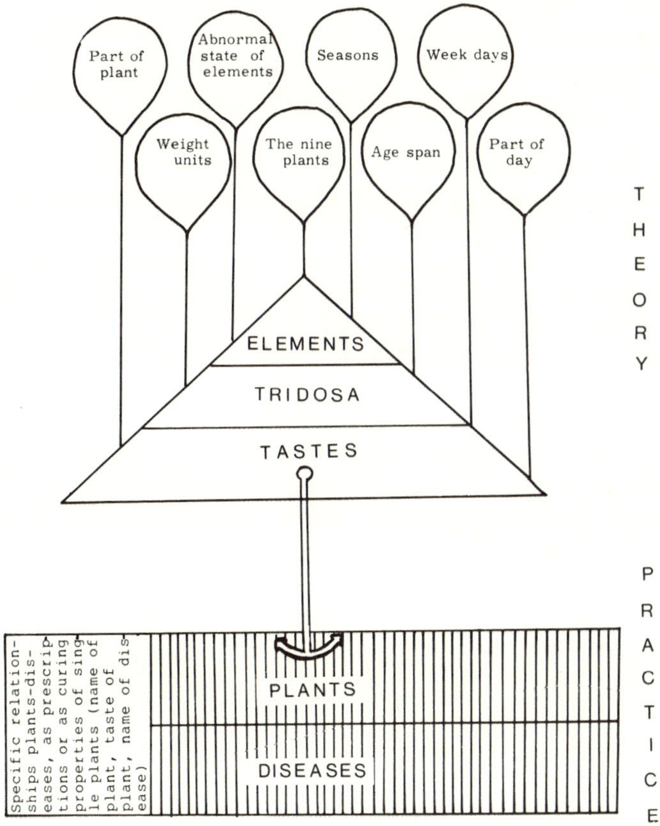

Fig. 7. A sketch of the relationship between theory and practice in the royal medical tradition.

tion to explain bits and pieces of the Thai royal medical tradition. In order to be able to compare the two traditions they must—for the time being—be kept apart, so that one can see how and to what extent the Indian borrowings have been incorporated into the Thai royal tradition.

3

The Medical Tradition of Northern Thailand

3.1. INTRODUCTION

Northern Thai traditional medicine is a living, local medical system, with a history that disappears in the mists of the past. It is nonscholarly without any kind of institutional didactic instruction. It is a popular-traditional system with a father-son or master-pupil educational system for its practitioners. It seems to be indigenous to Northern Thailand, although there are similar traditions in surrounding areas like Laos and the Shan States of Burma. Today the tradition is found among the Thai-speaking peoples of Northern Thailand (khon myaŋ), and is mostly confined to the rural parts of this area. Since the turn of the century Western medicine has gradually taken away many of the patients from the rural traditional doctors, thus undermining their economic base. Furthermore the urban variant of traditional medicine, emanating from Wat Pho in Bangkok, has during the last few decades attracted many of the potential students of traditional medicine, thus diminishing recruitment to the rural medical tradition. In this situation the possibility for survival of the unauthorized local medical tradition of Northern Thailand is slim. Still we feel that the tradition is worth studying, not only because during its long existence it has acquired experience in the treatment of diseases which may be valuable for medical science, but also because it is an integral part of Northern Thai culture and social history and thus worthy of study in itself.

3.2. TRADITIONAL CURERS

The herbalist is but one of several types of traditional curers in Northern Thailand. Below we give a brief description of the other types of curers we found practicing in the area we studied.

A. The general term *mɔ̌ɔmyaŋ* (local doctor) refers to three types of curers—the herbalist, the blower, and the sender—who all have in common that they are part of an exclusively male tradition, with "fixed words" as its basic characteristic. Outsiders have to pass an initiation ceremony to enter this tradition. In principle, one and the same person may be herbalist, blower, and sender, although normally these functions are divided among different persons.

A-1. The herbalist (mɔ̌ɔphɛ̌ɛnboolaan) covers almost the whole disease panorama, using his arsenal of herbs and other natural substances as the basis for his therapeutics. Incantations form an integral part of the tradition.

A-2. The blower (mɔ̌ɔpàw, mɔ̌ɔkhwagsuj) specializes in wounds and broken bones. He reposes the broken bones, stiffens the area around the fracture with sticks tied together, and then blows incantations and applies alcohol to the fracture. The blower may also stop bleeding with incantations.

A-3. The sender (mɔ̌ɔsòŋ) performs a series of ceremonies aimed at reintegrating people—including sick ones—into the community, through ceremonies calling on the spirit-essence of a person (hɔ̂ɔŋkhwǎn) or by sending away bad luck (sòŋkhrɔ́ʔ).

B. Aching muscles (mŷaj) are often treated with massage (nûad, teg sẽn ʔen), which is normally performed by one's relatives or children. Famous masseurs and masseuses (mɔ̌ɔnûad) are few and far between, and we have not come across anyone making a living from it. In spite of the fact that massage is a very common treatment, we have seen no signs in Northern Thailand that this art is passed on through a tradition, nor did we find any medical manuscripts dealing with the art of massage. Most people seem to learn it from personal experience.[1]

C. The traditional midwives (mɔ̌ɔtamjɛɛ) are predominantly female, specializing in child delivery. At present most women prefer to give birth with the aid of Western-trained midwives, or in hospitals. In areas where these facilities are within reach, the traditional midwives are thus rapidly disappearing. Our team did not investigate the practices and beliefs of the traditional midwives.

D. The swinger (mɔ̌ɔkwǎjkhãw, phǐimɔ̃ɔnŷŋ) is a female practitioner who finds the cause of minor children's ailments through divination.

E. The mediums (máakhìi, tîinâŋ) are part of a predominantly female tradition who, through possession of omniscient male spirits, find the cause of diseases, and who may even attempt curing certain diseases with "rubbing" ceremonies (cédhɛ̀ɛg). People with psychological and social problems often turn to the mediums for help and advice.

We found that, besides childbirth, broken bones, and mental diseases, the herbalists dominated the traditional disease arena.[2]

The difference among these curers and in their ranges of activity cannot be fully understood unless one has an overall understanding of the types of spirits that inhabit the supernatural world of the Northern Thais. It is not the task of this study to go into de-

1. Riley et al. (1979) have studied massage in the royal tradition.

2. Toothache is regarded as an inevitable phenomenon which has to follow its natural course, until the rotting teeth fall out by themselves. No traditional treatment is offered, beyond pulling the teeth out.

tail about this background knowledge, although certain aspects of the supernatural are discussed in section 3.8.9. Causality concepts.

3.3. HERBALISM

The fundamental characteristics of the herbalist tradition are:

A. It is male. We have not come across any women practicing the tradition. Women may collect plants, make and sell herbal medicines (although they seldom do), but they never diagnose diseases or actually treat the sick. Furthermore, women do not know the appropriate incantations, and even if they knew them, the incantations would lose all power if recited by the "impure" sex. In addition, the prescriptions are often long and complicated, and it therefore has become necessary to write them down. Traditionally it was during novice- or monkhood that literacy was acquired. Women could not be ordained, and thus did not acquire this art—one more barrier to their participation in the medical tradition.

B. It is closed. The knowledge of the tradition is not passed on freely to people outside the tradition.[3] In order to get a share of this knowledge, one has to be accepted as a pupil (lûug sid) by someone already in the tradition, who will then function as a teacher (khuu). An initiation ceremony (wãj khuu) has to be performed, and the teacher is given a fee. This ideal procedure is not followed among well-established herbalists, who may exchange, sell, or give away prescriptions or knowledge to one another without any formalities being involved.[4] The medical tradition as such considers Vishnu (pídsanu?) to be the tradition's original teacher, and once a year homage is ceremoniously paid to him.[5]

---

3. Among the nonspecialists there exist various degrees of medical knowledge, partly in the form of a general understanding of diseases and their causes, and partly as a knowledge of simple prescriptions against clear-cut symptoms ("good advice"). The food prohibitions are generally known to everyone. Our investigation focused on the knowledge and practice of the medical specialists, although we have of course incorporated information from the "folk-medicine" level, especially through interviews with patients.

4. The members of our team did not have to go through any of these formalities either, even though we suggested it.

5. The Wat Pho traditional school regards Kumarajiva, the legendary physician of the Lord Buddha, as their ultimate teacher.

3.4. THE HERBALISTS—PERSONAL HISTORIES OF MAIN INFORMANTS

Po Liang Tan Thammakhrong, born 1900, died 1979, native of Wang Tong area just north of Lamphun town. Son of a farmer who also practiced as an exorcist (mɔ̌ɔlâjphǐi). Resident of Ban Myang Nga at the time of our investigation.

Po Liang Tan had no schooling until he entered novicehood at the age of ten. He remained a novice for five years, becoming literate in Northern Thai during that period. Afterwards he helped his father with farm work, and started flirting with girls. At the age of nineteen he was bitten by a mad dog during one of his nocturnal escapades, but was cured by means of incantations by a local doctor. He then began studying with the doctor, and gradually began practicing. At first he only treated bites of mad dogs, but by and by he got into the trade of making and selling traditional drugs, and later on he also expanded his range of curing activities to other diseases. When his teacher died, the patients naturally turned to Po Liang Tan instead. At twenty-two he married a fourteen-year-old girl. This first marriage lasted only a few years, and was followed by four other marriages. At about thirty he left on a long journey lasting over three years, which took him all over Northern and Northeastern Thailand, even to Vientiane and the Cambodian border. During this odyssey he made a living buying and selling anything, including medicines, and also diagnosed and treated the sick people he met on his way. Returning to the North he brought back an increased medical experience and many new prescriptions, written down in scrapbooks. Po Liang Tan took up farming again, but also started speculating in land, and turned to itinerant trading when occasion demanded, all the while continually practicing traditional medicine.

In 1936 he applied for an official license, forwarding a letter of recommendation from another traditional doctor with his application. The ministry accepted the application, without apparently requiring any kind of examination. The license seems to have served Po Liang Tan in two ways, besides keeping the police away.

Traditional pharmacies must be supervised by a traditional doctor with a license in order to operate legally. Po Liang Tan rented out his license to a pharmacy in Lamphun, becoming its formal operator, for which he collected an annual fee and gained access to raw materials for his drugs "on the cheap."

Later on, in 1967, when a branch of the Wat Pho traditional medical school was opened in Wat Nong Chang Khyn some ten kilometers north of Lamphun town, Po Liang Tan was chosen as its president, precisely because he had an official license. At that time he seems to have had no extensive knowledge of the theories of this branch of traditional medicine with roots in the royal court, but these theories did influence him to a certain extent during the few years the school existed. Po Liang Tan now knew, for example, the four and the five elements, and the body constituents that belonged to each of these elements, although he never mentioned the elements when discussing concrete diseases and their etiologies.

In 1978–1979 Po Liang Tan still practiced traditional medicine. He received the patients in his living room, where he kept his arsenal of drugs, and he also made drugs himself. His garden was full of medicinal plants, but he bought most of his raw materials in traditional pharmacies in Chiangmai and Lamphun. The frequency of consultations was uneven, averaging one to three patients a day. Po Liang Tan was a general practitioner, but he was particularly famous for his treatment of tumors (săan), including his method of moving the tumors from one place in the body to another. (For details, see the section on "săan.")

Po Liang Tan was a very sociable person, with a particular gift for telling stories, and making people laugh.[6] He was an untiring informant, sharing freely with us all his wisdom and knowledge. Po Liang Tan died in 1979, half a year after we had left Thailand.

Po Liang Nan Mi Wannaphrom, born 1901, native to Northern Thailand, resided near Pratu Li, just outside the southern moat of Lamphun town.

Nan Mi lived most of his life in temples. First as a temple boy and novice for eleven years, beginning when he was eight, and then for another thirty-three years as a monk, until he left the monkhood in 1961 for health reasons. Nan Mi was continually plagued by var-

6. In fact, Viggo Brun knew him very well from earlier sojourns in Myang Nga village, when Po Liang Tan was his main informant on local oral tradition.

ious diseases throughout his lifetime, and he took—nay, indeed fed on!—traditional herbs, because his self-imposed dietary restrictions excluded almost any kind of normal food. His interest in medicine was due to his ailments, which he wanted to learn more about in order to be able to cure them. Nan Mi had experienced the following diseases: bàheŋkhúd, bàheŋ khanthámaalaa,[7] nĩw, pòoŋ, and nedsaa, just to mention the most important. Besides curing himself, Nan Mi also treated patients, although we did not see many.

While a monk Nan Mi traveled extensively and he visited Bangkok several times. He often employed disease names of Bangkok-Thai origin, and his collection of medical manuscripts contained both Northern Thai and Central Thai prescriptions. Nan Mi died in 1981.

Mo Camnong Tonkid, born 1919, native of Saraphi district, Chiangmai.

Mo Camnong ran a small pharmacy in the market of Saraphi, selling mostly traditional drugs, some of which he himself made. He also treated patients now and then. His father, Mo Som, was a traditional doctor, and so was his uncle, who was of Burmese origin. Camnong studied traditional medicine with his father and uncle, and also in the temple during his monkhood. In 1949 he passed the examination in traditional pharmacy and, two years later, one in traditional medicine, receiving his official license in 1951. Mo Camnong in this way gained extensive knowledge of both the local Northern Thai medical tradition, with some Burmese variations, and the official traditional medicine of the Wat Pho school. One of the things that made him such a valuable informant was that he did not intermingle this knowledge, but was able to keep the traditions apart and to compare them. Furthermore, he was concise and simple, with a natural knack for discovering the distinctive features of the traditions and, finally, he was modest, admitting when he did not know something, and never making up stories. When we were in difficulties, a few hours with him usually helped to sort things out, and tie up loose ends. Mo Camnong died suddenly in 1983.

7. Nan Mi used the term *bàheŋ* with its modern Bangkok-Thai meaning: "tumor, cancer." The Northern Thai cognate is *sǎan.*

3.5. THE KNOWLEDGE

The tradition consists of knowledge of (1) the diseases, their symptoms, etiology, and pathogenesis, (2) the materia medica, (3) the incantations, and (4) how these elements should be combined.

3.5.1. Acquisition of knowledge

The Northern Thai medical tradition, is, as we have mentioned already, nonscholarly without any kind of institutional didactic instruction. The medical knowledge is passed on partly by word of mouth and partly in handwritten manuscripts in the Northern Thai language. The herbal doctors acquire their basic medical knowledge by establishing a teacher-pupil relationship with someone who is already within the tradition. A student of traditional medicine will normally establish many of these relationships, and thus acquire knowledge from many different teachers, while the teachers most commonly just pass on certain parts of their total knowledge to each student.

Obviously nobody covers the total knowledge of the whole tradition. Very often the medical interest of a future herbalist will start because he himself is sick with one particular disease and is cured by a practicing herbalist. He will afterwards ask the herbalist for the prescription that cured him; that is, become his disciple, and then slowly begin practicing on patients with this particular disease. By and by he will collect more prescriptions against the disease and, if his interest, experience, and reputation allow it, expand his range of cure, acquiring new knowledge and other prescriptions by becoming a disciple of other herbalists. Practitioners thus start out as specialists but will, as time goes by, widen their range of curing activites and thereby become more and more generalists.

It is rather uncommon to find herbalists who operate as general practitioners, accepting all kinds of diseases. Our main informant, Po Liang Tan, was an exception in this respect. We should also note that indigenous practitioners may adopt whatever seems useful from cosmopolitan medicine, and we have come across herbalists who also distributed Western medicine (pills) to their patients.

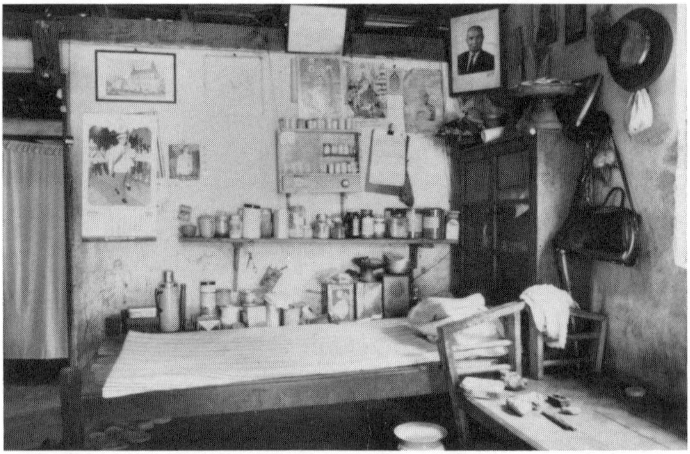

Po Liang Tan received and treated patients in the living room of his house.
(Photo: Terje Bjørnland)

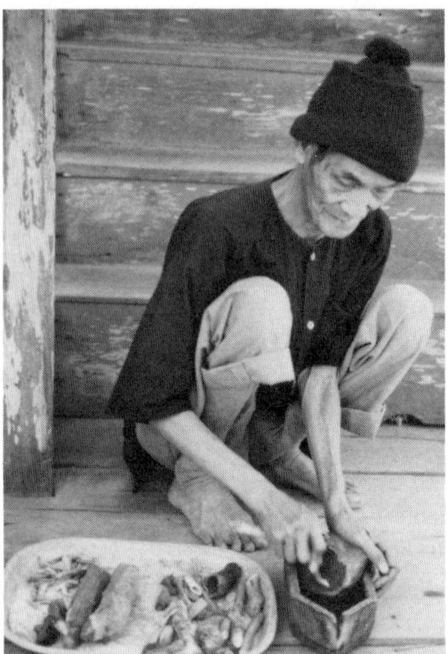

Po Liang Nan Mi prepares a jaa fŏn, that is, a medicine ground against a stone in water.
(Photo: Terje Bjørnland)

Mo Camnong in front of his pharmacy in Saraphi market.
(Photo: Terje Bjørnland)

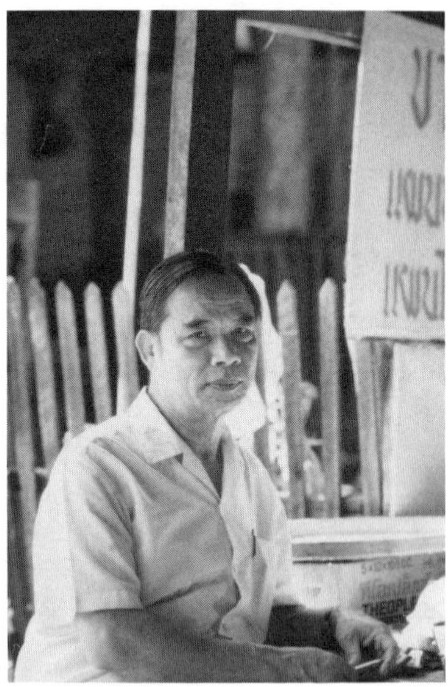

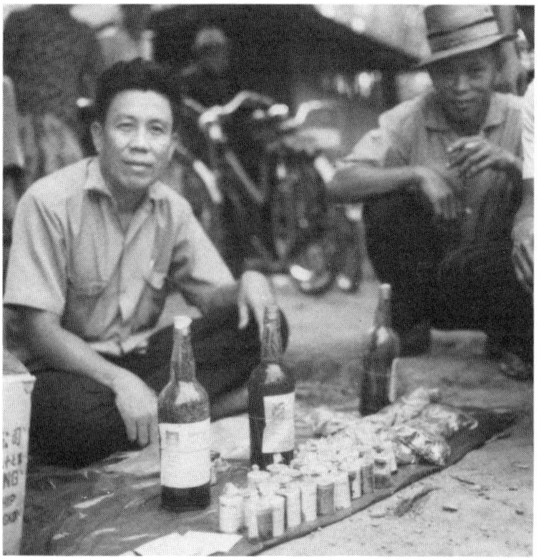

Selling traditional medicines in the market.
(Photo: Viggo Brun)

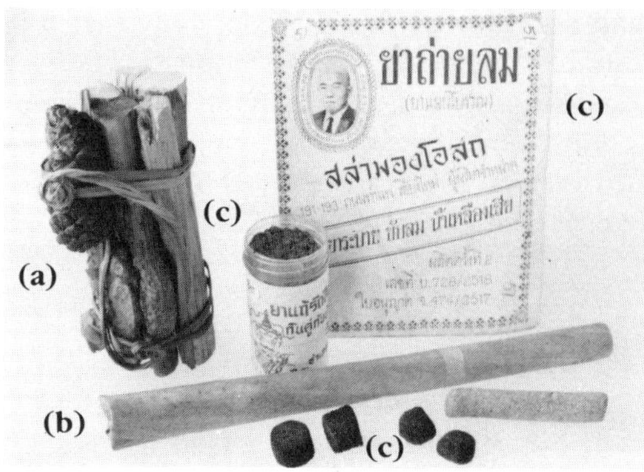

Some traditional drugs and some ready-made traditional-style drugs for sale everywhere: (a) used as decoction, (b) to be smoked, (c) taken orally.
(Photo: Terje Bjørnland)

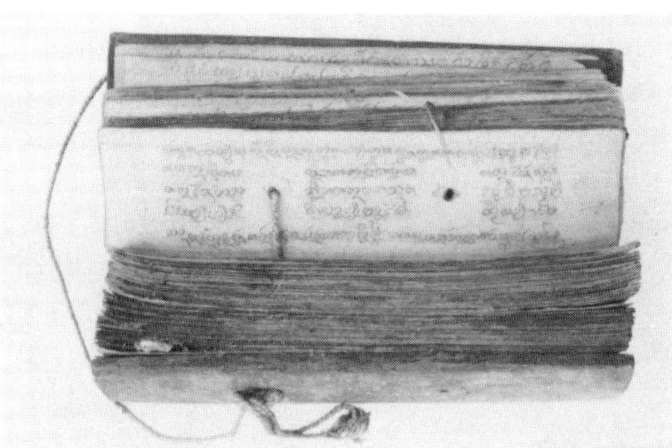

Northern Thai medical manuscript.
(Photo: Terje Bjørnland)

3.5.2. The Medical manuscripts

In an attempt to check and compare the oral information with the information in the medical manuals, we had five manuscripts copied, all written in the Northern Thai alphabet. The manuscripts belonged to people from (1) Sankamphaeng, Chiangmai, (2) Pong Noi, Tambon Sutheb, Chiangmai, (3) Yang Noeng, Saraphi, Chiangmai, (4) Pa Daet, Saraphi, Chiangmai, and (5) Lamphun town. These manuscripts were either copied for us by their owners, or borrowed and copied by a hired copyist.

The contents of the manuscripts almost invariably turned out to contain simple sequences of independent prescriptions, written in no apparent order. We did find, however, some cases of more detailed descriptions of main disease groups, such as tùm, bàheŋ, módtakhyd, and saníbàad. In our corpus they stand out as something exceptional, but they do show that there have been attempts made to systematize small sections of the disease panorama, even if inconsistently and incompletely. Furthermore, astrology may be used in connection with determining the origin and development of diseases, and thus astrological data are also reproduced in some medical manuscripts.

3.5.3. Prescriptions

Each prescription is a separate entity. These entities are transferred piecemeal from one person to another. Transfer of a greater corpus of prescriptions at one time occurs also, as when someone acquires a whole manuscript. Our experience, however, points to the occasional transfer as being the most common. An herbalist is always eager to collect new prescriptions and he will write them down chronologically as he gets them. This explains why the manuscripts actually take the form of collections of prescriptions.

On the whole, there exist literally thousands of different prescriptions in the Northern Thai medical tradition. An herbalist often possesses hundreds of prescriptions, although only a small fraction of them—the ones that are considered particularly effective—are in daily use. We should also note that there exist many different prescriptions against the same disease.

Due to a lively trade with neighboring regions over the centuries, it is certain that a lot of prescriptions have found their way into the tradition from other areas of Northern Thailand, from other regions like Northeastern and Central Thailand, and also from neighboring countries like Laos and Burma.

The information in the prescriptions is always arranged in the same way: First comes a brief heading with the name of the disease(s) and the symptom(s), followed by an enumeration of the materia medica in the prescription (and sometimes their relative weight), and finally an explanation of how the components should be treated and administered to the patient.

We transcribed all the prescription headings in the manuals—altogether some 1,300. Our first aim was to ensure that we had not missed any important disease concepts, and for this limited purpose the prescription headings were very useful. As for the content of each of the disease concepts, however, the majority of the headings were too short to be of much value. The following examples illustrate this:

> Medicine against all kinds of sànίbàad, take ... (jaa sànίbàad sapaʔ taŋ muan)
>
> Medicine against phaaj entering the joints, take ... (phaaj khãw khɔ̂ɔ)
>
> Medicine against jerking fever, take ... (jaa khãj satog)
>
> Medicine against all kinds of "blood-and-wind," take ... (jaa kɛ̃ɛ lŷad lom taŋ muan)
>
> Medicine against white tongue, take ... (jaa kɛ̃ɛ lín khăaw)
>
> Medicine against the 120 kinds of mahòog, take ... (mahòog 120 cămpûag)

Some prescriptions, however, do describe the diseases in enough detail to give a rough indication of what they are, and can thus supplement the oral information.

Certain prescriptions have a wide range of curing properties, and will thus cover several diseases and symptoms. These prescriptions contain an implicit classification of the diseases. We have made attempts to classify the diseases based on a limited number of prescriptions—about a hundred—and the result provided us with indications which later helped us to arrive at a more substantial systematization of the whole disease panorama. (See section 3.8.12 Disease classification: Conclusion.)

Our conclusion is that each prescription by itself is not a valuable source of information about the disease concepts and the disease system, but a large corpus of prescription headings does present us with useful patterns. On the whole, though, there can be no doubt that the student of the diseases will first of all have to rely on oral information and observations.

3.5.4. Prescriptions and materia medica

All prescriptions are mixed drugs composed of two, five, twenty, or even more than a hundred different ingredients. Plant material makes up the heavy part of the drugs, although some animalia and minerals are also commonly used. The composition of the prescription obviously has an economic value to the owner, and is thus guarded with great care. While the healers talk freely about the diseases and the curing properties of single plants, there is an aura of secrecy surrounding the way these components are mixed to form prescriptions. Stories of herbalists who only reveal nine out of ten components in a prescription to their pupils—the most important one being left out—are frequently heard. The opposite situation also occurs, when a pupil tries to lure prescriptions out of his teacher by making him drunk! We had certain difficulties obtaining prescriptions from most informants, although our main informant had no reluctance whatsoever about sharing them with us.

The prescriptions—together with the incantations—make up the core and the most stable part of the medical tradition. The content of these has been fixed once and for all, and must not be tampered with. The omission of even a small part renders them useless. Additions of new ingredients is, however, permissible.

In spite of veneration for the tradition and for the teacher, changes in old prescriptions—both intentional and unintentional—have occurred and, furthermore, a few entirely new ones have been created. There exist now, for example, prescriptions against diabetes (bawwǎan)—an entirely new disease concept.

A further elaboration of prescriptions and their ingredients is presented in chapter 5.

3.5.5. Incantations

The incantations are an integral part of the tradition as a whole. They are sometimes "blown" on to the drug while it is being prepared to enhance its effect, sometimes recited while the herbalist is administering the drug or performing other curing practices—especially the "rubbing away" rituals (cédhɛ̀ɛg),[8] or they are simply blown on to the patient without being accompanied by drugs at all. According to our informants there are basically two types of incantations: (a) those taken from the Buddhist scriptures (sidphákhun) and thus in the Pali language, and (b) those (khaathǎa ʔaakhom) in vernacular languages, mainly Northern Thai. The incantations were not a part of our study, but we noted the fact when they formed a part of the treatment.

3.6. THE HUMAN BODY

Although the Northern Thais have an extensive vocabulary for the exterior parts of the body (see figs. 8–10), they have few terms for the internal organs (see fig. 12). This is owing to the fact that the traditional doctors do not perform any surgery or dissection on the human body, and therefore their knowledge of the internal organs and the way they function is, from a Western point of view, cursory and often wrong.

The skeleton consists of bones (dùug) and joints (khɔ̂ɔ). The distance between two joints is called khɔ̄ɔ when the distance is

8. This is actually a rough form of massage. A spot on the body is rubbed with something hard. The direction of the rubbing is always toward the hands or the feet, that is, out of the body.

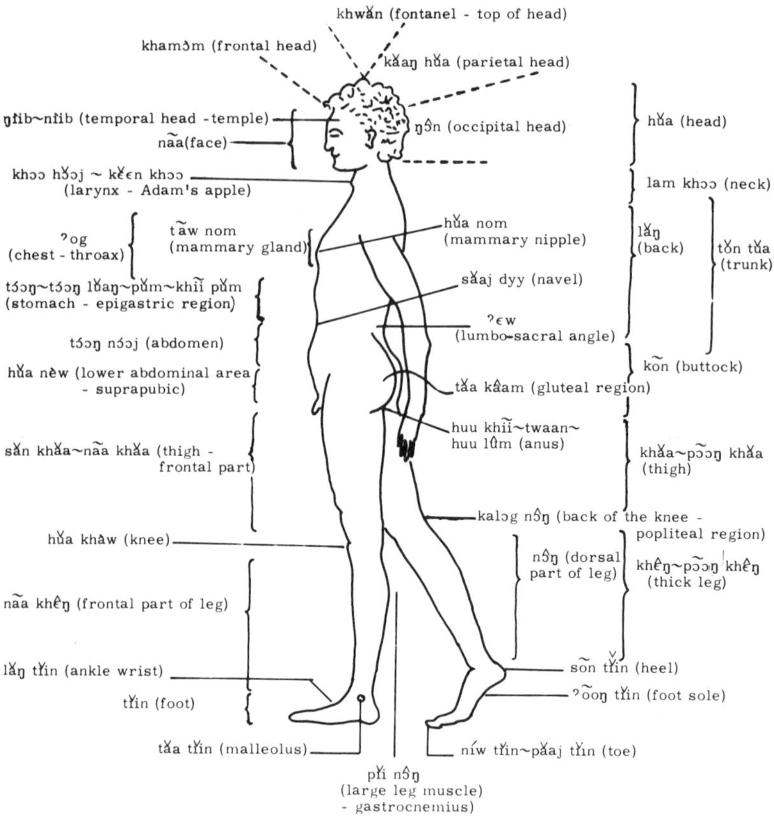

Fig. 8. Medical vocabulary: human body—exterior I.

short, as in the fingers (e.g., khɔ̃ɔ níw); when the distance is long, it is called pɔ̃ɔŋ, as in the legs (e.g., pɔ̃ɔŋ khɛ̂ŋ, pɔ̃ɔŋ khǎa) (see figs. 8 and 10).

The flesh, muscles, and tendons. Although there are specific words for flesh (nýa cín), muscles (kãam), and tendons (ʔen = sẽn ʔen), these concepts are generally not kept apart, but are normally referred to collectively as "nýa" or "kãamnýa."

The circulatory system. It is recognized by all that blood (lŷad) is present in the body in vessels (sẽn lŷad), but there is no clear concept that these vessels form a system, that the blood is cir-

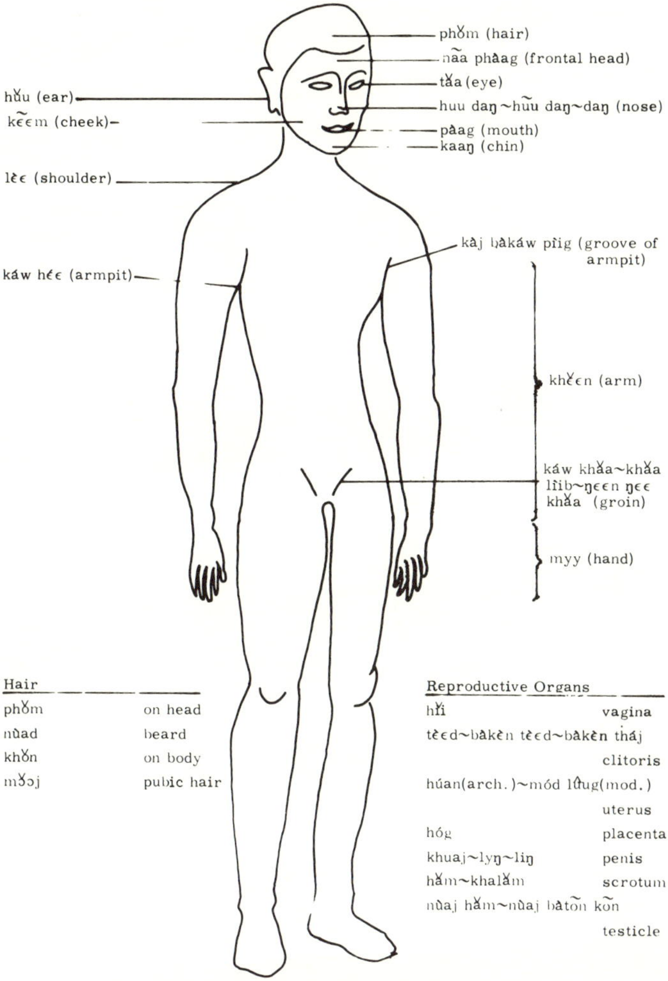

Hair	
phǒm	on head
nùad	beard
khǒn	on body
mɔ̌ɔj	pubic hair

Reproductive Organs	
hǐi	vagina
tɛ̀ɛd~bàkɛ̀n tɛ̀ɛd~bàkɛ̀n tháj	clitoris
húan(arch.)~mód lûug(mod.)	uterus
hóg	placenta
khuaj~lyŋ~liŋ	penis
hǎm~khalǎm	scrotum
nùaj hǎm~nùaj bàt͠on k͠on	testicle

Fig. 9. Medical vocabulary: human body—exterior II.

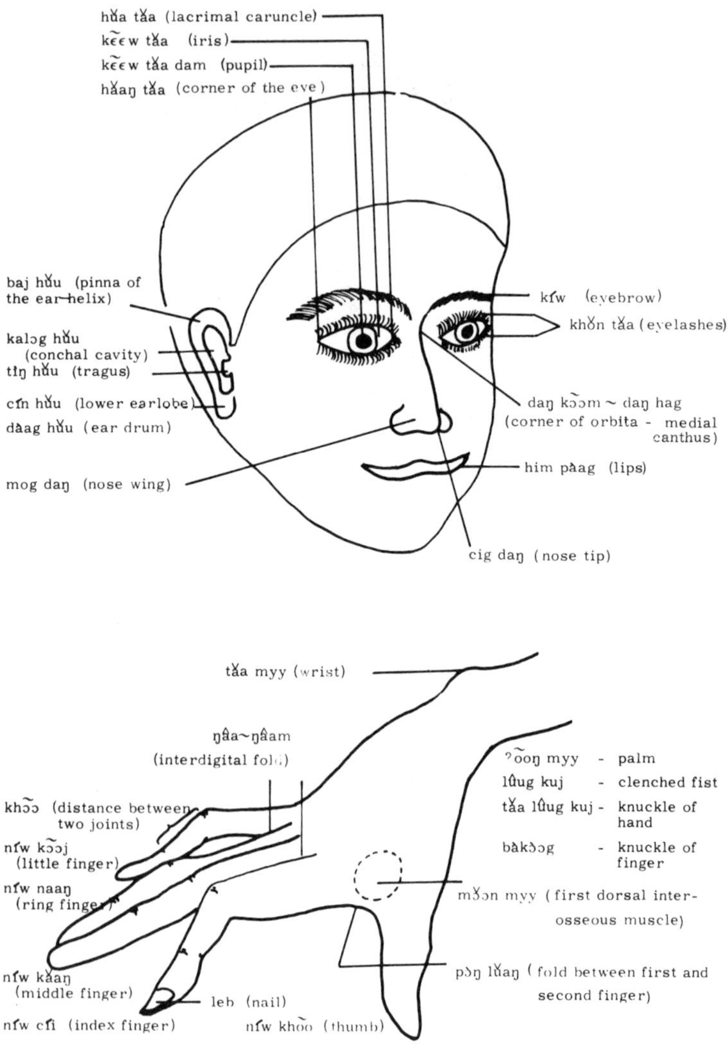

Fig. 10. Medical vocabulary: human body—exterior, details.

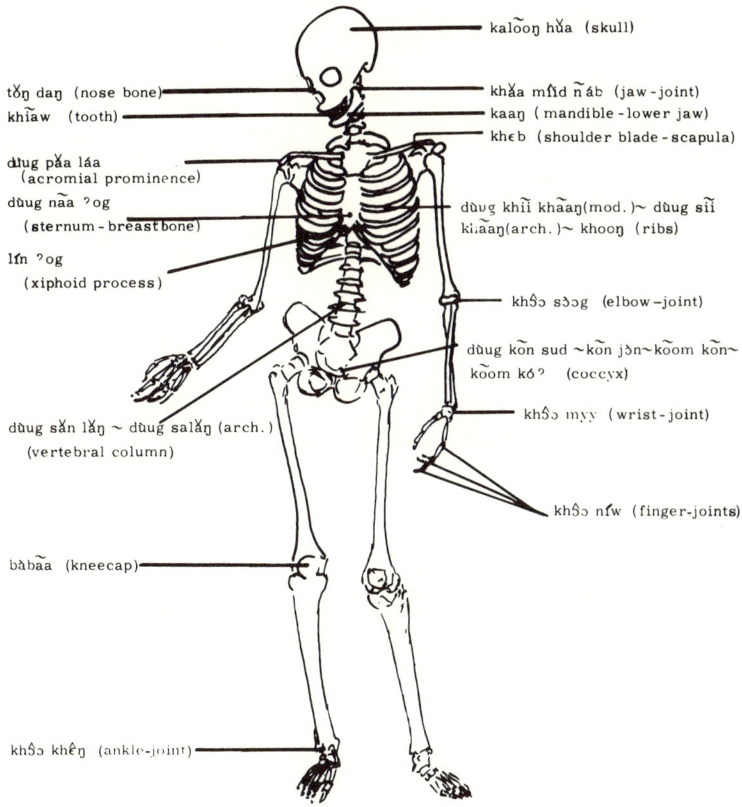

Fig. 11. Medical vocabulary: human body—bones and joints.

culating in it, and that the heart pumps the blood around.[9] Still, some herbalists maintain that an important part of a diagnosis is to take the pulse (cab sîibpacɔɔn). However, we never saw any of them actually taking any interest in the pulse in concrete cases of disease. As far as we have noticed, the pulse is not mentioned in the medical manuscripts either.

9. Blood-letting is generally not practiced, although we have heard of instances when leeches have been applied to suck out spoiled blood.

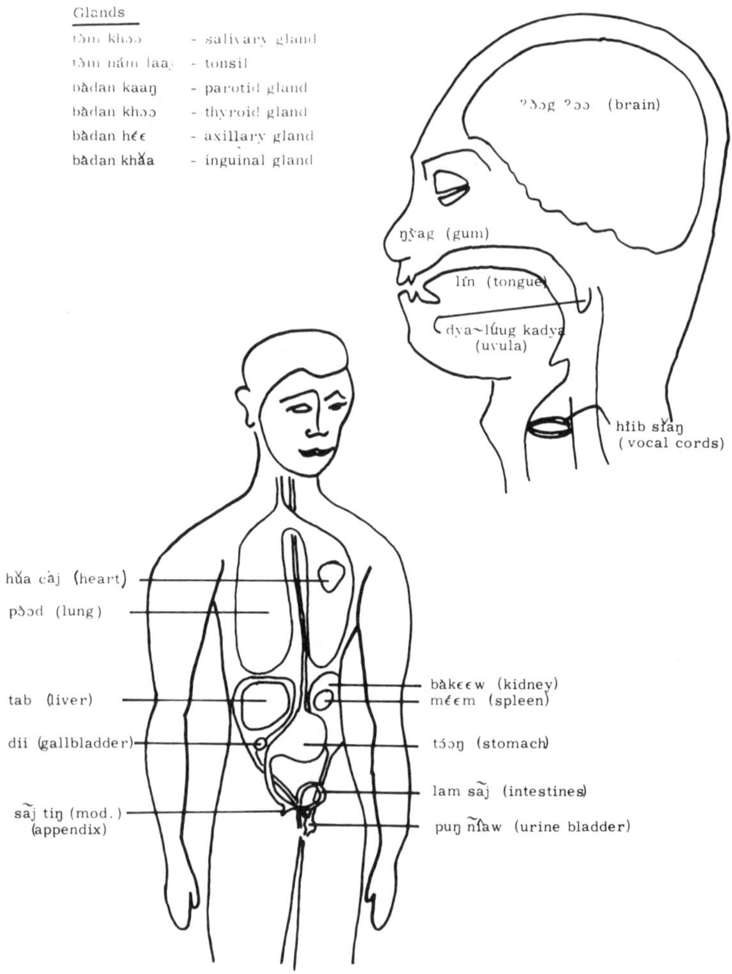

Fig. 12. Medical vocabulary: human body—internal organs.

The heart (*bŭa căj*) is considered vital, but its position in a circulatory system is not well understood. Changes in the heartbeat following changes in the mood are well known.

The liver (tab), *gallbladder* (dii), *kidneys* (bàkɛɛw), and the *spleen* (mɛ́ɛm = máam) are all known by name and vaguely by location, but besides the kidneys, which are associated with urination, there are no clear concepts of how these organs function. It is known that they can swell and become hard. In a Northern Thai context the liver (tab) is considered the most important internal organ, while we have seen that in royal traditional medicine it is the gallbladder (dii) that is prominent, being the only internal organ included in the tridosa theory.

The digestive system. As we shall see later, many diseases occur in or can be traced back to disturbances in the digestive system, and ultimately to food. People in the North place great importance on a well-functioning digestive system. The types and location of pain in the stomach region, and the type of stool (color, smell, consistency, accompanying matter, frequency, etc.) are important diagnostic criteria, and food prohibitions are an important part of the treatment of many diseases.

The sensory faculties are well known, but not the way they function. The nerves and the nervous system are not part of traditional medicine, and the modern term *sẽn pràsàad* (nerves) has only recently been introduced to the area, with the connotation of "having a nervous disease."

3.7. TRADITIONAL MEDICAL TERMINOLOGY

Because explorers of the Northern Thai medical tradition will have to learn the terminology used to describe diseases, symptoms, and signs, and this invariably turns out to be a very time-consuming task, we have found it appropriate to pass on the most pertinent medical vocabulary we have come across. It should be evident that there are local and individual variations in the usage of the terms, and thus our understanding of them is not necessarily the only correct one. The lists are not complete, and it has been necessary to leave out whole semantic groups, such as color and smell (relevant for diseases) and tastes (relevant for medicinal plants and foods).

I. *Secretions and Discharge from the Body*

kǎan lŷad	Excessive bleeding (e.g., from mouth, nose, vagina). See also the disease kǎan lŷad.
nám laaj	Saliva.
nám tə́əj	Salivation from the mouth, slobber.
nám laaj pěn pùag	Frothy sputum, foam.
khĩi tə̂ə = khĩi tə̂əg	Phlegm.
sěemahaʔ	Mucous discharge.
salèed	Mucous sputum in the throat of a dying person.
khĩi	Discharge (colloquial for feces, excrement). Syn.: ʔaacom.
khĩi mûug = nám mûug	Snot.
nám tǎa	Tears (lacrimation).
khĩi tǎa	Eye secretion.
khìw nãa khìw tǎa	Running eyes and nose.
khĩi hɛ́ɛ	Perspiration in armpits.
ñîaw	Urine.
nám kǎam = nám ʔasuciʔ	Semen.
nám khaaw	Leukorrhea.
nám khaaw pǎa	Lochial discharge.
nɔ̆ɔŋ	Pus.
nám lɯ̌aŋ	Serous secretion.

II. Abnormalities

A. Skeleton and muscles

dùug hag	Fracture.
thɔ̆ɔŋ	To strain (muscle).
samɛ́ɛŋ	To twist (ankle).
kóon	A sprain, distortion.
pɛ́d = pɛ́d mɔ̃n = palɛ́d	To dislocate (joint).
khɛ̌ŋ	Hard; opposite: ʔɔ̀ɔn, nuan.
tyŋ	Tight (muscles); opposite: maaj.

B. Veins

ʔen fuu	Protruding vein.
ʔen khɔ̀ɔd	Varicose vein.

C. Sensory faculties

tǎa láaw = tǎa keg = tǎa lə̃ə = tǎa líi = tǎa kɛg	Squint, be cross-eyed.
tǎa bɔ̀ɔd	Be blind.
tǎa bɔ̀ɔd nám sǎj	Be blind even if eyes look normal.
hǔu nùag	Be deaf.
bãj = ʔə̆ə	Be mute.

III. Symptomatic Expressions

A. Weak, tired, completely worn out (lassitude)

kǐn khãaw bà lam	Loss of appetite.
ʔɔ̀ɔn	Be weak.
mɔ̂ɔj	Be drowsy, tired.

nỳaj	Be weak and tired.
ˀid	Tired, exhausted.
hǐw	Tired, weak, fatigued, exhausted.
salâab = tɔ̂ɔd tǐin tɔ̌ɔd myy = tɔ̂ɔd nýa tɔ̂ɔd tǔa	Be debilitated, not able to get up.

There are in fact many expressions for being debilitated, weak, and sickly; for example, phɔ̌ɔm hɛ̃ɛŋ lɛɛŋ nɔ́ɔj—pěn dɔ̃ɔŋ pěn phɔ̌ɔm—ˀɔ̀ɔn ˀɔ̀ɔn ˀɛ̀ɛd ˀɛ̀ɛ—khĩi hób khĩi hãj—khĩi cũu cĩi—khĩi pĩa—khĩi cɔ̌ɔj—khĩi pĩa khĩi cɔ̌ɔj—khĩi pĩa khĩi ñɔ̂m—khĩi pĩa khĩi jɔ̃ŋ mɔ̃ŋ sɛɛ—pěn pĩa pěn kɔ̂n. Similar expressions are also found in section 4.2.1 under khǎaŋ saaŋ.

B. Ache, hurt

kaaj	Feel irritation on the skin (general).
khan	Itch.
sɛ̀ɛb	Feel burning pain, scorching pain.
ned	Paresthesia; sensation of tingling, prickling, or numbness.
khed khĩaw	Icy pain in the teeth.
khad	Have aching joints and bones, rheumatic pain.
khob = mŷaj	Have aching muscles, feel stiff and sore.
ceb = pùad	To hurt, have pain, heavy acute pains.
kĩw = bid líw	Have colic, have strong, irregular abdominal pains, premenstrual pains.

lom beŋ	Niggling pain (of puerperal labor), labor pains.
sìab	Have sharp, lancinating pain (e.g., from abdomen toward heart or from loin upwards).
kɛɛn	Feel a beating or throbbing pain.
kɛɛn tɔ́ɔŋ	Have stitch in the side (as after running).
tɔ́ɔŋ tẽn	Regular throb in the stomach.
tɔ́ɔŋ pùan = tɔ́ɔŋ pàn	Rumbling in the stomach (as when hungry).
tɔ́ɔŋ fə́ə	Flatulence.
ceb tɔ́ɔŋ	Have stomachache, colic.
kád	Feel persistent, constant dull pain (as in full bladder or woman's breast full of milk).
hád	Have compressing pain.
háaw	Have muscle cramps (especially in the legs).

C. Neurologic complaints

cág = satog	Have clonic cramps (especially in arms and legs), have convulsions.
khamên	Have a tic.
kìaw	Have spastic cramps in muscles and joints.
ceb hŭa	Have headache.
maw hŭa = mua maw = mŷŋ mâŋ	Feel dizzy.
căj bà dii	Be ill at ease, feel like fainting.

pỳan	Be restless, ill at ease, unable to sit still.
pěn piʔ = pěn lom = lyym khiŋ	Faint (piʔ is also used as a disease term).
kôon = lóm	Collapse (as when fainting).
tâaw	Fall headlong (as when stumbling).
cǔaŋ = cwǎŋ = cwǎaŋ = kǔaŋ = kwǎŋ = phɔ̃ə	Delirious, raving.
bà húu khiŋ = bà húu (syg) tǔa = tǎaj lyym	Unconscious.
tǎaj phàag	Hemiplegia.
tǎaj phaaj	Die in childbed (mother).
tǎaj kǒm	Die in the prenatal period or during labor (mother and child).
tǎa mua	Be dim-sighted.
tǎa laaj = tǎa mŷyd tǎa laaj	Have blurred vision.
tǎa wàn tǎa laaj	Have excessive lacrimation.
hǔu ʔỹy = hǔu tyy	Have dull hearing.

D. Respiratory and digestive phenomena

hǎaj cǎj	Breathe.
hǎaj cǎj fŷyd	Breathe with difficulty.
hǎaw	Yawn.
hɔ̀ɔb	Gasp.
ʔaj	Cough.
thòm = pùn	Spit.

khaaj	Hawk and spit out.
khamug khamûn = khajɔg khajɔ̂n	Feel nauseated.
ʔuaʔ = hâag lom	Retch.
saʔỹyn	Hiccup.
ʔəʔ = ʔə̀ə = ʔə̂ə	Belch.
tóon	Burp (of babies).
sōm pàag	Acrid regurgitation.
hâag	Vomit.

Vocabulary related to skin (secretions from the skin, wounds, efflorescences of the skin, verbs for to swell, retract, spread, rot, and decompose, etc.), see section 4.2.8. Skin diseases.

Degrees of fever, see section 4.2.7. Infections and fever diseases.

3.8. THE DISEASE SYSTEM

3.8.1. Introduction

In this section we discuss certain prominent traditional medical concepts and characteristics, and then proceed to apply them as criteria for a classification of the local disease concepts.

The idea behind the classification has been to plot the disease concepts on a "map" in such a way that curves drawn around diseases with common characteristics will appear as straight and neat as possible. We believe that if we can achieve this when applying a series of different cognitive medical concepts as criteria, we will in fact arrive at a classification that will reflect the classification implicit in the local medical tradition itself.

We proceeded in the following way: First we defined the borders between each disease concept. Working like lexicographers, we sought out differences (see section 4.2). The next logical step was to uncover the relationship between the disease concepts; that is, to look for similarities. On the basis of relative similarity among the diseases, we plotted them out tentatively on a map, with distance reflecting the degree of similarity; that is, the closer the concepts were plotted, the more they had in common, in one way or another.[10] The final step was to choose a number of criteria from the tradition itself, and apply these to the disease map by drawing curves around the diseases that had each of the criteria in common. When the curves turned out to be sinuous or discontinuous, we pushed the diseases around—like magnetic labels on a metal board—to straighten out the curves. Applying many different criteria one by one, we finally arrived at the present location of the diseases (see fig. 13). (The final classification of the diseases and the major dividing curves appear in fig. 24.)

We must warn, however, that our map is a rough and simplified one, mainly because some of the disease names on the map are in fact not one disease but a generic term for a group of diseases and cover a number of subentities with different characteristics. This applies to concepts such as khǎaŋ, lídsaduaŋ, sǎan, módtakhyd, bàhòog, fii, and tùm, just to mention the most obvious examples. We have indicated that subentities of generic terms belong to different classes of diseases, simply by letting the curves run right through these concepts.

Obviously, the way we have plotted the diseases merely reflects the weight of the various criteria we have selected. Below, we go through each of the criteria, which include central medical concepts in the tradition. The medical concepts that have been used as criteria are those referred to in figures 14–23, and they are presented in a sequence of decreasing weight as to the construction of the disease map.

10. In order to help the reader find his way on the map, we have superimposed a coordinate system. In the index accompanying figure 13 the disease terms are arranged alphabetically and the location of each term is indicated by references to the two axes of the coordinate system.

3.8.2. Location

The location of a disease is an all-important factor in disease circumscription. According to this principle, diseases in (a) the skin, (b) the digestive and urinary systems, (c) the respiratory system, and (d) within or around the apertures of the body have been encircled in figure 14.

3.8.3. Wind

The wind (lom) is an integral constituent of the body, similar to the air and wind around us. It is extremely volatile and is easily influenced both in terms of quantity and quality. There may be too much or too little wind in the body, and it may ascend (lom khỹn) or descend (lom loŋ), or a concentration of wind may get stuck in a specific location in the body (lom tid) and, finally, the wind may turn poisonous (lom píd). The wind in one of these abnormal states causes a multitude of symptoms, like swellings, pressure, aching and pains, jerks and spasms, loss of balance, fainting and loss of consciousness, paralysis, and asocial behavior.

There is a close connection between wind and blood (lŷad), and the wind may somehow spread around anywhere in the body with the blood. The concepts lŷadlom and lomlŷad are often given as causal factors of diseases.[11]

Diseases in which an abundance of wind is a prominent symptom affect the faculty of balance—including loss of balanced social behavior—and the movement of the limbs, and results in headache and fainting, pressure in the heart, breast, and stomach regions, and jerks and spasms. Typical diseases of this kind are bàheŋkhúd, píʔ, sànίbàad, khãj satog, lom sakun, and lom phid dyan (see fig. 15). Certain foods and smells are often given as the immediate reason why the wind ascends.

A deficiency of wind will also affect the mobility of the limbs, but in a negative direction, that is, toward immobility and paralysis. Diseases of this kind are ned, nedsaa, and ʔammápâad. A deficiency

11. See also Yoddumnern 1976:7, 9.

	A	B	C	D	E	F
7		mỹn	khĩĩ khòog khĩĩ hid	khĩĩ sĩan khĩĩ khàag	cɔ̃ɔ khĩĩ kɔɔ khĩĩ tûud	
6		phãm	bàheŋ	hýan phaj hɔ̌ɔ tùm pɨ́d	khĩĩ móo khúdtálâad tùm dɛɛŋ	kõoŋ
5		tɔ́ɔŋ kə̃əm sǎan	sɨ̌w cáaŋ khɔɔ fɔ̂ɔg	fɨ̌i tùm fɨ̌i sǎan	tùm lɨ́i tùm had tùm sǎj tùm sug pɨ́d lɔ́ʔ	lɨ́dsaduaŋ dàad khãj pàa
4	khǎa maan maan nám	hâa wɔ̂ɔg	lɨ́dsaduaŋ khǎaŋ khãnyy	bàhòog	nĩw mɔ́dtakhyd khĩĩ hâag sɔ̌ɔŋ kɔɔŋ	ŋúan tǎa lɨ̌aŋ khãj hâag sàag khãj sàní-bàad lýa
3	pɔɔŋ	khĩi khûu phaaj	mâw khǎaŋ khǎaŋ saʔab	tooŋ saaŋ	pɨ́am dɔ̃ɔj	khãj wád jàj pãaŋ tǎa dɛɛŋ
2			kǎan kɨ́aw	bàheŋkhúd piʔ	sànɨ́bàad lom phid dyan	láduu khǎaw
1			nedsaa	lom sakun ʔammápâad	khãj satog pòoŋ	

ʔammápâad	D1	khi͠i khàag	D7	phaaj	B3
bàhòog	D4	khi͠i khòog	C7	phaj	D6
bàheŋ	C6	khi͠i khûu	B3	pha͠m	BC6
bàheŋkhúd	D2	khi͠i kɔɔ	E7	piʔ	D2
cɔ͠ɔ	E7	khi͠i móo	E6	pîam	E3
dɔ͠ɔj	E6	khi͠i sîan	D7	pîd lɔ́ʔ	E5
fǐi	D5	khi͠i tûud	E7	pòoŋ	DE1
fǐi kǎan see tùm lîi		khɔɔ fɔ̂ɔg	C5	pɔɔŋ	A3
fǐi sǎan	D5	khúdtálâad	E6	sǎan	B5
hâa wɔ̂ɔg	B4	kìaw	C2	saaŋ	D3
hɔ̌ɔ	D6	ko͠oŋ	F6	sànîbàad	E2
hýan	D6	láduu khǎaw	F2	sɨ̌w cáaŋ	C5
kǎan	C2	lîdsaduaŋ	C4	tǎa dɛɛŋ	F3
khǎa maan	A4	lîdsaduaŋ dàad	F5	tooŋ	D3
khǎaŋ	C3	lom phid dyan	E2	tɔ́ɔŋ kə͠əm	B5
khǎaŋ khan͠yy	BC5	lom sakun	D1	tùm	D5
khǎaŋ saʔab	C3	maan nám	A4	tùm dɛɛŋ	E6
kha͠j hâag sàag	F4	mâw	D34	tùm had	E5
kha͠j pàa	F5	módtakhyd	F4	tùm lîi~fǐi kǎan	E5
kha͠j sànîbàad lýa	F4	mɨ̌n	BC7	tùm pîd	D6
kha͠j satog	E1	nedsaa	C1	tùm sǎj	E5
kha͠j wád jàj	F3	ni͠w	E4	tùm sug	E5
khi͠ihâag sɔ̌ɔŋkɔɔŋ	EF4	ŋúan tǎa lɨ̌aŋ	F4		
khi͠i hid	C7	pa͠aŋ	F3		

Fig. 13. Disease reference map and alphabetical index.

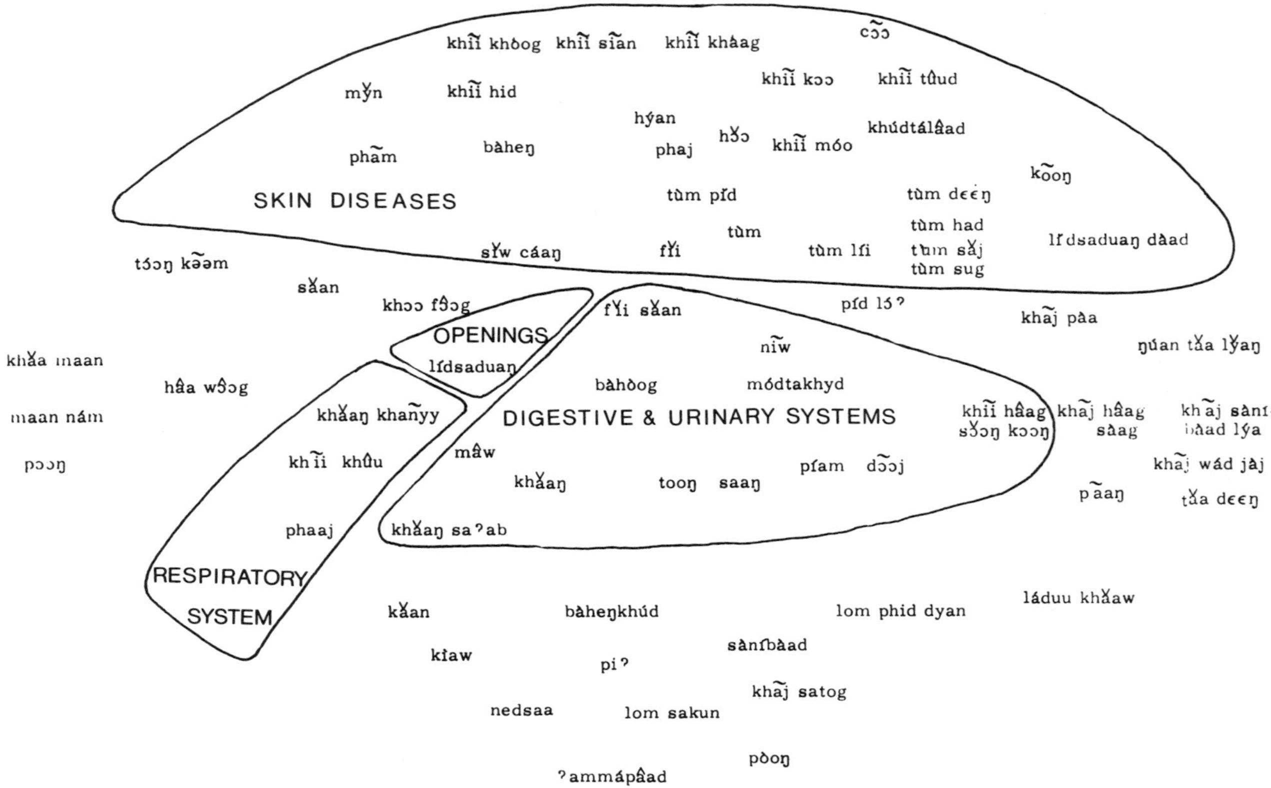

Fig. 14. Disease groups based on location.

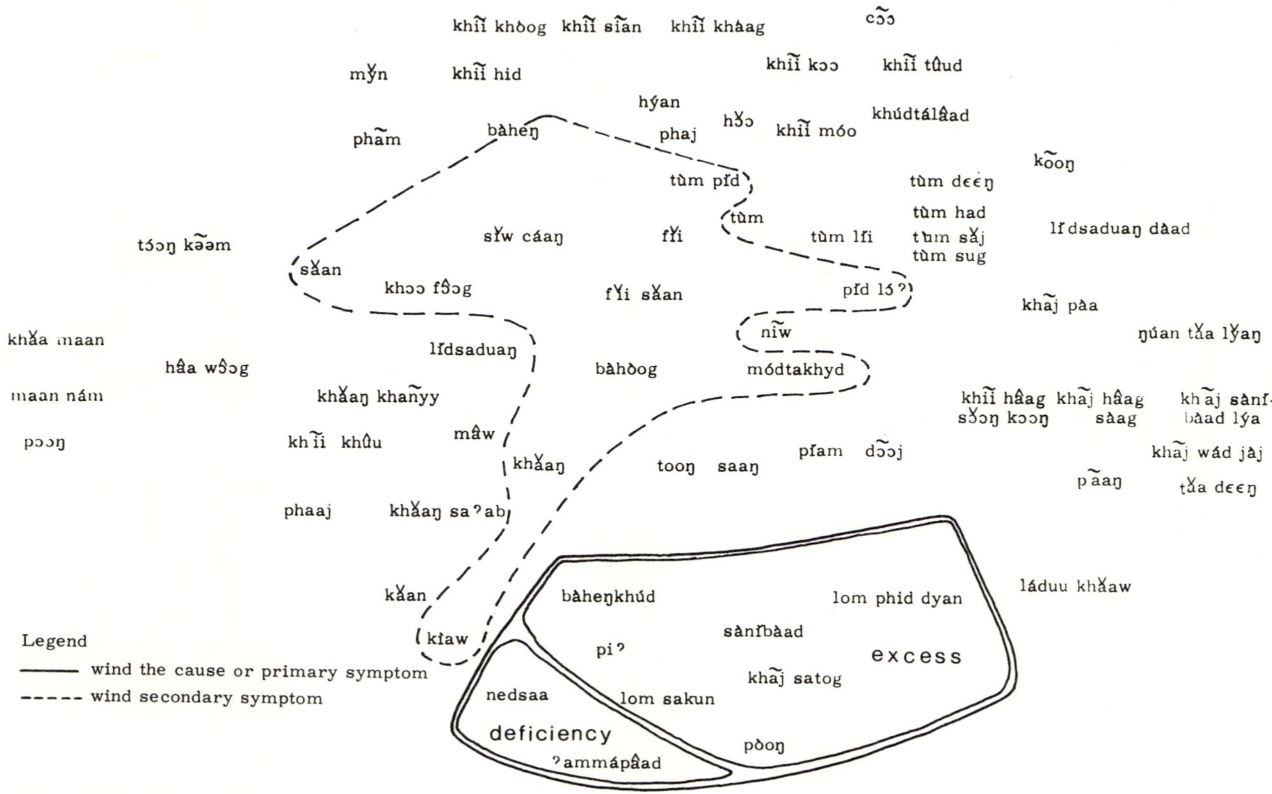

Fig. 15. Wind diseases.

of wind causes the blood to harden, and hot foods and remedies are prescribed to enhance the wind and to dilute the blood.[12]

The wind may also turn "poisonous" (lom píd), and is then considered very dangerous. If a poisonous wind ascends (lom píd khỹn), it will result in sudden loss of consciousness, normally followed by death. A poisonous wind is common with diseases like tùm píd, píd lɔ́ʔ, and sǐw cáaŋ, but is a possible complication with other diseases as well.

The wind may also appear, in addition to the compulsory symptoms, as a secondary symptom or complication in diseases like bàhòog phanládii, módtakhyd lom, certain khǎaŋ diseases, fǐi sǎan, kìaw, many bàheŋ, sǎan, fǐi diseases, and khɔɔ fɔ̂ɔg. In fact, a disease may be cured as such, but the wind may still remain.

The tradition contains a huge number of prescriptions curing wind in one of its many appearances. These prescriptions usually contain numerous ingredients and are used together with other more specific medicines.

The wind is regarded as the most vital constituent of the body, and is referred to as the essential pathophysiological explanation of a variety of diseases. It is tempting to say—as K. Sassady does for the Laotian medical system—that the Northern Thai medical tradition is basically a pneumatic system.[13, 14]

3.8.4. Blood and lymph

The blood (lŷad) is recognized as the basic fluid in the body, although—as we mentioned earlier—the concept of a circulatory

12. Mulholland has found that in Central Thai tradition a growing understanding of a circulatory system has given blood a more distinct meaning—to the point of erecting it as a new humoral element of the body, and to some extent replacing the concept of wind. Mulholland 1979*a*:103.

13. Sassady 1962:38–39.

14. Wind illnesses in Northern Thailand have also been studied by M. A. Muecke (1979). Her findings correspond largely to ours. Her study includes wind illnesses only, and therefore she does not demarcate borders between wind illnesses and other traditional disease entities. Muecke includes spirit-caused diseases and "madness" into the category of illnesses caused by wind, whereas we keep these disorders apart.

system is not well understood. The blood may be found in various states: it may be normal (lŷad dii) or it may turn stale and become spoiled (lŷad sĭa) and then cause diseases, as is also frequently mentioned in the manuscripts. The blood may also become hot or cold, and there may be too little blood in the body.

Blood is brought up as an important disease factor in many contexts:

> The condition of the blood is regarded as the major characteristic in the diseases kăan and kìaw.
>
> Bad or spoiled blood is said to be the cause, or one of the causes, of bàheŋkhúd, kìaw dam, ʔammápâad, khĩi móo, khúdtálâad, and săan dɔ̀ɔg bug. One informant also maintained that certain skin diseases may be caused by spoiled blood, in which case an expelling medicine (jaa thàaj) should be used.
>
> In some diseases the blood may turn poisonous (lŷad pĕn píd) as a complication, as in the major bàheŋ-types and some dangerous kinds of săan, like săan dɔ̀ɔg bug and săan khanthámaalaa.
>
> The disease piʔ lŷad is, according to one informant, caused by the blood "not being thick enough," an explanation coalescent with the popular biomedical expression of the condition of anemia, which is a central part of the concept of piʔ lŷad. A contamination of cosmopolitan medical ideas may thus have occurred.
>
> Diseases like phadoŋ lŷad and bàheŋ lŷad are simply said to "come from the blood."
>
> The disease săan bàkham hɔ́ɔj is said to spread around in the body via the blood.

As can be noted, the blood is said to be the cause of several typical wind diseases, like piʔ, bàheŋkhúd, and ʔammápâad. This underlines what we have already pointed out; namely, that there is a close connection between the wind and the blood, and that the two influence each other.

The presence of exudant blood gets considerable attention as a clinical sign or symptom, and it is a major characteristic of diseases like khǎaŋ pú? and lídsaduaŋ lŷad (coughing or vomiting blood, nose-bleeding), and in bàhòog lŷad, módtakhyd lŷad, and kĩw loŋ dam loŋ dɛɛŋ (where the stools are accompanied by blood).

Finally there are diseases for which the word for blood (lŷad) is part of the disease name: phadoŋ lŷad, móo lŷad, bàheŋ lŷad, sǎan lŷad, lídsaduaŋ khǎaŋ lŷad, lídsaduaŋ lŷad, bàhòog lŷad, módtakhyd lŷad, pi? lŷad, and kǎan lŷad.

In figure 16, diseases particularly associated with blood in one context or another have been encircled. Although there is a considerable overlap with the wind group in figure 15, there are typical diseases in both groups where the concepts of wind and blood are not intermixed.

The lymph (nám lỹaŋ) refers to watery secretions, as from wounds or skin eruptions, and is regarded as a specific fluid of the body. The lymph may, like the blood, become spoiled (sĭa) and is then a potential cause of diseases, but one may also contract a disease by touching the lymph of a sick person. According to one informant, the lymph moves along the skin outside the veins without mixing with the blood. Another informant also associated nám lỹaŋ with swollen glands in the armpits and groin—an idea that may have been borrowed from cosmopolitan medicine.

3.8.5. Poison

The word *píd* means poison or venom in a concrete sense, like snake venom (píd ŋuu) or poison from mad dogs (píd mǎa wɔ̃ɔ). Eating meat of animals dead from diseases, or in epidemics, introduces píd into the body, resulting in the disease tùm píd or in food poisoning in general. Also, infected wounds and carbuncles may produce píd, as in the diseases píd lɔ́?, sĭw cáaŋ, and tùm líi.

Some bàheŋ and sǎan diseases have poisonous blood (lŷad pěn píd) as an inherent symptom, while in other diseases poisoning may occur as a complication, as it does in several types of fĩi, in fĩi sǎan, and in kǎan.

Diseases in which poison occurs also produce wind as a secondary symptom (except in tùm líi, kǎan, and pòoŋ), whereas there

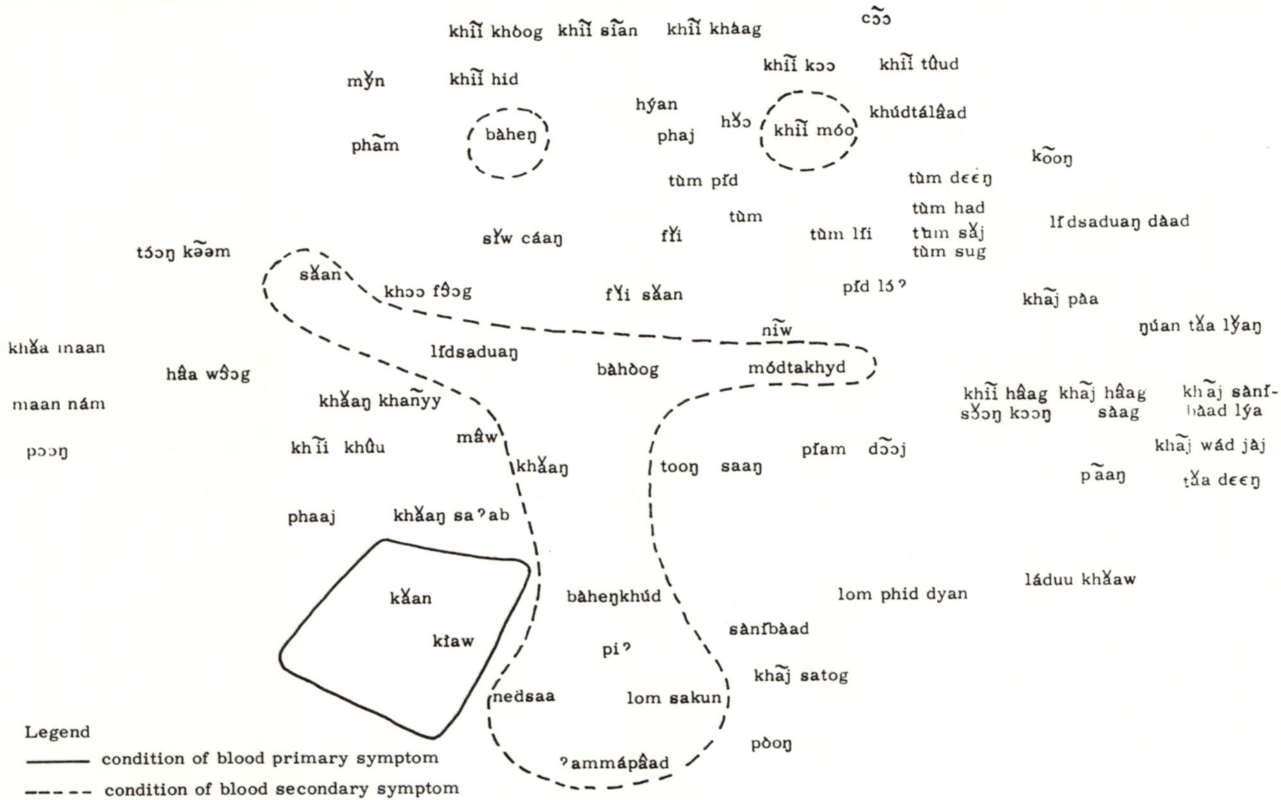

Fig. 16. Diseases in which the condition of the blood is a prominent symptom.

is no overlapping between the blood diseases and the poison diseases, except in the case of kǎan.

But píd also refers to the less tangible concept of "something with the attribute of poison," which is not easily conceived in concrete terms. Spirits may for example insert píd into the body (píd phǐi sàj), as in the case of pòoŋ. The wind and the blood may also turn poisonous (lom píd, lŷad pěn píd).

The presence of píd normally results in pain, and the disease is regarded as acute or critical and should be treated with great care. First of all the píd should be prevented from spreading by means of dietary restrictions and incantations (khaathǎa pàw píd). The medicines administered aim ultimately at expelling the poison from the body (thàaj píd, thìib píd). If the treatment is not successful, the píd, together with the wind, will cause sudden attacks, normally followed by immediate death.[15]

In figure 17, the poison diseases have been encircled. They include diseases that may suddenly turn fatal. Most of them (except tùm líi, kǎan, and pòoŋ) also produce wind as an important secondary complication (see figure 15), while none of them includes blood as a characteristic symptom (except kǎan and bàheŋ). Most of the poison diseases also require food prohibitions as part of the treatment (except bàheŋ, tùm líi, and kǎan).

3.8.6. Hot-cold

The opposition hot-cold (hɔ́ɔn-jen) is an important classificatory principle in the medical tradition. Both plants and medicines, and reactions of the body, are classified as hot, cold, or something in between (kǎaŋ). Certain diseases are also regarded as hot or cold, although most diseases fall outside the dichotomy altogether (see figure 18). The dichotomy functions as a physiological explanation model of both the diseases and the reactions of the drugs in the body. It is the patient's perception of heat or coolness in his

15. The distinction between píd and ŋúan is discussed in section 3.8.9 under B-6.

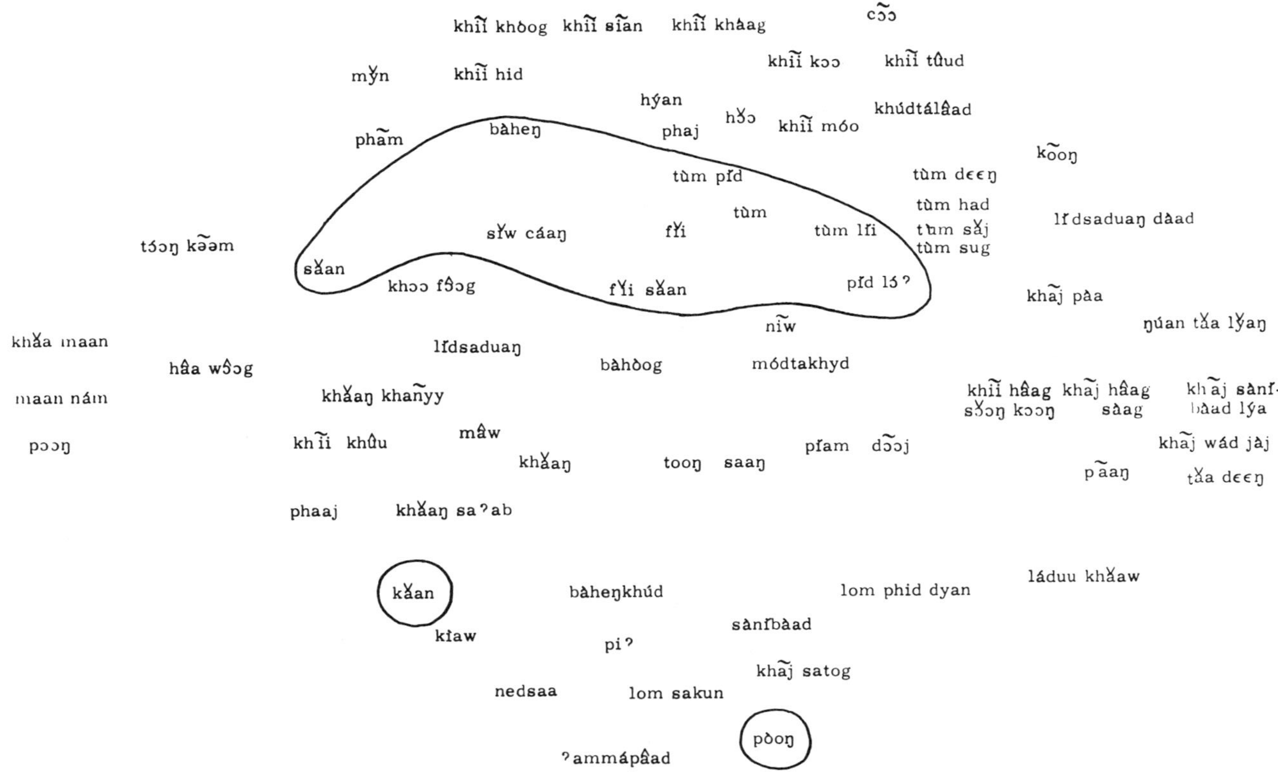

Fig. 17. Diseases with píd (poison) as prominent symptom.

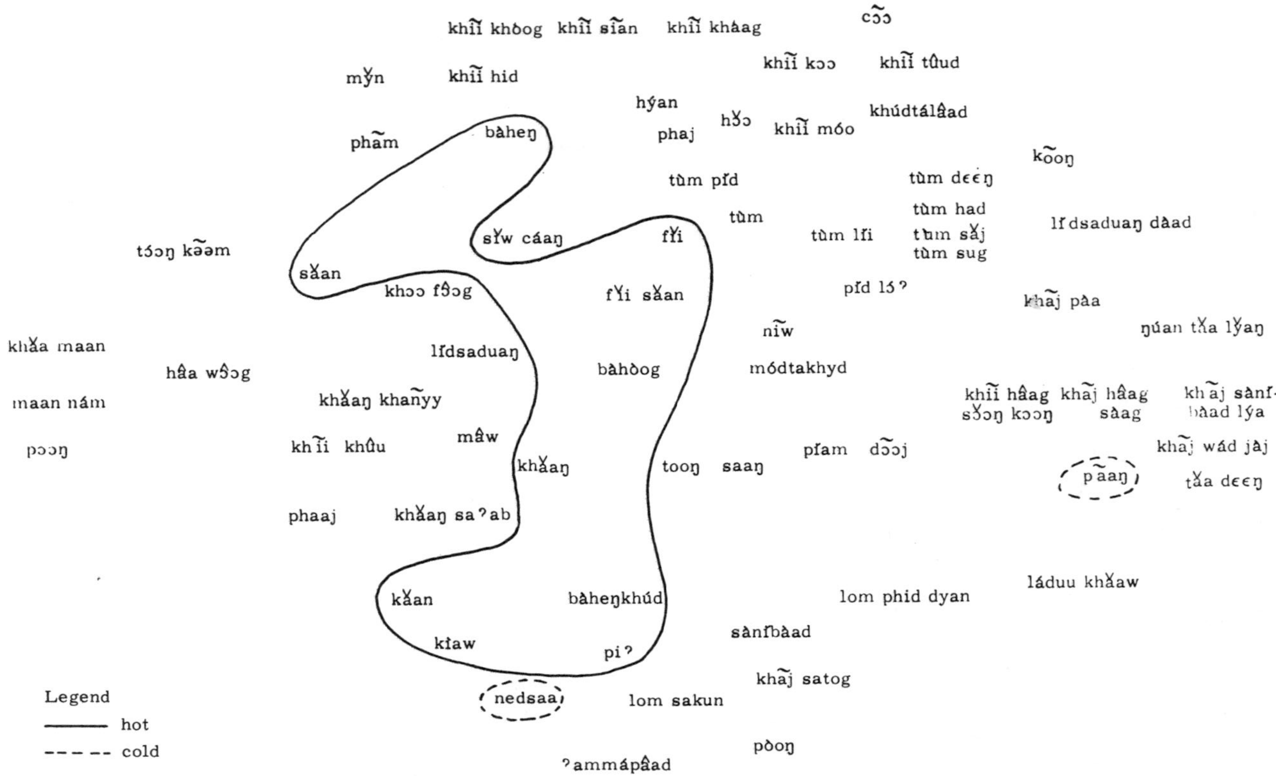

Fig. 18. Hot and cold diseases.

body that is decisive for this classification. Uncomfortable hot symptoms characteristic of hot diseases are painful and cause burning sensations due, for example, to an inflammation, be it in the mouth (khǎaŋ), the urinary tract (khǎaŋ loŋ liŋ), the intestines (bàhòog, kĩw bàhòog), or the skin (bàheŋ, fĩi). The most typical wind diseases are perceived as hot. Exceptions are diseases with loss of sensation, paresis, or immobility, which are regarded as cold (see ned, nedsaa, ʔammápâad). A fever disease may turn out to be hot, cold, or neither hot nor cold. The conditions khãj ceb hũa (fever and headache) and khãj hɔ́ɔn naj (perception of an internal heat) are typically hot, whereas a shivering fever (khãj nǎaw sàn), for example, makes the patient feel cold and is consequently classified as cold. When a patient has the disease kìaw dam, his skin feels cool, but he feels hot inside, so the disease is classified as a warm disease.

The blood may also be classified as either hot or cold. Hot blood is associated with a fast pulse or may produce excessive bleeding or spontaneous hemorrhages. Menstruating women emanate a destructive heat from their bodies, caused by hot blood. Cold blood is associated with a slow pulse and produces hardness, stiffness, or loss of sensation.

One of our informants classified all crude drugs—both single plants and mixtures of plants—into hot, cold, or indifferent. (See the column headed "Physical quality" in the list of Medicinal Plants in the Appendix.) A hot medicine will cause a hot reaction in the body inducing an internal heat which in turn will eliminate the opposite feeling of coolness. It also induces thirst, stimulates the appetite, and restores vigor (tonic) and usually provokes diarrhea as a part of the hot reaction (purgative), although an indifferent medicine may act as a purgative, as well. A typical hot reaction to a medicine, when it is applied externally, is caustic, producing redness and a burning sensation (inflammation). A cold drug-mediated reaction reduces the uncomfortable hot symptoms characteristic of hot diseases. The intermediate reactions caused by an indifferent drug are not measured by any dramatic or specific effects, but are deemed capable of diminishing a wide range of symptoms perceived as neither hot nor cold. A mixture of plants of the indifferent kind has probably a wider range of applications than the hot and cold remedies.

The same informant also postulated a connection between six main tastes—bitter (khom), sweet (wăan), sour (sõm), salty (kem), spicy (phed), and tasteless (cỳyd)—and the three temperature qualities, inasmuch as he usually classified a crude drug with a sour taste as cold, a spicy taste as hot, and bitter, salty, and sweet tastes as indifferent.

The hot-cold dichotomy forms a link between certain diseases and certain medicines, and is thus a guide for treatment. The general rule is that hot diseases are treated with cold medicines, and vice versa, although there are important exceptions. Hot diseases treated with cool medicines are piʔ and bàheŋkhúd (the treatment for these consists of taking the patient into the shade, applying water to his head, and letting him relax and cool off), fĭi diseases when these have developed wind and poison and thus have turned serious, and kăan. Excessive bleeding, like nosebleed and menstrual bleeding, is stopped with cold medicines that make the blood hard.

There are also quite a few hot diseases that require hot medicines for effective cure, like bàhòog, săan, fĭi săan, kìaw dam, and bàheŋ. Typical cool diseases treated with hot medicines are nedsaa and pãaŋ. When we apply the hot-cold criteria to our disease map, we notice that the hot diseases are nicely lumped together, although bàheŋ is separated from the rest. The two cold diseases are located far apart (see fig. 18).

Our information on the subject of hot and cold diseases and their treatment is sparse. Further studies with more consistent information may reveal alternative classifications and interpretations.

3.8.7. Left-right and female-male

The oppositions left-right and female-male are common classificatory principles in both medical and nonmedical contexts.[16]

We have come across several examples:

Some informants classified fĭi into female fĭi, those occurring on the left side of the body and not containing pus, and male fĭi,

16. R. Davis includes the opposition female-male into a larger dualistic framework of opposite concepts: low-high, south-north, west-east, feet-head, female-male, junior-senior, red-white (Davis 1974:197). See also Bradley 1865:86–87, and Riley et al. 1979:25.

those on the right side with pus. A fĭi naj tɔ́ɔŋ appearing on the left side is female, on the right side, male. When a săan is moved, the traditional doctor will move it to the left side of a woman, and to the right side of a man. And, finally, according to a manuscript, pains in the right half of the body are called lom saduaŋ, whereas pains in the left half are called lom săan.[17]

3.8.8. The concept of "mother"

Another pathogenic factor relevant to some diseases is the existence of a "mother" (mii mɛ̂ɛ, mii cŷa mii mɛ̂ɛ). The mother is a physical entity that settles down in the body, and from which the disease spreads. This mother must be "killed" (khãa mɛ̂ɛ) in order to eradicate the disease properly. The mother thrives on certain foods. When the mother eats these foods, it is like pouring fuel on flames: the mother, and therefore the disease as a whole, will flare up and grow exuberantly. Killing the mother involves (1) withholding the foods she thrives on, that is, one should follow the food prohibitions and thus weaken her, and (2) one should take the medicines that will actually kill her. When informants explicitly referred to the presence of a mother, we found that they had lídsaduaŋ or the skin diseases khĩi khòog, tûud, bàheŋ, or săan, all of which also require food prohibitions as part of the treatment, with the exception of khĩi khòog.

3.8.9. Causality concepts

On a general level, the answer to the question, What is the cause of this disease? elicited the replies: (1) "It comes from outside" (maa càag nɔ̂ɔg), (2) "It comes from inside" (ʔɔ̀ɔg càag naj maa, khỹn maa ʔeeŋ), or (3) "I don't know." More specific causal factors mentioned by the traditional doctors were:

A. *Traumatic causality,* resulting in wounds, fractures, and so on.

17. In Laos, fevers are classified into male (dry, not accompanied by sweat) and female (wet, accompanied by sweat). See R. Pottier 1971:267.

B. ***Intervention of material or immaterial agents alien to the human body.***

B-1. *Contact with external agents,* such as dirty water, metal chains, certain plants, washing powder, or sunshine may cause various skin diseases.

B-2. *Spoiled or wrong food.* Food is regarded as the fundamental cause of many diseases. The food may be spoiled or indigestible, causing disease, or it may be "wrong." (See section 3.8.8 on "mother.") Wrong foods (kǐn phid) aggravate an already existing disease, causing a minor symptom to turn into a more prominent and dangerous one. (See also section 3.8.10 Food restrictions.)

B-3. *Noxious odors* are given as a causal factor of some wind diseases, especially those attacking women.[18] Odors are commonly given as the ultimate cause of the disease lom phid dyan and, in the same way as food, wrong smells may cause the wind suddenly to ascend and create havoc in the body.

B-4. *Insect and animal bites.* Insect bites may cause itching and certain skin diseases and, due to the influence of Western medical concepts, insect bites are now also regarded as the causal factor of some fever diseases. It is well known that bites of mad dogs cause rabies.

B-5. *Intestinal worms* (khĩi tỳyg, tǔa tɔ̂ɔŋ), which are very common in Northern Thailand, especially among children, are regarded as a disease in themselves, and there are very effective herbal remedies causing diarrhea to expel intestinal worms, like máklya (Diospyros mollis), which unfortunately also may cause blindness as a side effect. In some diseases, like khǎaŋ tooŋ, khǎaŋ saaŋ, and dɔ̄ɔj (see section 4.2.1), where a Western diagnosis points at intestinal worms as the cause, the traditional herbalist only exceptionally refers to the worms as a major cause. Northern Thais

18. Women, both during menstruation, and before and after childbirth, for example, have to be very careful with both foods and smells. A description of the diet and dietary restrictions of women being in the above situation in the Lampang province is found in Yoddumnern 1976.

recognize several types of intestinal worms: tŷyg bɛɛn, tŷyg pɛ̂ɛb (flatworm, tapeworm); tŷyg khɔ̌ɔ (hookworm); tŷyg kǒm (pinworm, short roundworm); and tŷyg sẽn dãaj (long roundworm, Guinea worm).

B-6. *Diseases may be caused by spirits* (thùug phǐi ñíaʔ) or by means of black magic (thùug khon ñíaʔ, thùug tũu lɔɔŋ). These supernatural causes, or personalistic etiologies, as G. M. Foster (1976) prefers to call them, require further elaboration.

The Northern Thai pantheon is inhabited by a number of spirits that may cause a variety of diseases.

B-6.1. *Moral spirits* are basically protective (phǐi dii).

B-6.1.1. *Clan spirits* (phǐi pùu ñâa) are inherited through women, and may cause diseases in a clan member as a punitive action if she has "wronged the spirit" (sǐa phǐi), particularly if she has engaged in premarital sex. The disease is automatically cured when the wrong has been admitted and a ceremonial excuse has been offered.

B-6.1.2. *Noble spirits* (cãw naaj) are spirits of longtime dead nobles or warriors, who need mediums through whom they can talk and thus help mankind. These spirits are omniscient and can in principle answer all kinds of questions.

Normally the noble spirits act as decision makers for people, but they can also find the cause of diseases, particularly diseases caused by other spirits. The noble spirits act in a way as supervisors of the spirit world, and they know what the other spirits are up to. When a sick person comes to ask about the cause of his disease, the noble spirit will thus answer that it is this or that spirit, living there and there, that has caused the disease, because the patient did this or that. The spirit in question likes this or that food (± alcohol, ± sweets, ± chicken/pig/cow meat), which should be offered at this or that time at this or that place by a specialist or by the relatives of the sick person.

The noble spirits may also attempt to cure certain diseases, especially aching joints or muscles, through a "rubbing-away" ceremony (cédhɛ̀ɛg), and there are examples of spirits even venturing into the field of the herbalists by giving food prescriptions or mentioning herbal mixtures that are effective.

In one instance, these noble spirits themselves cause diseases; namely, when they want a new medium. The disease they induce in the person they want as the new medium is always of the same kind, resulting in the victim's behavior, usually a female, becoming totally asocial and unpredictable, and finally resulting in the victim withdrawing from social intercourse. The disease cannot be cured by any available method, and thus drags on for months or even years. The victim will finally die unless she accepts mediumship.

B-6.1.3. *The village spirit and the temple spirit* (sẽw bãan, sẽw wád) are basically protective spirits but may, like the clan spirit, cause light diseases, like sudden attacks of fever, in retaliation for some disrespectful behavior.

B-6.2. *Amoral spirits* (phǐi háaj, phǐi pàa, phǐi kàw phǐi dəəm) are the many nameless and hungry spirits living anywhere in the immediate village neighborhood or in the forest. It is this type of amoral spirit that most frequently causes troubles to human beings, including diseases. Diseases attributed to amoral spirits are of two kinds:

B-6.2.1. Diseases affecting the relationship between the patient and concrete persons in the patient's immediate social environment. The spirit itself possesses the patient (phǐi khãw, phǐi kǐn, phǐi ñam, phǐi loŋ), who all of a sudden becomes disrespectful in language and behavior, and completely unruly, disregarding all social norms. The curing process for these uncontrolled fits of rage or despair consists of calling on someone to whom the spirit is willing to reveal its identity and asking what kind of offerings it wants.

If the spirit is fierce and does not want to comply and leave the patient after an offering has been promised, the only way left is to force it out (khěe), which normally is done with a whip. The important point here is to note that the spirit is amoral, and that the patient has not intentionally done anything to offend the spirit, and thus is in fact totally unresponsible for what he or she does during the possession. In this way personal frustration and tension between individuals are given permissible outlets, without the patient being left with any kind of guilt or stigma.

B-6.2.2. Diseases with sudden onset, resistant to treatment, or of an epidemic nature. Fever, swellings, and aching joints or muscles are often prominent symptoms of these diseases.

We are here only concerned with this last kind—the "normal" diseases caused by spirits—which may be cured by normal herbal methods but where magic becomes the essential part of the curing process. Diseases of this type are caused by something being inserted into the body by the spirits (phǐi sàj, phǐi pɛ̌ɛŋ). This "something" is a kind of poison (píd, ŋúan), which the spirits "sow" (thùug phǐi wàan ŋúan wàan píd); *píd* can be conceptualized as a liquid or a vapor, which can spread around the body (see section 3.8.5 Poison); *ŋúan*, however, must be understood as something lumpy (pěn kɔ̃ɔn). This term is used with words for tumors, as in ŋúan sǎan, and carbuncles, as in ŋúan fǐi, although ŋúan may also be found with a meaning very close to píd, as in ŋúan tǎa lɯ̌aŋ, below, where there are no lumps present. We have come across two diseases for which ŋúan is part of the name, both having fever as a prominent symptom:

a. *ŋúan sǎan~fǐi ŋúan sǎan* is characterized by a hard lump in the stomach plus fever, in contrast to fǐi sǎan (naj tɔ́ɔŋ), where there is no fever, but the patient feels hot inside.

b. *ŋúan tǎa lɯ̌aŋ,* another name for khãj tǎa lɯ̌aŋ (yellow eye fever).

The curing process of diseases caused by spirits involves the following steps:

1. Ask a specialist about the cause (thǎam mɯ̂a thǎam mɔ̃ɔ).
2. Give offerings to the spirit in question (bɔ̀ɔg kàaw bon líaŋ).
3. Perform rubbing-away ceremonies (cédhɛ̀ɛg) or cutting-away ceremonies (tad phom tad phaaj), thus relieving the patient of the poison (thɔ̃ɔn píd, thɔ̀ɔd píd), which is afterward ceremonially sent away (sòŋ).

The diseases and symptoms for which spirits are thought to be the main cause are *phaaj* (tuberculosis); *pòoŋ* (polio, arthritis); and *khãj* (fever). Many fever diseases, especially of the malaria types, which the patient has caught in the forest, are traced back to an unspecified "forest spirit." Symptoms like *aching joints* (khad hŭa-khàw khɛŋkhăa), if unresponsive to treatment, may be attributed to a spirit (phĭi ñam).

Also sudden, *unexpected deaths* may be attributed to spirits (phĭi hag khɔɔ), as in the case of *kăan* and certain *lom* diseases. In addition *epidemic* diseases, like certain types of *tùm* and *fĭi*, are said to be caused by unspecified spirits (see fig. 19).

Spirits can also frighten people and cause gooseflesh (khŏn lúg), as in sàníbàad sadũŋ (startled sàníbàad), which is also called sàníbàad phĭi pɛ̆ɛŋ (spirit-caused sàníbàad).

B-7. *Black magic.* Foreign matter may be introduced into the body not only by spirits but by humans as well (thùug khon ñíaʔ, ŋúan khon sàj, thùug lɔɔŋ). This requires the art of *black magic* (săjásàad). The objects in question are often metal objects, pieces of skin, or lumps of hair, which are magically introduced into the stomach of the victim. In the Lamphun area people fear (and admire) the Karens and the Khamu for their powerful incantations, although Northern Thais also practice this art. The objects can be removed only by incantations more powerful than the ones used to insert them. And if a person with such power is found, he can in fact not only extract the object, but may send it back to attack its owner.

In the case of leprosy, *curses* may be one possible way of transferring the disease (see khĩi tûud, below).

C. *The climate, the seasons, and the age and sex* of a person are loosely referred to as etiological factors on a very general level, and they may also influence the development of a disease. The Thais have found that some diseases are common during the cold season (hýan), while others occur in the rainy season (hɔ̆ɔ, khĩi móo nɔ̀ɔ) or the hot season (kìaw). Some diseases show preference for men (bàhòog), while others attack mainly women (lom phid dyan, láduu khăaw, maan nám). Age may also be a triggering factor for certain diseases, if other preconditions are present. Although not a causal factor in itself, the prevalence of certain diseases in restricted age groups, such as children, for instance, is an important characteristic of a number of diseases. Typical children's diseases

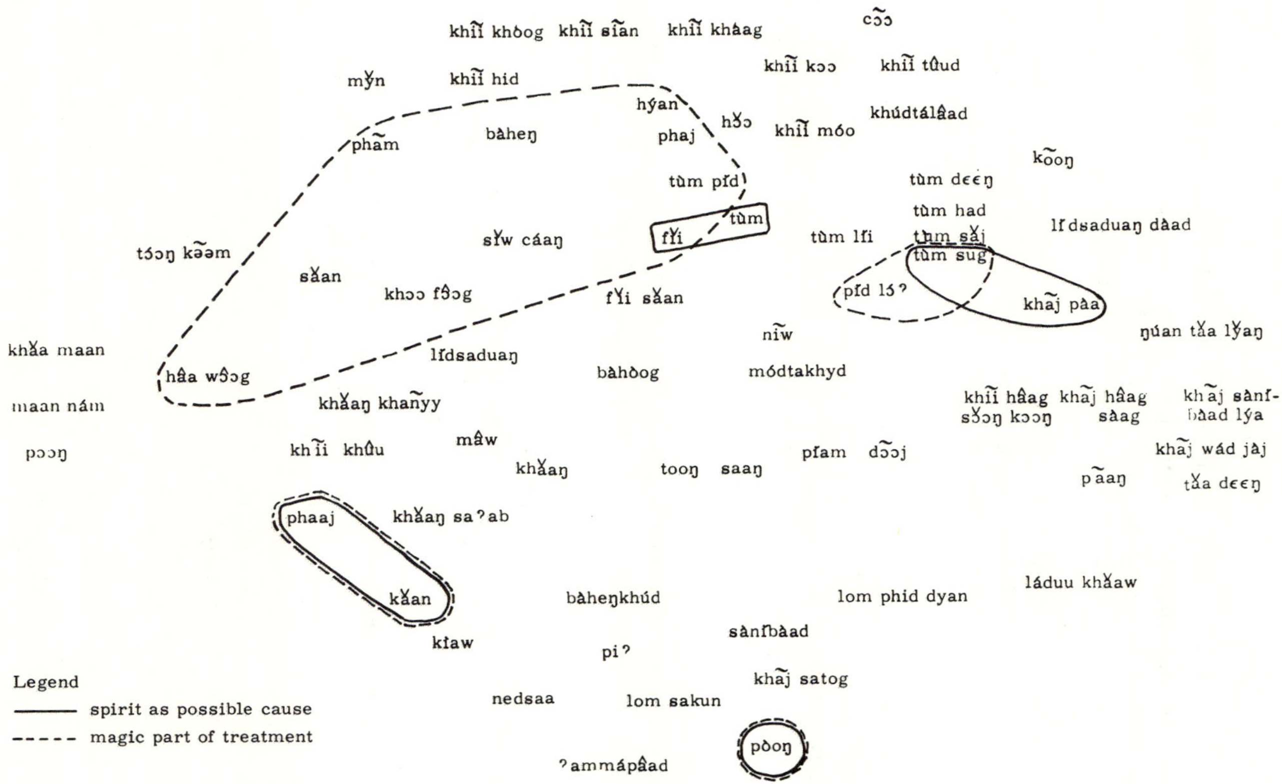

Fig. 19. Diseases connected with spirits and magic.

are, for example: khǎaŋ, khǎaŋ khañyy, hâa wɔ̂ɔg, mâw, dɔ̄ɔj, píam, pãaŋ, tùm had, tùm dɛɛŋ, tùm sǎj, tǎa dɛɛŋ, khǎa maan, bàheŋ khàj pǎa.[19] When arranging the disease map we have attempted to plot child diseases as close to one another as possible (see fig. 20).

D. *Karma.* In some cases people regard diseases as a consequence of their earlier actions and thus refer to karma (kǎm) as the ultimate cause. When people are getting old they are particularly apt to use karma as an all-round explanation for the inevitable and often incurable diseases they have to suffer. But also when younger people get diseases, references to specific actions of that person which may explain the disease are frequent. For instance, a man caught a hawk that had killed some of his chickens. After tying its legs, he dipped it slowly into boiling water, legs first, till it finally died. This fellow was later attacked by a heat wave which mounted from his feet to his head and killed him. There exist many stories of this kind.

However, while karma may be referred to as the original cause of a disease in retrospect, it is rarely brought up initially as the triggering factor.

E. *Concept of contagiousness.* Some diseases are regarded as transmittable (tid), either through direct contact or from ancestry. For example, touching the skin eruptions of a diseased person may cause a transfer of the disease; that is, in hýan, hɔ̌ɔ, phaj, and khĩi khàag. Ancestral diseases are said to be "coming from the parents" (tid càag pɔ̂ɔ càag mɛ̂ɛ), "passing through the blood" (tid tǎam lŷad, sỳyb tǎam lŷad), or "passing through the mother's milk" (tid tǎam nám nom). Such diseases may include a word for "family" or "clan" like lom sakun, piʔ sakun, phaaj khakǔn. Other examples of inheritable diseases affecting the next generation are khĩi tûud, phaaj, and some types of módtakhyd. These are regarded as difficult or impossible to cure (see fig. 21).

19. In some few cases a disease is called one thing if attacking children and another if attacking adults. Examples are, for children: khāj satog and khǎaŋ khañyy; for adults: sàníbàad and khĩi khûu.

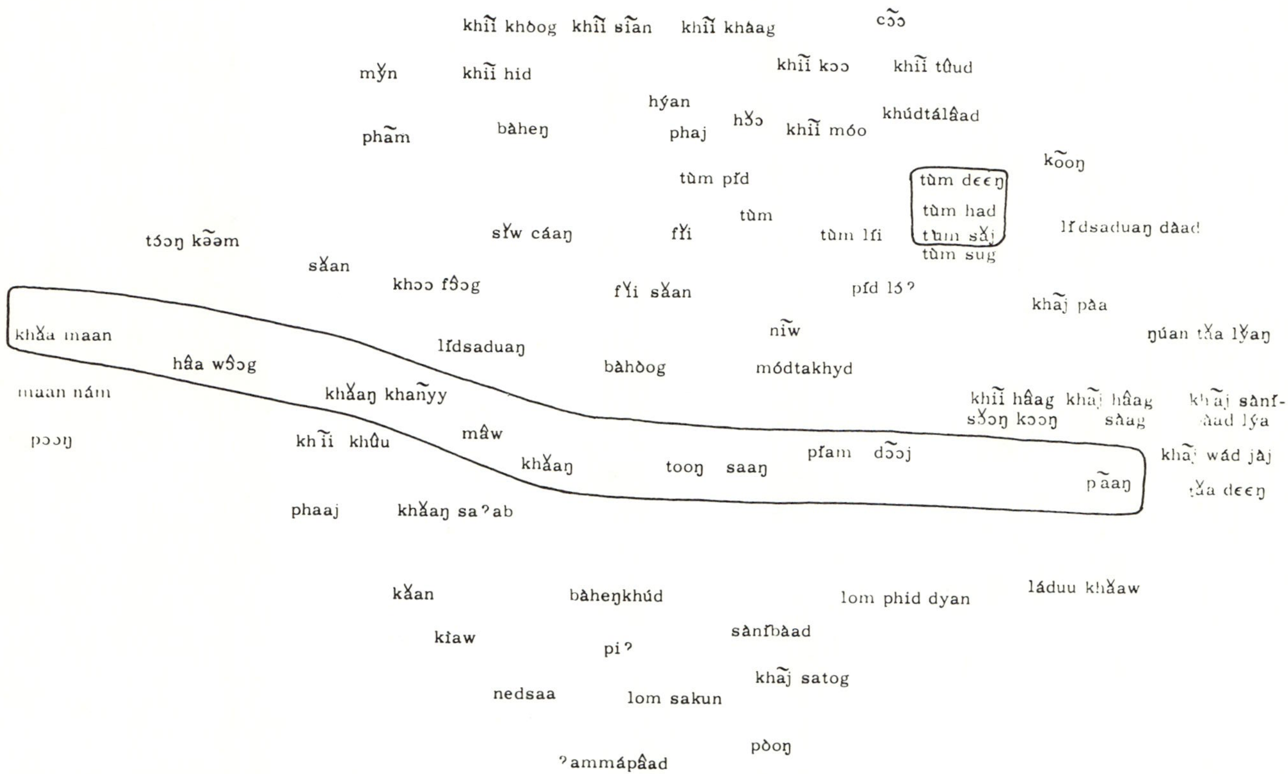

Fig. 20. Children's diseases.

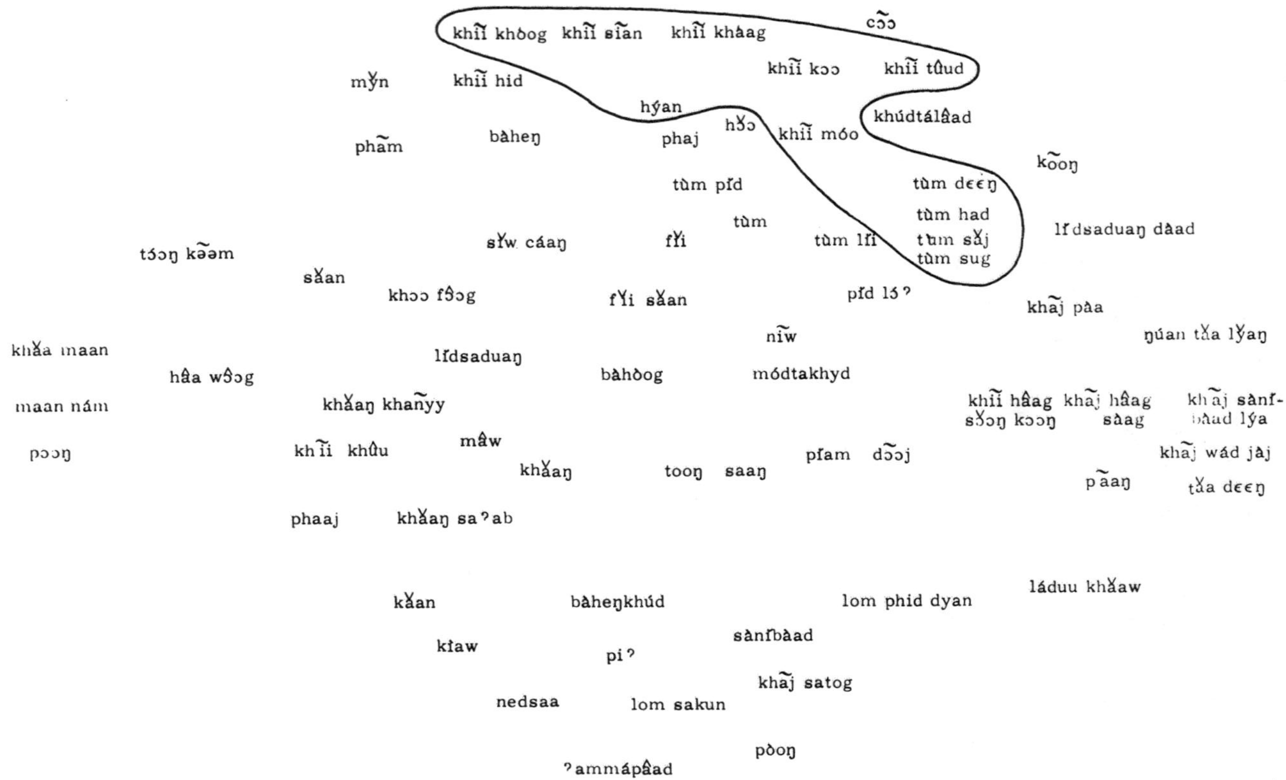

Fig. 21. Contagious diseases.

F. *Internal factors.* The core pathogenic medical concepts such as wind, blood and lymph, poison, "mother," and the hot-cold opposition are also commonly brought up as causes of disease.

Conclusions

As will be noticed, the recorded causality concepts include both the naturalistic and the personalistic (see Foster and Anderson 1978). Some diseases are attributed to a single causal factor, while others reveal multiple causalities. A distinction among a primary cause ("root" cause), or *etiology*; the factors producing disease, or *pathogenetic factors*; and triggering factors, or *predisposing factors*; is usually not made. In diseases with multiple causalities, there may exist contrasting levels of causality, but they are seldom consistent among the practitioners. Diseases with an internal, pathogenic factor (point F) as a cause are most likely to elicit further explanations. Questions such as What then causes the internal heat to arise, or Why is the wind ascending, and so forth, quite often were answered by bad smell, bad or indigestible food, climate, or age as further causal factors. The personalistic explanation models may exist together with the naturalistic ones; however, the former are even more common as explanations among the populace than among the practitioners.

3.8.10. Food restrictions

Food prohibitions (kān ʔaahǎan) play a very important role in traditional medicine, and with quite a few diseases they represent the crucial part of the treatment. Traditional doctors lose no opportunity stressing the importance of keeping strictly to the prohibitions, which normally is quite unnecessary as the patients will invariably do so anyway. The general food prohibitions are in fact common knowledge, although the herbalist may add some specific prohibitions to the general ones. On the whole the food prohibitions seem to be a stable part of the tradition with few variations.

We have recorded the food prohibitions when they occur after a disease has erupted. The diet in general and its relation to the diseases were not included in our studies.

The general food prohibitions consist of several units:

Meat (nýa): cow or water buffalo meat, pig meat, or chicken meat. It will be specified whether all three, just two, or only one of these enter into the prohibition. Chicken meat is the least harmful, although it may result in itching.

Frogs, and fish with skin (scaly fish are not prohibited) like kob (frogs), khìad (toads), pǎa dug (catfish), pǎa jìan (eel), pǎa tɔ́ʔ (a kind of catfish).

Seafood (khɔ̌ɔŋ thálee), fresh or canned (pǎa kapǒŋ), like pǎa thuu (a kind of mackerel), pǎa myg (octopus), kũŋ (shrimps), hɔ̌ɔj (shellfish), pǔu (crabs), tàw (turtle).

Pickled food (khɔ̌ɔŋ dɔɔŋ).

Certain vegetables. The prohibition will point out which ones in each case. We have recorded the following vegetables being prohibited: phag laʔ,[a] phag pǎŋ,[b] bàtɛ̌ɛŋ,[c] bànám,[d] bànǔn,[e] bàtãw,[f] bàkhỷa hyyn,[g] bàkhỷa cɛ̃ɛ,[h] phag bũŋ,[i] saliam,[j] phag wɛ̂n.[k]

In addition there are *specific foods* and beverages that are prohibited for various reasons, like egg (khàj), banana (kũaj hɔ̌ɔm tɔɔŋ), coconut (bàpáaw), and liquor (spiritus) (lãw).

Finally there are prohibitions that refer to *taste*; for instance, sweet things (khɔ̌ɔŋ wǎan), sour things (khɔ̌ɔŋ sõm), fat things (khɔ̌ɔŋ man, khɔ̌ɔŋ càaw khɔ̌ɔŋ cỳyn). The categories "seafood" and "pickled food" correspond to salt and sour tastes, respectively, while liquor and egg are regarded as hot. One informant said that sour things result in an abundance of pus, and should therefore be avoided when suffering from wounds or vesicles (see fig. 22).

[a] Acacia insuavis (mêed 1965:343); [b] H Boerhavia diffusa—hog weed (mêed 1965:339); [c] Ex-CH Cucumis sativus—cucumber (mêed 1965:333); [d] Ex-CH Lagenaria siceraria—gourd (mêed 1965:334); [e] Artocarpus integrifolia—jackfruit (McF 1944:140); [f] Lagenaria siceraria—melon (mêed 1965:334); [g] Hibiscus esculentus—ladies' fingers, okra (mêed 1965:331); [h] H-US Solanum xanthocarpum (mêed 1965:331); [i] Ipomoea aquatica (McF 1944:484); [j] T Antelaea azadirachta var. siamensis (mêed 1965:350); [k] Desmodium triflorum (mêed 1965:343).

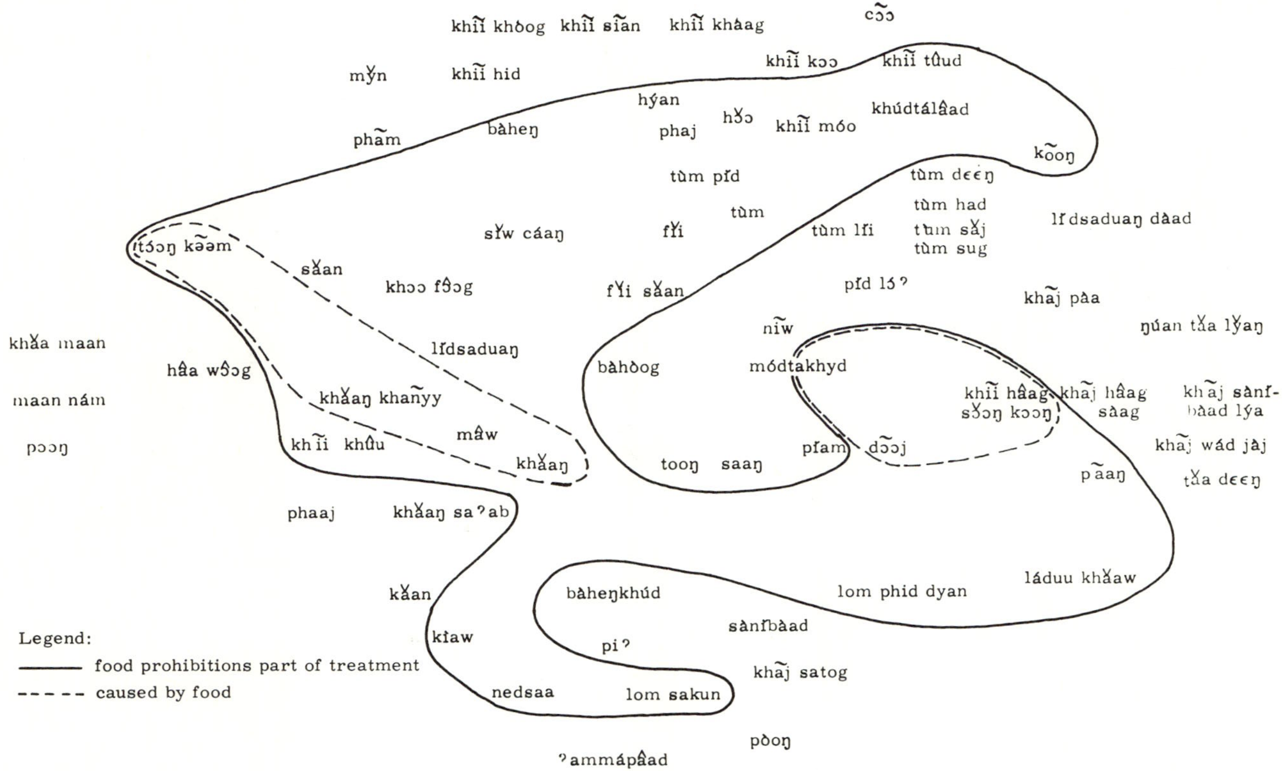

Fig. 22. Diseases connected with food.

One reason given for including cow meat on the list was that it is often contaminated by disease. This prohibition stops people from eating lâab, an appreciated dish in the North, consisting of raw minced meat with blood and lots of chilies and other spices.

One informant said phag bũŋ was prohibited for anyone taking medicine because it causes the "force of the medicine to deteriorate."

Some of the prohibitions are included because of *sympathetic magic.* In the case of tumors (sǎan), for example, everything resembling a tumor is prohibited; for example, everything that has a head (hǔa) or a round fruit (nùaj); everything that multiplies by means of root sprouts and everything that has fingers (mii myy) and thus could help the tumor to develop roots; everything with sap (jaaŋ), which could cause the tumors to become ripe and develop pus.

In table 2, a summary of food prohibitions for some twenty diseases is given.

Other diseases for which we have recorded food prohibitions as part of the treatment, without any specifications as to what types of food were prohibited, are khúdtalâad, fĩi hǔa khwãm, fĩi khĩi kàj, sǐw cáaŋ, lom sakun, láduu khǎaw, and fĩi sǎan.

3.8.11. Overlapping terminology and unclear concept borders

In a number of cases our informants disagreed about the content of a disease name (i.e., they used the same name for different concepts), or about the name of a concept (i.e., they used different names for the same concept). This inconsistent use of the terminology often reflects confusion about the concepts themselves, because the border between them is not clearly established, thus resulting in some degree of overlapping, that is, similarity. For example, the considerable confusion that surrounds the content of the terms *khĩi kɔɔ, khĩi tûud, khĩi móo,* and *khúdtálâad* qualify them for relative closeness on the disease map. The overlapping terms have been encircled in figure 23, where we use "confusion" as a criterion to arrive at a system.

3.8.12. Disease classification: Conclusion

Our findings hitherto in chapter 3 are summarized in figure 24, where the diseases have been classified into eight major groups. Using the criterion of location, we arrived at the following classifications: skin diseases, diseases of the digestive and urinary systems, diseases within and around the apertures of the body, and diseases of the respiratory system. Then the traditional concepts of wind and blood were employed, thus leaving two groups on the right and left sides of the disease chart, to which the features of tumors and swellings and the modern concept of infection are applicable denominators, respectively. The result is eight groups of diseases which neatly divide the disease chart among them. The other criteria that we discussed above have not been directly employed in the final classificatory step, but none of them contradicts our conclusion. On the contrary, they almost invariably support the present location of the diseases on the map.

We will not claim to have uncovered *the* cognitive Northern Thai disease system. Our classification is not "God's Truth." It belongs, in R. Burling's words, to the "hocus pocus" tradition.[20] Still, we have not randomly conjured up this classification. We have in fact made sincere efforts to arrive at a system that would reflect the nature of the tradition.

First, most classificatory criteria we use are prominent characteristics of the herbalist tradition in Northern Thailand. We selected them, but did not invent them.

Second, we have used a relatively large number of criteria, all quite different from one another. Thus, the very fact that it has been possible to arrive at a relatively neat system, mainly on the basis of different, indigenous criteria, we believe to be—if not a proof—then at least a strong indication that the results do reflect the basic nature of the tradition.

Third, the system we have arrived at corresponds to a disease classification based on the information in the prescription headings.

20. Burling 1964.

TABLE 2

FOOD PROHIBITIONS IN CONNECTION WITH CERTAIN TRADITIONAL DISEASES

	Foods prohibited					
Name of disease	*Meat*	*Fish, frog*	*Seafood*	*Pickled food*	*Vegetables*	*Other*
khăaŋ						Sweet and fat food
tùm khăaŋ						Sweet and fat food
khĩi khûu					phag bũŋ,[a] nám tãw,[b] bàfág khĭaw[c]	
khăaŋ lídsaduaŋ		x		x	bàkhỹahyyn[d]	Egg
pãaŋ						Sweet, fat, and sour food
nedsaa	C, P	x	x		x	Coconut
kõoŋ	C, CH	x	x	x		
hýan	C	x		x		
phaj	C	x		x		
khĩi móo	C	x		x	bàkhỹahyyn[d]	
khĩi tûud	C	x		x		Liquor
tùm píd	C, CH		x		phag bũŋ[a]	Liquor
bàheŋ	C, CH	x	x	x	bàkhỹahyyn[d]	Liquor, egg, banana
khɔɔ fɔ̂ɔg	C, CH, P	x	x	x	bàfág kɛ̃ɛw[e]	
săan	C	x	x	x	tɛɛŋ kwaa,[f] pĩi kũaj[g]	Liquor, egg, things with "head, sap or hands"
hɔ̆ɔ	C, CH			x	bàkhỹahyyn[d]	
módtakhyd (veneral)						pǎa tɔ́ʔ dam (a kind of black catfish), liquor

TABLE 2 (*continued*)

	Foods prohibited					
Name of disease	*Meat*	*Fish, frog*	*Seafood*	*Pickled food*	*Vegetables*	*Other*
ceb tăa (painful eyes)					jɔ̂ɔd fág kɛ̃ɛw[h]	
dùug hag (fractures)						Sour food

Legend: C = cow or water-buffalo meat; CH = chicken; P = pork.
[a]Ipomoea aquatica (Convolvulaceae) (McF 1944: 484). [b]Ex-CH Lagenaria siceraria (Cucurbitaceae) (mêed, 1965: 334). [c]Ex-CH Cucurbita moschata (Cucurbitaceae) (mêed, 1965: 335). [d]Ex-H Hibiscus esculentus (Malvaceae) (mêed, 1965: 331). [e]Ex-CH Cucurbita moschata (Cucurbitaceae) (mêed, 1965: 335). [f]Cucumis sativus (Cucurbitaceae) (McF, 1944: 376). [g]The blossom of the banana tree (Musa sp.-Musaceae) (McF 1944: 58). [h]The tip of the Cucurbita moschata (Cucurbitaceae) (mêed 1965: 335).

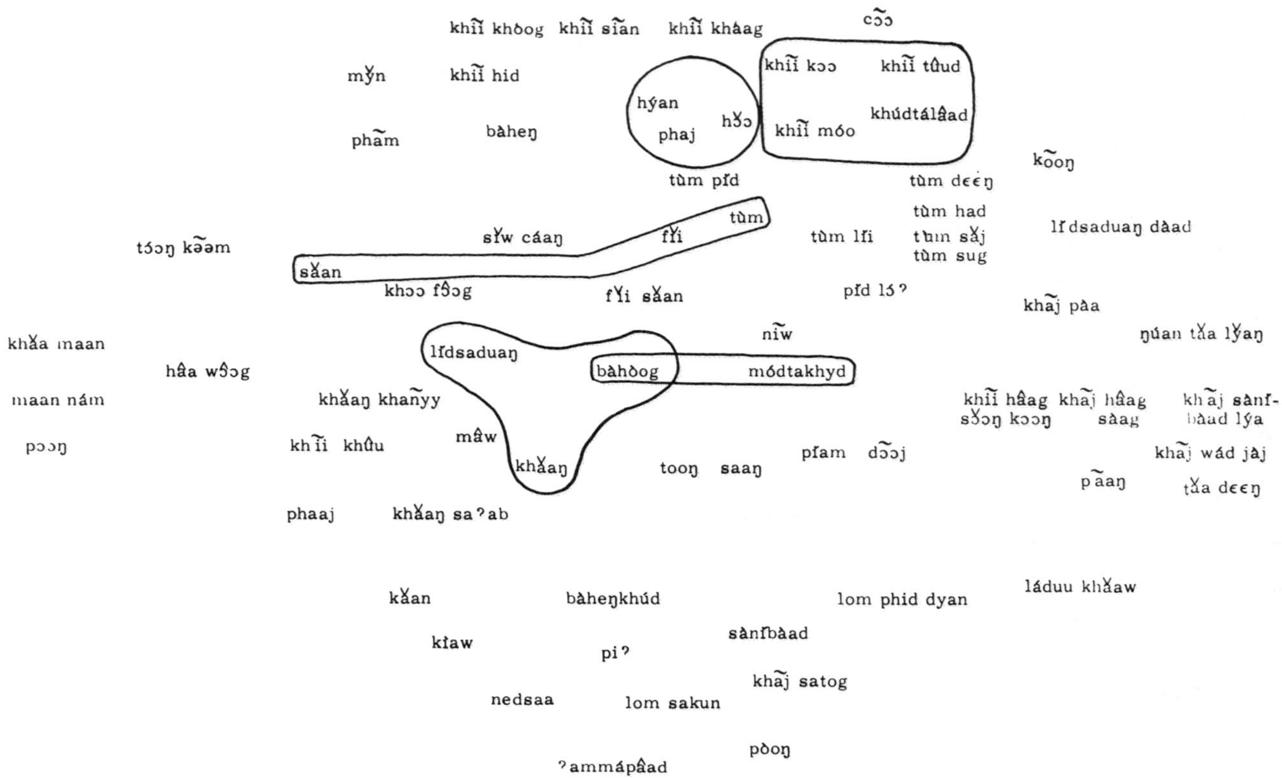

Fig. 23. Overlapping terminology.

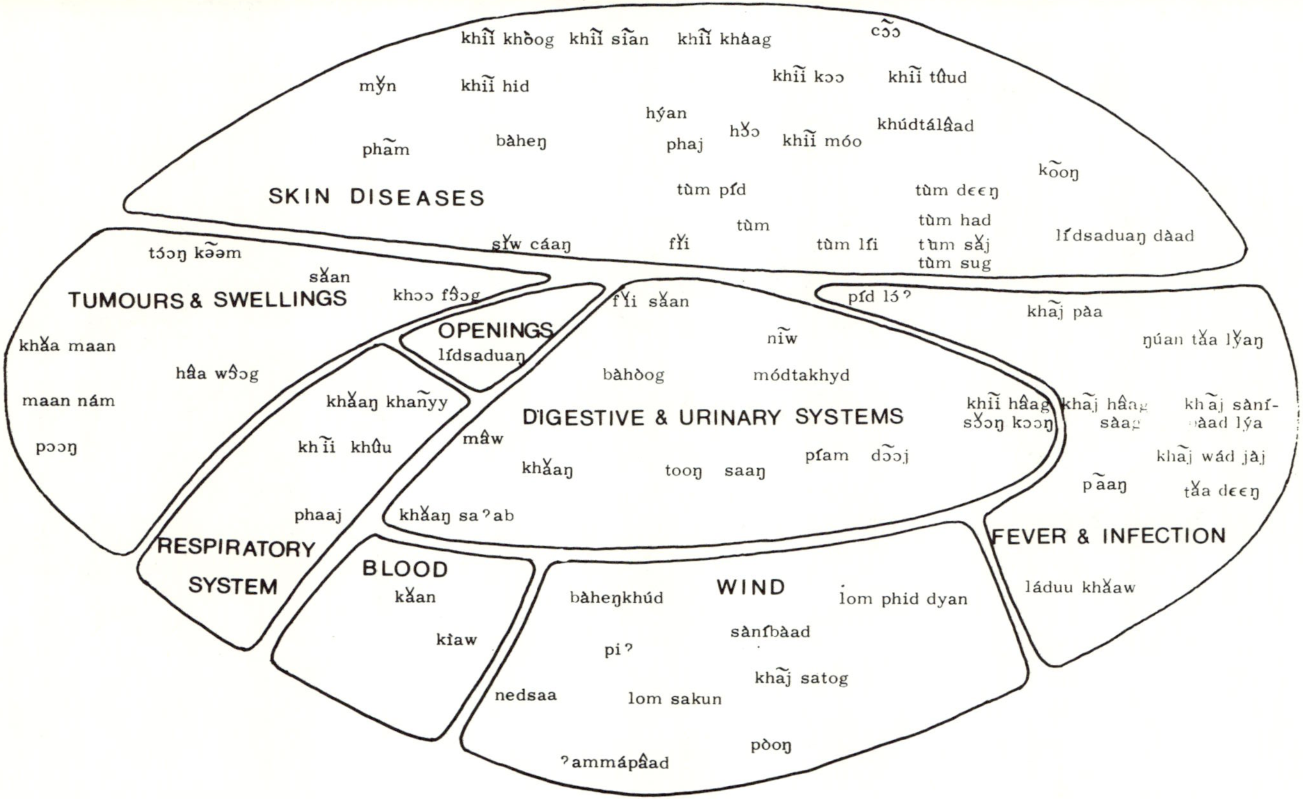

Fig. 24. Major disease groups.

This point needs some elaboration. Many prescriptions are used against several diseases; for example, prescription A may cure diseases *a, b,* and *c,* prescription B may cure diseases *a, c, d,* and *f,* prescription C may cure diseases *c, d, e, f, m,* and *n.* The prescriptions are in fact a classification of the diseases: those cured by one and the same prescription are grouped together. The reason for this is that they have some medical characteristics in common. Still, this classification is not clear-cut and consistent because the prescriptions do not classify the diseases in the same way. We believed, though, that we could go a long way toward eliminating this problem if we used a statistical approach. The idea behind this approach is the following: If, on the basis of a statistically representative number of prescriptions—a few thousand, for example—the diseases were plotted on a map, and a line were drawn around the diseases cured by each prescription, the result might turn out as shown in figure 25.

The "map" should be read in the following way: The ten circles correspond to ten prescriptions, the six letters correspond to six different diseases, and the circles enclose the diseases which each of the prescriptions is said to cure. In our example, there are thus two prescriptions curing disease *a* only, one curing *a* and *d,* one curing *a* and *b,* and so on. The important point is to look for the patterns that emerge, that is, the clusters of circles. We see that diseases *c, e,* and *f* seem to form a group, and that *a* forms another

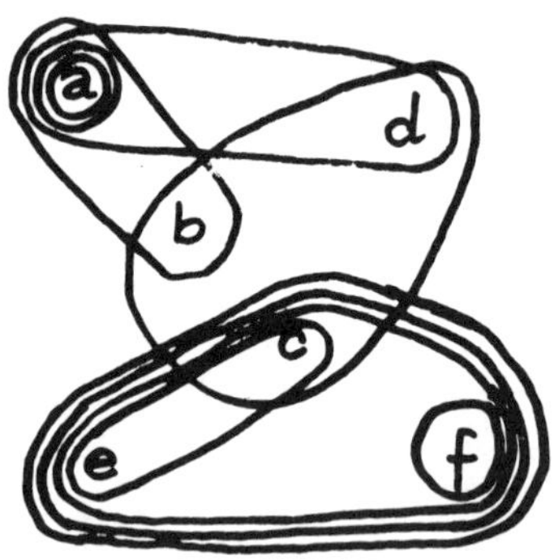

Fig. 25. Outline of disease classification based on the curing range of the prescriptions.

group by itself. However, there is not sufficient evidence to put diseases *b* and *d* in either of the two groups.[21]

We tentatively applied this method to about a hundred random prescription headings, and the patterns of disease groups (not presented here) that were beginning to emerge did indeed resemble the disease groups presented in figure 24. We therefore feel rather confident that our classification must roughly reflect an underlying classification implicit in the tradition itself.

We realize that our classification is a flat one—lacking the depth of taxonomies and hierarchies. The fact is, though, we do not believe that there exists any all-encompassing taxonomic system for the Northern Thai diseases. There are traces of hierarchies in a few sectors of the disease map, each covering disease groups such as sǎan, bàheŋ, and fǐi, but each of these hierarchies is very shallow and does not include more than one inclusive term and just a few specific ones. The underlying principle of these shallow taxonomies reveals nothing of theoretical interest. Thus we believe the shallowness of our system to be a characteristic of the tradition itself.

The presentation of the local disease concepts in the next chapter (section 4.2. Disease Panorama) follows the classification as summarized in figure 24.

21. Suggestions for statistical analysis of the components of the prescriptions are found in chapter 5.

4

Northern Thai Disease Concepts

4.1. DISEASE CONCEPTS AND DIAGNOSIS

A disease concept may include both symptomatic, pathogenic, and etiologic characteristics. In cosmopolitan medicine most diseases are described and circumscribed with reference to all these criteria. The growing experiences and knowledge as to pathogenesis and etiology of illnesses have brought forward a classificatory system that puts the main emphasis on these criteria in disease circumscription rather than on the symptomatology.

In a local medical tradition, such as the Northern Thai one, the situation is different. The medical knowledge is empirical, growing out of practical experiences, and diseases are mainly conceptualized in symptomatic terms. Etiological and pathogenic data, when present, are either inconsistent or of a very general nature and indeed of little importance in most disease circumscriptions. Consequently, compared with cosmopolitan medicine, the Northern Thai traditional disease concepts turn out to be "collective diseases," or syndromes, each concept having various etiologies and pathophysiological mechanisms (see section 4.2).

In a medical system it is important to distinguish between the verbally communicable *disease concept* on one hand, and the *diagnosis* of a disease in the medical practice on the other. A diagnosis is a label on a disease, assigned to a patient in one particular, clinical case. This label is the result of a diagnostic procedure during which all available information from the diseased is appraised with reference to the medical knowledge of the diagnostician. Depending on which components of a disease concept are selected by the diagnostician, he may give different designations of a disease in an actual clinical case. Consequently, a given disease may get different diagnostic designations from one clinical case to another. Obviously, the possibility of new and different designations of a given disease increases with the intervention of several diagnosticians of the tradition. An example from our own investigations of disease concepts and diagnostic practices should illuminate what can happen.

In theory there are four main types of the skin disease bàheŋ (primarily assigned to various vesiculobullous dermatites), namely bàheŋ fáa máan, bàheŋ khàj pǎa, bàheŋ ʔɔ̄ɔm, and bàheŋ tēn—each of which was conceptualized and circumscribed in almost the same way by all our informants. In medical practice, however, the fully expressed clinical picture, including all components of any one of these ideal types of bàheŋ, was naturally enough never (or quite seldom) met with. The diagnostician would use a more descriptive and typical designation of the disease, applicable to the one particular case of bàheŋ at hand. During our investigations we observed fourteen patients suffering from bàheŋ. Only one was given a diagnosis coalescent with one of the four names above. Instead, we recorded, among others, diagnostic entities such as bàheŋ khan (itching bàheŋ) and bàheŋ mǎa ñy̌aŋ, a bàheŋ with an intense itching, like the itching produced by the hairs of the leguminous plant mǎa ñy̌aŋ (= Mucuna pruriens). Another entity recorded was bàheŋ lŷad (blood bàheŋ), which is a pathogenic diagnosis pointing to the pathophysiological process behind the condition, that is, the blood being out of order. The two former diagnoses emphasize the characteristic itching condition of those cases observed, thus making them symptomatic designations. These three diagnostic entities, two symptomatic and one pathogenic, are all components and inclusive parts of the disease concept of bàheŋ. And they also describe components of (and may possibly be applied in) clinical cases of any of the four verbally communicated disease concepts specified above.

C. O. Frake (1961) in his study of disease diagnosis among the Subanum people of the southern Philippines introduced the term *diagnostic category* to embrace all his recorded diagnostic entities from that area. His definition and characterization of a diagnostic category and its relation to and interconnection with a disease were clearly stated: "A diagnostic category is a conceptual entity which classifies particular illnesses, symptomatic or pathogenic components of illness, or stages of illness. The course of an illness through time and its symptomatic components at any one time do not always fit into a single diagnostic category. Consequently, a single illness may successively or simultaneously require designation by several disease names. Although not all illnesses can be diagnosed by a single disease name, every disease name can diagnose a single illness."

Consequently, the system of disease concepts is one thing, the system of diagnostic designations is something else. The number of possible diagnostic categories far exceeds the number of actual disease concepts as verbally defined by the tradition itself. In some way, the number of diagnostic entities is indefinite, as was also observed and expressed by Frake (1961): "... at the most specific level we have recorded 186 human disease names (apart from referential synonyms), and the productivity of Subanum disease terminology permits the formation of an indefinite number of additional names."

In our survey of the disease panorama in Northern Thailand, we have presented the verbally communicated disease concepts, as outlined by the practitioners. The many recorded diagnostic entities are only commented on in connection with these current disease concepts. Referential synonyms, that is, mutually inclusive or equivalent terms, are listed at the heading of each recorded disease concept.

We would here like to insert that in some cases it has been

experienced by the practitioners that some identical clinical pictures may need quite different therapies, a fact that has been encoded into medical theory by the recognition of different diseases giving exactly the same symptoms (see loŋ liŋ). In those cases an on-the-spot diagnosis is impossible. The diagnosis has to be proved by the therapeutic response to the actual prescriptions. The therapy is given *ex juvantibus,* and the diagnosis is established ex post facto.

We have found it justifiable to try to elucidate the content of the indigenous diseases with biomedical terms and also, when possible, to support it with clinical observations and some "educated guesses." It is important to have in mind that when it is suggested or observed that a traditional disease entity corresponds to a disease concept of cosmopolitan medicine it is not the same as saying that one concept is equivalent or totally included in the concept of the other system. As the disease concepts of cosmopolitan medicine and the Northern Thai medical tradition are rather incongruent, most interrelationships will be of a partial type, the concept of the one system only partially matching the concept of the other system. The relations are many-to-many rather than one-to-one or one-to-many. It should be emphasized that an evaluation and interpretation of the local disease concepts by means of cosmopolitan medical concepts cannot be satisfactorily made by means of recorded information or direct observations of diseased persons by biomedically trained interpreters alone. It is also necessary to know the totality and prevalence of the illnesses (in cosmopolitan terms) that affect the people of the area and to evaluate the disorders against the available disease concepts of the tradition. Thus one has to be sure that all local disease concepts have been recorded and adequately conceptualized. Only then can a meaningful interpretation of the relationships between the diseases of the two medical systems be made. It is evident that such an ideal approach would require years of work. In order to get started, however, we have presented our preliminary information, observations, conclusions, and suggestions, well knowing that in many respects our data are still cursory and incomplete.

4.2. DISEASE PANORAMA

4.2.1. Digestive and urinary complaints

khǎaŋ

khǎaŋ[1] is considered the mother of all diseases, and can thus develop into a host of other diseases.[2] Generally speaking the cause of khǎaŋ is food (for babies it is mother's milk), particularly an excessive intake of sweet or fat food (khɔ̌ɔŋ wǎan, ʔaahǎan man, khɔ̌ɔŋ caaw khɔ̌ɔŋ cy̌yn), or an unbalanced diet consisting of meat or fish only, and not enough rice. This will produce a heat in the body (hɔ́ɔn naj) and a wind (lom) responsible for the symptoms. khǎaŋ primarily attacks children, although adults may also get it.

The mouth is the main place of occurrence of this disease, although it may spread to virtually any part of the body.

khǎaŋ will often "descend or fall down into the stomach" (khǎaŋ tog tɔ́ɔŋ, khǎaŋ loŋ tɔ́ɔŋ), where it produces a wind (lom khǎaŋ) that is hot (khǎaŋ faj, khǎaŋ mãj), and cause the stomach to rumble (khǎaŋ tɔ́ɔŋ tẽn) and become warm (khǎaŋ hɔ́ɔn tɔ́ɔŋ hɔ́ɔn pǔm). The khǎaŋ-wind will try to escape from the body, either by ascending (khǎaŋ khy̌n) and cause:

–ʔəʔ hǎaw ŋâab (burping and yawning)

–khǎaŋ hâag~khǎaŋ hâag khǎaŋ toon (vomiting)

or it may descend (khǎaŋ loŋ) through the intestines and then cause:

–khǎaŋ khãw lam sãj (khǎaŋ entering the intestines)

---

1. In Bangkok-Thai dictionaries, *khǎaŋ* is translated as "egg" (McFarland 1944), "expose to the warmth of a fire, making hot, making ripe" (in this sense referred to as a Northeastern Thai term) (maaníd 1971).

2. Diseases that may develop from khǎaŋ: lídsaduaŋ, bàheŋkhúd, sàníbàad, hâag sàag, phaaj, fĩi, sǎan, nĩw, tɔ́ɔŋ kə̃əm, bàheŋ, kìaw, módtakhyd.

–khăaŋ luʔ tɔ́ɔŋ (loose defecation—diarrhea)

–khăaŋ khĩi khăaw (white mucus or fat accompanies the stools)

–khăaŋ faj bàhòog~bàhòog lom khăaŋ (the hot wind dries up the stools making them hard)

–khăaŋ mûub mâab (sunken stomach and short breath—see píam, below)

–khăaŋ ñîaw khũn~khăaŋ loŋ liŋ~khăaŋ naj puŋ ñîaw (muddy urine)

khăaŋ may also pass via the blood, and the khăaŋ-wind may ooze out through the flesh. It then manifests itself as skin diseases, causing patches of brown, itching rashes to appear anywhere on the body, called khăaŋ lŷad, khăaŋ khan, or tùm khăaŋ.

The khăaŋ medicines aim at driving out the hot wind from the body. These medicines have a rather general curative property, and are commonly used together with other more specific medicines. khăaŋ medicines are commonly found for sale in the markets, and the khăaŋ prescriptions are perhaps the most numerous in the manuscripts. We came across nearly one hundred.

There are many kinds of khăaŋ:

khăaŋ pàag sug pàag pỳaj (ripe and decomposed mouth khăaŋ)~khăaŋ pàag sug pàag pɔɔŋ (ripe and swollen mouth khăaŋ)~khăaŋ pàag ʔoo pàag mĕn (stinking mouth khăaŋ). This disease results in a painful white rash on the tongue, causing the surface to decompose (pĕn khũm pĕn fãa). It is caused by excessive consumption of sweet or fat food. Common among children, but adults may also get it (see also mâw).

khăaŋ námlaaj ñɔ̌ɔj (tickling saliva khăaŋ)~khăaŋ námlaaj púʔ (saliva gushing forth khăaŋ) results in a slight fever and a swollen, fissurated tongue with a red rash, accompanied by abundant secretion of saliva.

khăaŋ lín lɔ̃n (easily peeled tongue khăaŋ). The tongue turns ash-grey, but the surface remains normal. Results in loss of taste.

khăaŋ ŋỳag (gum khăaŋ)~khăaŋ tùm káw khĩaw~khăaŋ tùm khob khĩaw~khăaŋ khwag is a painful disease attacking the gums, which swell and turn into stinking wounds with outflow. The teeth fall out. May spread to other parts of the mouth. Also called khăaŋ lídsaduaŋ and khăaŋ lammánâad.

khăaŋ hɔ̂ɔn khɔɔ (hot throat khăaŋ) means a red, swollen, and painful, burning throat. (Generally speaking, a hot or burning mouth or throat, or feet or hands, may be called khăaŋ faj [fire khăaŋ] or lom khăaŋ faj.)

khăaŋ lammánăad[3]~săan lammánâad~lammánâad. This term is borrowed from Bangkok Thai *rammánâad,* and is now used for an advanced stage of khăaŋ ŋỳag. It attacks the roots of the teeth and causes palpable swellings in the joints of the jaws and under the ears. It appears as painful, white-spotted wounds in the gums and is accompanied by fever. Dietary restriction is part of the treatment, together with magic and oral medicine. (See also hâa wɔ̂ɔg.)

*Diagnosis**: These "mouth"-khăaŋ, centered around some inflammatory conditions of the gums, tongue, tonsils, pharynx or throat, are commonly seen, and are frequently a result of a vitamin deficiency (especially of vitamin B).

khăaŋ saʔab attacks the vocal cords (kĭn hìib sĭaŋ naj khɔɔ), causing at first hoarseness, then gradual disappearance of the voice, emaciation and constriction of the throat. The patient will die, but it can take years.
*Diagnosis**: Laryngeal cancer.

khăaŋ púʔ (gushing forth khăaŋ) is a general term that in-

3. The condition of slight swellings on the lateral parts of the upper neck under the mandible lasting only some three or four days is called badan kaaŋ or kaaŋ pɔɔŋ (swollen jaws). If these swellings are not responsive to (magical) treatment they are considered to be khăaŋ lammánâad.

cludes symptoms like coughing blood, nosebleeds (khǎaŋ púʔ lŷad), and abundant secretion of saliva (khǎaŋ námlaaj púʔ).

khǎaŋ lídsaduaŋ is a general term that may be used for lesions of (a) the gums (see khǎaŋ ŋŷag), (b) the corner of the mouth (see lídsaduaŋ pàag), (c) the nose, also called khǎaŋ daŋ mĕn (see lídsaduaŋ huudaŋ), (d) the eyes (see lídsaduaŋ tǎa), (e) the throat, resulting in vomiting blood, general weakness, and pale skin (see khǎaŋ púʔ), and (f) the skin. The treatment includes food prohibitions.

Comments: The diagnosis khǎaŋ lídsaduaŋ was applied in three cases of skin diseases; that is, one case of pustular acne vulgaris of the face and neck, one case of discoid lupus erythematosus with lesions of the lips (verified by biopsy), and one case of a chronic widespread dermatitis with lesions of the lips (cheilosis) and enanthema of the mouth, probably due to a vitamin-B deficiency (dry beriberi). These three distinct and unrelated diseases (in the Western sense) are grouped together on the basis of localization in and around the mouth (the site of predilection of most khǎaŋ), and the fact that the lesions "were eating the bottom of the skin," typical for lídsaduaŋ.

khǎaŋ tooŋ~tooŋ~tuaŋ. A children's disease resulting in slightly loose stools, stomachache, a little fever, emaciation and weakness, and pale skin. One informant mentioned three kinds of khǎaŋ tooŋ: tooŋ wáʔ, tooŋ luuŋ, and tooŋ bua. If not responsive to treatment, this disease will change into the more chronic khǎaŋ saaŋ.

khǎaŋ saaŋ ~ saaŋ~pŭm sǎj tǎj lŷaŋ~khǎaŋ lŭaŋ[4] is a children's disease with the same symptoms as khaaŋ tooŋ, except that the stomach is inflated, the limbs get lean, and the skin and eyes turn yellowish. The child whines.

4. In Bangkok Thai, *rôog saaŋ* is defined as "a follicular pharyngitis or laryngitis common to Siamese children" (McFarland 1944:308). Sassady understands the Laotian term *saang louang* as "diarrhée jaune (enterite)," while *kang louang* should correspond to glossitis (Sassady 1962:66, 71).

Comments: The diseases tooŋ and saaŋ are very similar, and the two are often mentioned together and with the term *khǎaŋ:* for example, pěn tooŋ pěn saaŋ, khǎaŋ tooŋ khǎaŋ saaŋ, khãj khǎaŋ khãj tooŋ, tooŋ kǔm khǎaŋ kǔm.

Quite a few flowery expressions are commonly used to describe various manifestations of the two diseases, but refer particularly to saaŋ: hǔa hɔ́ɔn kõn jen (hot head cool buttocks), pǔm lǔaŋ kõn teb (big stomach flat buttocks), khĩi pǔm lǔaŋ (big stomach), khĩi pǔm ʔɛ̃ɛ ñɛ̃ɛ, khĩi pǔm ʔə̃ə ñə̃ə, puŋ loo hǔa too kõn hèw, puŋ loo kõn pòoŋ, khǎaŋ tãŋ, pěn pĩa pěn kɔ̂m.

Prescriptions against tooŋ and saaŋ are only found once or twice in the manuscripts, but they are probably treated with one of the numerous khǎaŋ prescriptions.

Diagnosis:* The clinical pictures of khǎaŋ tooŋ and khǎaŋ saaŋ among children are typical for infestations of intestinal worms. The symptomatology of khǎaŋ saaŋ is indicative of a heavy infestation of Opistorchis spp. (liver-fluke in its advanced stage), which is still abundant among children in Northern Thailand.

> ***khǎaŋ lŷad*** (blood khǎaŋ). This term was applied in medical practice in two cases: the one representing an infantile eczema (atopic dermatitis), the other an intertriginous dermatitis (candidiasis), both attributed to wrong food.
>
> ***khǎaŋ khan~tùm khan*** (itching khǎaŋ). The term was used in a case of a generalized allergic dermatitis, which might have been due to oral intake of a herbal remedy.
>
> ***khǎaŋ nám nom*** (mother's milk khǎaŋ). Diagnosed in a case of infantile eczema in an eight-month-old boy.
>
> ***khǎaŋ khañyy*** (See section 4.2.3.)

Some *modern concepts* included in the traditional concept of khǎaŋ are:

–khɔɔ thìib (diphtheria)

–ʔaj dãn (whooping cough—pertussis)

We have also recorded some *unspecified* terms of khǎaŋ:

–khǎaŋ naj mód lǔug (khǎaŋ in the uterus); (see also lídsaduaŋ mód lûug

–khǎaŋ kǐn sēn ʔen (khǎaŋ that eats the muscles)

–khǎaŋ kǐn dùug (khǎaŋ that eats the bones)

–khǎaŋ khêŋ khɛʔ (weak leg khǎaŋ)

The term *khǎaŋ* is often prefixed to names of other diseases; for example, lídsaduaŋ tǎa~khǎaŋ lídsaduaŋ tǎa; lídsaduaŋ kǐn ný̌a~khǎaŋ lídsaduaŋ kǐn ný̌a; khǎaŋ kɛ̌ɛm kìaw; khǎaŋ kɛ̌ɛm sǎan. In these contexts the term is an etiologic designation and indicates from where the disease originated.

mâw

A mouth disease that attacks babies up to one year of age resulting in a furry white coating of the tongue and the palate. It is painful and the child cries. It can spread down into the throat, thus preventing the child from eating, so that it will die of hunger.

Cause: Mother's milk.
Treatment: Lustral water.
Comments: It may develop into khǎaŋ.
Diagnosis: Oral moniliasis.

dɔ̄ɔj

dɔ̄ɔj is a term used when children are weak and cry easily. It is commonly accepted to be a result of intestinal infestations of worms. It is said to be caused by eating meat and fish only (cf. dɔ̄ɔj cín dɔ̄ɔj pǎa).

píam

píam~khīi píam is a condition known only by some herbalists and is identified variously as tɔ́ɔŋ mûub mâab (see khǎaŋ mûub mâab, above) or pāaŋ.

luʔ

luʔ~luʔ tɔ́ɔŋ~khǎaŋ luʔ tɔ́ɔŋ is a term for diarrhea leading to weakness without other prominent symptoms. luʔ by itself is not considered dangerous, but if accompanied by pains in the abdomen (kĩw) or fever (khãj) it is diagnosed as kĩw luʔ tɔ́ɔŋ or khãj luʔ tɔ́ɔŋ and may be fatal.

Cause: Wrong food.

Cure: We have recorded medicines used against luʔ alone, but the manuscripts also contain medicines that should simultaneously cure luʔ, kĩw, and kìaw.

Comments: luʔ together with other symptoms also make up concepts such as:

–luʔ + khãj, which may also be referred to as khãj thajfɔɔj (typhoid fever)

–luʔ + kĩw, which may also be referred to as bid (dysentery)

–luʔ + kád, which also may be referred to as khǎaŋ khãw lam sãj (khǎaŋ in the intestines)

(See also discussion under kĩw and thajfɔɔj.)

khâj khĩi khâj hâag

Soon after a meal the patient gets nauseated, vomits, and may have slight diarrhea. There is no fever.

Cause: Toxic or spoiled food.

Diagnosis: Food-intoxication.

kǐn phid (to eat wrong food)

This expression is used for a clinical picture of headache and dizziness in combination with nausea and a desire to vomit, these symptoms being attributed to a wind ascending to the head. This is not a specific disease, as it may occur in connection with different disorders. The syndrome, however, whether accompanied by other complaints or not, needs a specific remedy called jaa kɛ̃ɛ kǐn phid (promoting vomiting—emetic) to get rid of ingested "wrong food," which is held responsible for the syndrome.

kǐn sàlɛ̌ɛŋ (to eat indigestible food)

This condition is manifested by vomiting and diarrhea occurring after a meal, understood to have been caused by the intake of some spoiled, indigestible food. The remedy, jaa kɛ̃ɛ kǐn sàlɛ̌ɛŋ (medicine to get rid of the indigestible food), acts thus as a genuine detoxicant.

kĩw

kĩw is a term for a twisting type of abdominal pain accompanying some intestinal diseases. When the intestines are obstructed by fecal matter, blood, or mucus, a kĩw-wind (lom kĩw) appears, resulting in kĩw-pains. These twisting pains may accompany diseases such as bàhòog and khǎaŋ.

> *kĩw bàhòog* (kĩw + bàhòog) is described as kĩw-pains together with frequent defecations with mucus or blood or both in the stools (cf. bàhòog lŷad). Ineffectual straining efforts to empty the bowel are typical.
>
> A variety is *kĩw loŋ dam loŋ dɛɛŋ* (black and red kĩw) where the kĩw-pains are accompanied by black stools, with strong smell, or by fresh blood.
>
> *kĩw lom khǎaŋ* is the condition of watery diarrhea of a fish-like odor together with kĩw-pains.

kĩw is nowadays recognized as an important symptom of modern disease concepts such as typhoid, cholera, and dysentery. When kĩw-pains are accompanied by strong diarrhea and/or fever, it may be variously called:

–khãj thajfɔɔj (typhoid fever), a loan-word from Bangkok Thai

–ʔàhìwaa (cholera), a loan-word from Bangkok Thai

–bid (dysentery), a loan-word from Bangkok Thai

–kĩw tûan (epidemic kĩw)

One informant used the term *kĩw* when referring to certain menstrual pains.

Comments: kĩw as it is expressed in connection with infectious intestinal diseases might be translated by the pathophysiological term *tenesmae,* typical of severe enteritis. Other indigenous diseases with enteritis are bàhòog lŷad, lídsaduaŋ naj lam sãj, and khǎaŋ luʔ tɔ́ɔŋ.

In the manuscripts, remedies against kĩw are also used against luʔ and kìaw.

bàhòog

bàhòog is a group of intestinal diseases. The delimitation against lídsaduaŋ and khǎaŋ of the intestines is vague, but important criteria for the diagnosis bàhòog are:

–twisting pains in the lower abdomen (kĩw) and aching in the lower back and pelvic region

–changes in the consistency and looks of the feces, being looser or harder than normal and mixed with blood, mucus, or fat

–emaciation that leads to difficulties to go on working

There are three types of bàhòog:

bàhòog lŷad (blood bàhòog). The symptoms are twisting pains in the abdomen, frequent defecations, usually four or five a day, of loose fecal matter mixed with red blood and mucus. There is a frequent desire to defecate, followed by the feeling that the evacuation is incomplete. The patient becomes thin and emaciated, and his eyes and skin turn pale and yellowish, while the nails and lips turn black. May result in death.

bàhòog phanládii~bàhòog khĩi kwǎaŋ~bàhòog khĩi khɛ̃n~phandii~phandyg~khǎaŋ phaladyg~khǎaŋ khĩi khên. The patient is constipated, and there may be up to five days between defecations. Feces are hard and mixed with mucus or fat (mûug). There is constant pressing pain in the abdomen and pelvic region, but also twisting and piercing pains at irregular intervals. The patient may get weak and dizzy and his sight may dim. These latter symptoms are caused by an ascending wind accompanying the disease.

bàhòog kõn pûud (protruding anus bàhòog). This is the situation when the intestines are pressed out through the anus resulting in a warm, smarting pain (sɛ̀ɛb hɔ́ɔn). The patient goes to the toilet two to four times a day, the feces are a little loose, and mixed with fat, mucus, and/or blood. Provoking factors are hard work and strong, spicy food. Consequently it is more frequently seen among men than among women. The patient can eat normally and still work.

Comments: According to one informant this disease should better be termed *lídsaduaŋ kõn pûud* as the localization of the lesions is just inside the anus, and is evidenced by the protruding intestine. Furthermore, the patients can still work and eat without discomfort and thus do not fulfill the criteria for a real bàhòog. lídsaduaŋ twaan is sometimes used in a very broad sense to include bàhòog kõn pûud, but normally the two concepts are kept apart. One informant emphasized that bàhòog kõn pûud normally is preceded by the other two types of bàhòog.

The eight bàhòog prescriptions we have collected from the herbalists support the above subdivision. There are prescriptions against bàhòog in general, defined as: twisting pains in the stomach, intestines coming out of anus, and bloody stools. There are also, however, specific remedies for bàhòog kõn pûud, bàhòog phanládii, and bàhòog lŷad.

When we turn to the manuals (where the spelling is máhòog) the bàhòog concept becomes both wider and more blurred. In addition to the above-mentioned types of bàhòog, one also finds: máhòog lom bid, máhòog lom khad, máhòog lom cuʔ, máhòog lom săan, máhòog lom khăaŋ, khăaŋ máhòog, khăaŋ faj máhòog, and máhòog faj. None of these terms is specified, but the names suggest an emphasis on the pain and aching aspect of the disease, and also associate it with diseases such as khăaŋ and săan.

Diagnosis: The Western counterparts of bàhòog probably include a wide spectrum of intestinal diseases. Most cases certainly represent dysentery and its complications, like prolapse of the rectum (bàhòog kõn pûud), but other chronic infections and parasitic infestations are also responsible for the symptomatology. (See also luʔ and kĩw.)

loŋ liŋ

loŋ liŋ (down into the penis) is the situation when a (male) person gets mucopurulent discharge from the penis. This symptom may either be classified as khǎaŋ loŋ liŋ, lídsaduaŋ loŋ liŋ, or módtakhyd loŋ liŋ, depending apparently on an ex post facto diagnosis. If the symptom responds to a khǎaŋ loŋ liŋ medicine, it is regarded as khǎaŋ loŋ liŋ, and so forth.

módtakhyd

módtakhyd covers two disease concepts: a modern one—which is heavily influenced by the current use of this word for venereal diseases in modern Bangkok Thai—and a traditional one.

A. *The traditional concept* is most clearly seen in the manuscripts where many prescriptions against módtakhyd are found. We have chosen to subdivide the many types of módtakhyd found there into three groups—a subdivision that corresponds neatly with that of some of our informants.

1. *módtakhyd lŷad* (blood módtakhyd) covers symptoms connected with abnormal urination and defecation, like módtakhyd ñîaw dɛɛŋ (red urine—haematuria); módtakhyd loŋ mûug loŋ lŷad (blood and mucus in the feces); módtakhyd ʔɔ̀ɔg twaan (módtakhyd in the anus), when a red, itching rash appears around the anus (candidiasis). If the stools turn hard afterwards, módtakhyd lŷad may have developed into bàhòog.
2. *módtakhyd lom*~lom módtakhyd (wind-módtakhyd) covers symptoms like módtakhyd tɔ̃ɔŋ tẽn (rumbling stomach); módtakhyd sìab khỹn kǔaŋ ʔog kǔaŋ cǎj (piercing pains ascending

in the breast toward the heart); módtakhyd loŋ sǎw (radiating pains down the legs); módtakhyd khamên paj taŋ tǔa (ticks all over the body); módtakhyd hɔ́ɔn ʔog hɔ́ɔn cǎj hɔ́ɔn tǎam phǐw nǎŋ (hot chest hot skin módtakhyd); módtakhyd khan (itching módtakhyd, affecting the skin). It was said that a lom módtakhyd may develop into fǐi dàad. If this wind is pressed out through the eyes it may result in blindness.

3. *módtakhyd ñîaw khǎn*~módtakhyd ñîaw fỳyd~módtakhyd ñîaw khad (módtakhyd with difficult urination) covers symptons like módtakhyd ñîaw dàŋ nám mûag (muddy urine—pyuria); módtakhyd ñîaw dàŋ nám khâŋ (urine with [the color of] shellac—pyuria), and módtakhyd loŋ liŋ (módtakhyd in the penis), which causes pus and/or blood to come out with the urine (urethritis), often accompanied by pain in the back and difficult and painful urination (cystitis, nephritis). There is a general consensus that módtakhyd ñîaw khǎn may develop into nǐw. (See also khǎaŋ loŋ liŋ, lídsaduaŋ loŋ liŋ.)

The connection between the traditional concept of módtakhyd and other disease groups is frequently seen in the manuscripts where we find prescriptions that cure both módtakhyd, bàhòog, maleŋkhúd, khǎaŋ, and lom khûu; for example, lom módtakhyd kɛ̌ɛm khǎaŋ (kɛ̌ɛm = mixed with), módtakhyd kɛ̌ɛm maleŋkhúd kɛ̌ɛm khǎaŋ, lom khûu lɛ́ʔ lom módtakhyd. One prescription was directed against both "nǐw and the various kinds of bàhòog and módtakhyd."

As can be seen, the traditional disease entity módtakhyd has a broad and variable content. In its original sense it covers a lot of pathological conditions mainly in the urogenital and gastrointestinal systems, but also some entities affecting the skin. Through the influence of cosmopolitan medicine the concept of módtakhyd among contemporary medical healers has been narrowed down to the complaints from the urogenital region that may be indicative of some venereal diseases.

B. *The modern concept* of módtakhyd—also called módtakhyd phǔu jǐŋ (módtakhyd from women)—covers several diseases:

1. *nɔ̌ɔŋ naj* (pus inside the penis)~módtakhyd nɔ̌ɔŋ (módtakhyd with pus)~módtakhyd khǎaw (white módtakhyd)~ñîaw khãn (urinating with difficulty). Urination difficult and painful. Pus in the urine. May develop into ʔɔ̀ɔg dɔ̀ɔg.
Cause: "Women."
Diagnosis: The Western concept is urethritis, including the symptoms of gonorrhea.

2. *módtakhyd pěn phɛ̌ɛ* (módtakhyd with wound)~khuaj pud (the penis falls off). Wounds on the penis-head appear, but urination is not painful. The disease may eat its way inward, causing the penis to fall off (módtakhyd khuaj pud), and is then fatal. It may also develop into fǐi mûaŋ.
Cause: "Women."
Diagnosis: Ulcus molle, syphilis, lymphogranuloma venereum, carcinomatosis.

3. *fǐi mûaŋ*~fǐi bàmûaŋ~fǐi módtakhyd. Painful, swollen lymph nodes appear in the groins and eventually suppurate with discharge of pus. Accompanied by fever and pain in the back. Does not affect penis. Now regarded as a venereal disease.
Diagnosis: This condition of bubonic plagues constitutes the stage inguinal adenitis in lymphogranuloma venereum (see also fǐi).

4. *ŋɔ̌ɔn kàj* (comb of cock). Appears on the penis-head.
Diagnosis:* Condylomata ("venereal warts").

5. *ʔɔ̀ɔg dɔ̀ɔg* (blooming flowers)~dɔ̀ɔg dãaj (flowers [on a] thread)~khãw khɔ̂ɔ (enter the joints). Normally the joints are attacked first. Then tùm appear on the body or on the face. The skin may turn dark. No fever. May develop into khĩi tûud (leprosy).
Diagnosis: Secondary stage syphilis?
Comments: Among most practitioners today módtakhyd is re-

garded as equivalent to venereal diseases.[5] It is then used in a broad sense as is the case in the following "modern" explanation: "Sometimes a módtakhyd makes the patient blind, and sometimes it results in eruptions all over the body. It may attack the joints or cause the penis to ulcerate and swell. In the latter case it is often fatal. módtakhyd may also cause blindness or tùm on newborn babies."

The diseases in the gastrointestinal tract earlier recognized as módtakhyd seem now to be classified among bàhòog or lídsaduaŋ.

In the following chart a comparison of the traditional, current entities and their probable Western counterparts is summarized:

Northern Thai system		Cosmopolitan system
módtakhyd phũu jĭŋ		*Venereal diseases pro parte*
nɔ̆ɔŋ naj	Mucopurulent discharge from the urethra	1. Gonorrhea (urethritis) 2. Unspecific urethritis
fĭi mûaŋ	Bubonic plagues	1. Lymphogranuloma
módtakhyd pĕn phɛ̆ɛ	Ulcers on the penis	1. Ulcus molle 2. Syphilis 3. Lymphogranuloma venereum 4. Carcinomatosis
módtakhyd khuaj pud	Penis eaten up	1. Carcinomatosis

fĭi săan

The common understanding of this disease or group of diseases is that it attacks some internal abdominal organs such as the

5. According to C. Spire, venereal diseases—which were hardly known in Laos when he was there in 1902—had only recently been introduced to that country from Thailand. Spire records gonorrhea as pen nam nong koué (= discharge from penis?) and syphilis as sa duong, while Sassady understands sa douang to mean

stomach, intestines, kidney, or liver, and makes itself known by the symptom of abdominal pain associated with a lom píd hɔ̌ɔn (warm, poisonous wind) going upward or toward the back. The patient feels uncomfortable and loses appetite. It comes from khǎaŋ. If it attacks the stomach, in which case it is called fĩi sǎan naj tɔ́ɔŋ, the patient feels very hot inside, has a piercing pain going upward, and cannot eat.

Cause: Unknown.

Treatment: Oral remedies. The medicines are hot, "to fight the internal heat with heat." As the disease develops from khǎaŋ, a khǎaŋ medicine is also used together with food prohibitions.

Comments: The diagnosis is assessed on the basis of internal pain without other specific symptoms typical for other diseases of abdominal organs such as bàhòog, nĩw, and lídsaduaŋ. This unspecific syndrome may coincide with a variety of cosmopolitan medical entities. The circumscription of fĩi sǎan naj tɔ́ɔŋ fits very well with a typical clinical manifestation of an ulcerous lesion of the upper part of the gastrointestinal tract, for example, ulcus ventriculi, ulcus duodeni, or carcinomatosis.[6] One informant used fĩi sǎan in a deviating sense, also to include painful, nodular lesions of the skin, more commonly referred to as some kind of fĩi.

khĩi hâag sɔ̌ɔŋ kɔɔŋ

khĩi hâag sɔ̌ɔŋ kɔɔŋ~khĩi hâag sɔ̌ɔŋ hǒn~luʔ sɔ̌ɔŋ kɔɔŋ.

This disease entity comprises the symptoms nausea, vomiting, and diarrhea associated with fever and dizziness. As the name indicates, the patient empties himself through "two openings."

"venereal diseases" (Sassady 1962:77). Spire notes that little importance was given to syphilis, the reason being that it probably was confused with the diseases khi mo and khi ma heng, both of which were very common children's diseases that would cure themselves. (Spire 1907:25). The Laotian term *mut ta kut* is, however, found in the name for epilepsy: tham ma la mut ta kut (Sassady 1962:81). McFarland gives the following definitions for Bangkok Thai: múdtàʔ—urine; múdtakìd—fluor albus, leukorrhea; múdtakhâad—a disease characterized by pus and blood in the urine; hematuria (McFarland 1944:653).

6. Sassady understands the Laotian term *fi nai thoŋ* to mean "ulcère digestif" (Sassady 1962:72).

Cause: The intestines have become slippery due to intake of wrong food (ʔaahǎan phid).

Treatment: The therapy is both symptomatic and causative. A medicine is prescribed to stop the vomiting and diarrhea, and a different prescription is directed against the causative agent, the poisonous agent of the food (jaa kɛ̃ɛ kǐn phid). Some of the ingredients of the two prescriptions are the same.

Diagnosis: Acute aseptic gastroenteritis of different etiology.

nĩw

This disease is usually conceptualized nowadays in etiologic terms; namely, the condition of having concrements in the urinary tract. The following "modern" outline of nĩw was recorded from one of our respondents:

"There are two kinds of nĩw: (a) the stone is lying within the kidney, (b) the stone is lying outside the kidney, that is, in the urinary bladder. That you can see, if you go to the hospital and take X-rays. When you have nĩw, you get very much pain [in the abdomen] and often fever. The pain may come and go at any time of night or day. Some get cloudy urine, and sometimes small stones come out during miction. Stones that lie in the kidney cannot come out, as there is no passage out [the anatomical connection between the kidney and the bladder was unknown], so the patient needs a medicine that dissolves the stone. The modern doctors do surgery. Stones in the bladder are also dissolved by the nĩw-medicine, and when they get small, they may pass from the bladder through penis together with the urine. You can feel them coming out when urinating."

Cause: Stones in the urinary tract.

Treatment: Oral remedies, usually taken as a tonic several times a day. The medicine will dissolve the stones (litholytic remedies). It is widely believed that herbal prescriptions are very effective in dissolving the stones, although some herbalists admit that surgery is necessary in severe cases.

Comments: The diagnosis usually rests on the presence of paroxystic pains in the lower back and across the abdomen. From old times these characteristic pains have been linked to the existence of urinary concrements by the fact that some patients with this type of pain may eject gravel or small stones together with the urine. As urinary concrements are very common among rural people in Thailand, the stone etiology is probably the usual explanation for this symptomatology. It should be emphasized, however, that in practice the diagnosis never rests on the demonstration of concrements in the urinary tract. The fact that no other diseases with paroxystic, radiating pains in the abdominal region have been recorded indicates that the concept of nĩw at least also includes the typical pancreatic and biliary pain seen in diseases such as pancreatitis and cholelithiasis. Other diseases with abdominal colic might qualify for the diagnosis nĩw as well; for instance, pyelonephritis and pyelitis. (One patient with pyelonephritis was observed.) With the influence of cosmopolitan medicine and the frequent demonstration of abdominal concrements by X-rays of patients with nĩw, the concept of nĩw has now focused on the stone etiology.

4.2.2. Diseases in and around the orifices of the body

lídsaduaŋ

lídsaduaŋ is a general disease term applied to mucocutaneous lesions, the majority centered around the orifices of the body.

A. *lídsaduaŋ twaan* (lídsaduaŋ in the openings) refers generally to lídsaduaŋ, above, but under the influence of the modern Bangkok-Thai concept lídsaduaŋ tháwaan applied to hemorrhoids. The term is now often used in a more restricted meaning comprising recto-anal disorders only, and hemorrhoids in particular.

A-1. *lídsaduaŋ ŋɔ̂ɔg* (sprouting lídsaduaŋ) refers to mucocutaneous outgrowths within or just outside the orifices of the body. Now most commonly used for disorders affecting the ano-rectal region (see also bàhòog kõn pûud).

Some informants recognized several subtypes applicable to diseases in the ano-rectal region:

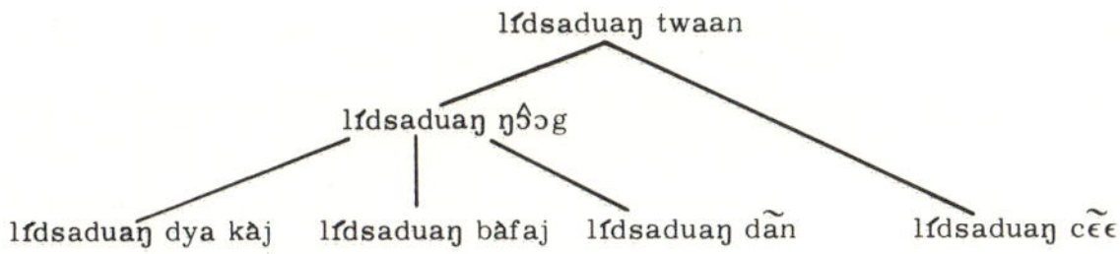

Fig. 26. Subdivision of lídsaduaŋ twaan.

lídsaduaŋ dya kàj (cock-spur lídsaduaŋ) is the condition of having a single nodule in the anus, which is pressed out during defecation, causing pain.

lídsaduaŋ bàfaj~lìib bàfaj~lìib fyaŋ. Two or more knotted nodules are present in the anus and are pressed out of the aperture during defecation, causing pain.

lídsaduaŋ dãn (hard lídsaduaŋ). One or more swellings or flat nodules appear on the mucous membrane of the rectum, which are pressed out during defecation, but not followed by pain.

A-2. *lídsaduaŋ cɛ̃ɛ* (small lídsaduaŋ) is the condition of several small itching and burning papules and vesicles around the anus.

A scheme of the different lídsaduaŋ twaan of the anus is found in figure 26.

Cause: From inside. The disease has a "mother" (mɛ̂ɛ).

Treatment: The different types of lídsaduaŋ twaan are treated with an oral as well as a topical medicine. The topical medicine applied within and outside the anus is "rather poisonous" and cannot be used to treat lídsaduaŋ twaan in other places, such as in the nose.

Diagnosis: Hemorrhoids, polyps (lídsaduaŋ ŋɔ̂ɔg), anal candidiasis, and eczemas (lídsaduaŋ cɛ̃ɛ).

B. *lídsaduaŋ naj lam sãj* (lídsaduaŋ in the intestines) may be localized anywhere in the intestines and manifests itself as sticky stools mixed with blood and mucus. The patient is usually still strong and can work. There is little or no pain in the abdomen, but as the disease spreads toward the anus opening, it may result in a hot, smarting pain during defecation.

Cause: From inside. The symptoms are due to small ulcers (phỳn tùm) on the intestinal walls.

Treatment: Oral remedies. Wrong food predisposes for the disease.

Diagnosis: Colitis, proctitis, (commonly a chronic shigellosis).

Comments: The disease may develop into lídsaduaŋ ŋɔ̂ɔg.

C. ***lídsaduaŋ buu liŋ***~lídsaduaŋ loŋ liŋ~lídsaduaŋ hǐi (lídsaduaŋ in the urinary tract)~lídsaduaŋ puŋ ñîaw (lídsaduaŋ in the urinary bladder) results in muddy urination and a hot, smarting pain during urination. The urination opening turns red, and skin on the penis tip may peel off.

Cause: From inside.

Treatment: Medicines taken by mouth.

Diagnosis:* Cystitis, urethritis.

D. ***lídsaduaŋ mód lûug*** (lídsaduaŋ in the uterus). No details. (See also khǎaŋ naj mód lûug.)

E. ***lídsaduaŋ buudaŋ*** (nose-lídsaduaŋ)~lídsaduaŋ kǐn nýa (lídsaduaŋ eating the flesh) starts as small, red "tùm" inside the nose. After a while small ulcers (phỳn) appear giving off constant secretion that smells bad. The secretion may get sticky. The disease is accompanied by headache, blurred vision, and dizziness, and it is impossible to breathe through the nose. Usually no fever. The disease may "eat" its way through the skin, causing open wounds and bleeding, and may finally also "eat" the nose bone, resulting in a flat nose.

Diagnosis: Rhinitis, sinusitis.

F. ***lídsaduaŋ tǎa*** (eye-lídsaduaŋ). Small white "tùm" or "phỳn" appear on the inside of the lower eyelid, causing an itching, smarting pain and running eyes. The border of the eyes turns red, swells slightly, and the eyelashes fall off. The disease does not attack the eyeball.

Diagnosis:* Sty (hordeolum).

Comments: For other eye diseases, see tǎa dɛɛŋ.

G. *lídsaduaŋ hŭu* (ear-lídsaduaŋ)~hŭu bɔ̀ɔ (the ear overflows [bɔ̀ɔ = well]) causes pain in the ear, and results in pus and secretion coming out.

Diagnosis: Otitis (media and externa).

H. *Skin-lídsaduaŋ*. Our main informant diagnosed a lot of skin diseases as ultimately belonging to the lídsaduaŋ group. The criteria used for the assessment of this diagnosis were the appearance of plaques with scaling and secretion, or just thick, indurated skin. lídsaduaŋ is said to eat deeper into the skin than khăaŋ and bàheŋ.

A short presentation of the different skin-lídsaduaŋ, and the observed Western dermatological counterparts, is given in section 4.2.8. Skin diseases.

I. *lídsaduaŋ lŷad* (blood-lídsaduaŋ) is also a general term used for bleeding from the orifices of the body, particularly from the nose and mouth. In the latter case it refers to coughing or vomiting blood that "comes from the lungs." The patient gets weak, his skin turns yellow, but he usually does not die (see also khăaŋ lídsaduaŋ and kăan lŷad).

Food prohibitions are normally part of the treatment of lídsaduaŋ diseases.

The twenty-six lídsaduaŋ prescriptions we found in the manuscripts for the most part confirm the picture of the diseases that the informants have given us. We find the above-mentioned types of lídsaduaŋ, such as lídsaduaŋ huudaŋ, lídsaduaŋ ŋɔ̂ɔg, lídsaduaŋ tăa, and lídsaduaŋ twaan. However, no reference is made to lídsaduaŋ in the urinary tract or to skin-lídsaduaŋ.

Furthermore, the manuscripts mention a lom saduaŋ (saduaŋ-wind) associated with pains in the right half of the body (starting from the stomach and spreading upward), and a fever followed by saduaŋ-fits (saduaŋ satóg). None of these conditions was mentioned by our informants.[7]

7. In Laotian, the term *sadouang* means "venereal diseases" or "syphilis." See note to módtakhyd.

4.2.3. Diseases affecting the respiratory system

khĩi khûu

Typical for this disease is difficulty in breathing, and coughing accompanied by a lot of whitish-yellow sticky mucus (khĩi tə̂ə). The patients often have to sit up in order to get their breath, but still they breathe hard and violently. It is usually not accompanied by fever. The attacks are likely to occur when it is going to rain. It attacks only adults.

Treatment: There are medicines to be smoked and medicines to be taken orally. According to the practitioners the medicines will usually give a permanent cure. Some herbalists also prescribe food prohibitions.

Diagnosis: The clinical picture of dyspnea, expectoration, and lack of fever points to asthmatic and chronic bronchitis as parts of the concept (cf. khǎaŋ khañyy).

Comments: Nine prescriptions have been collected from the practitioners, whereas the manuscripts have provided us with only two. In the manuscripts there are quite a few prescriptions against coughing (ʔaj), mucus of the throat and lungs (salèed, sěemahaʔ), and difficult breathing (hǎaj cǎj fŷyd, hŷyd hɔ̀ɔb).

khǎaŋ khañyy

khǎaŋ khañyy[8] is a disease occurring in children aged from six months to about ten years, rarely seen among adults. The child breathes with difficulty, resulting in a loud piping or squeaking noise (hɔ̃ɔ hɛ̃ɛ), because of the slime in the throat. It is also called khɔɔ daŋ (loud throat). Attacks not as serious as with khĩi khûu. The disease will disappear by itself when the child grows bigger. Caused by mother's milk or by excessive eating of sugarcane juice or fat food. Not recorded in the manuscripts. One specific prescription collected.

Diagnosis: The central symptoms, such as tracheobronchial stridor and dyspnea, may point to different respiratory diseases;

8. In Laos the term *kha nhu* is used for asthma (Sassady 1962:39).

however, false croup in children, laryngitis, and bronchial asthma are probably the core of this concept (cf. khīi khûu).

phaaj

phaaj~phaaj khakŭn~pĕn phom pĕn phaaj~pĕn hɛ̃ɛŋ pĕn phaaj. The patient does not really feel sick but loses freshness and becomes thin and emaciated as if being "dried out" in spite of a normally good appetite. The breathing is weak, and dry coughing is typical. The coughing may be accompanied by slime and even blood. The patient is unable to work and is usually found lying down. There is no fever. The disease is long-term, and may be fatal after years in bed.

Cause: The etiology is traced back to a phaaj-spirit, which is a kind of family spirit, as the term ***khakŭn*** (family) indicates. The disease follows and eats the blood. The phaaj-spirit also looks after the belongings of its owner. If one touches objects—especially metal objects—guarded by a phaaj-spirit, one will catch the disease. The basic ingredients in the indigenous explanation are that this disease is both contagious and that it may be inherited.

Diagnosis: It is commonly equated with wannárôog, the modern Bangkok-Thai term for tuberculosis, and it certainly includes some typical manifestations of pulmonary tuberculosis.

Treatment: There are medicines that are used against phaaj—we have recorded five—but magic is commonly resorted to, either through a brushing ceremony (pád) or a cutting-away ceremony (tad phom tad phaaj). The disease is regarded as very difficult to cure.

4.2.4. Wind diseases

bàheŋkhúd

bàheŋkhúd~lom bàheŋkhúd~bàheŋkhúd khăm~bàheŋkhúd lŭaŋ.[9] This disorder has many clinical manifestations, and many sub-

9. ***khúd*** in Bangkok Thai means "grow inward, crooked" (McFarland 1944:204).

types are recognized; all are treated with the same medicine. The central symptom of a lom bàheŋkhúd (bàheŋkhúd-wind) is pain due to a migrating wind that may settle down in different parts of the body. Usually the wind ascends to the head and causes headache, pressure on the eyes, and dizziness, which are obligate symptoms of most conditions attributed to the bàheŋkhúd-wind. If the wind fills the entire head, a terrible headache follows as the only symptom.

Comments: A more specific disease entity recognized by some informants is *bàheŋkhúd fáa mɛ̂ɛb* (lightening bàheŋkhúd) characterized by a sudden onset of an intense, piercing headache that may continue for one to three days. It may reappear three or four times a year, but if treated with traditional, cool oral remedies it will permanently disappear. The bàheŋkhúd-wind may blow out through the eyes (usually out of only one eye), leaving them painful and red, with photophobia and blurred vision, or with a partial or complete loss of vision. If the wind blows out through the ears, it may cause a painful sensation in the eustachian tube, a ringing or tinkling sound (tinnitus), or even deafness. A sudden loss of teeth may also be due to this wind. Furthermore, discoloration of the hair at an early age is another manifestation of the disease.

The bàheŋkhúd-wind that attacks the skeleton of the body gives painful bones and joints, and is called *bàheŋkhúd kǐn dùug* (bàheŋkhúd eating the bones).

bàheŋkhúd loŋ sǎw is caused by winds descending into the lower limbs and results in radiating pains in the legs or painful swellings of the lower limbs (see loŋ sǎw).

The skin disease *bàheŋkhúd dàad* is also a clinical manifestation of a lom bàheŋkhúd. This diagnosis was given to two patients, one with lichen ruber planus, another with seborrheic dermatitis. The diagnoses were based on the existence of thick, discolored, scaly (pale) plaques of the skin and general symptoms such as headache and fatigue.

Cause: bàheŋkhúd comes from the blood being out of order. "The blood turns black and the face red." This gives support to a serious wind (lom lǔaŋ, or "big wind") that rages around in the body.

Treatment: The disease is regarded as serious, usually chronic, and difficult to cure. There are several traditional remedies both for topical and internal use. Some practitioners now regard aspirin as an appropriate medicine in many cases.

Diagnosis: bàheŋkhúd is circumscribed by the existence of severe pain somewhere in the body, together with rather few objective signs that can explain these painful conditions. Some informants equate lom bàheŋkhúd with the modern Thai medical term *khwaam dan sǔuŋ* (high blood pressure), and in some cases the symptoms may in fact point to hypertension as a possible explanation. However, the concept is much more complex and borders on cosmopolitan diseases and syndromes such as headache (of different origin), migraine (bàheŋkhúd fáa mɛ̂ɛb), arthropathia (bàheŋkhúd kǐn dùug), ischialgia and lymphedema of the legs (bàheŋkhúd loŋ sǎw), and diseases of eyes and ears such as glaucoma, iridocyclitis, otitis, and so forth.

piʔ

piʔ is an archaic term, frequently found in the manuals (25 prescriptions), but not much in use anymore. piʔ produces blurred vision and a severe dizziness that may result in fainting and temporary unconsciousness. The manuals mention piʔ in connection with diseases such as sànībàad, khǎaŋ, and kìaw. Most practitioners mention three kinds of piʔ, although they are not always used consistently.

> *piʔ tǎa mŷyd* (dim-eye piʔ) is characterized by dizziness, swimming eyes, trembling heart, and weakness that suddenly occurs when standing up, working hard, or when exposed to sunshine. After a short rest in a shady place it disappears.
>
> *piʔ fáa mɛ̂ɛb* (lightning piʔ). The patient suddenly loses consciousness, usually in the same situations as for dim-eye piʔ. Normally it is not dangerous, and the patient wakes up after a while. (One informant also used the term for a comatose condition that may result in death; see lom sakun).
>
> *piʔ faj*~khǎj piʔ (fire-piʔ) appears in the same situations as mentioned above for dim-eye piʔ and is characterized by high fever, profuse sweating, short breath, vomiting (hâag lom—

vomit air), restlessness, and loss of consciousness. May end in death.

The expression piˀ lom piˀ lŷad (wind piˀ and blood piˀ) is often heard, and accordingly one informant divided piˀ into the following two main types:

> *piˀ lom* is caused by a wind, and results in unconsciousness lasting from minutes to hours due to hunger, hard work, or exposure to the sun. The victim feels warm.
>
> *piˀ lŷad* is caused by the blood, and results in unconsciousness as a result of extreme thirst or of "the blood not being thick enough." Fainting in connection with strong emotional feelings—as when terrified—is also a kind of piˀ lŷad.

This informant did not regard fainting after standing up abruptly as a type of piˀ, but called it simply pěn lom pěn lŷad, "to have wind and blood."

Other piˀ terms include *piˀ sakun, piˀ tanuu sǐŋ, piˀ sajob* (see lom sakun). The villagers now associate the term *piˀ* with "being hungry for something one cannot define."

Diagnosis:* The various piˀ comprise clinical conditions of vertigo and syncope of different etiologies. When accompanied by other symptoms and signs, other diagnostic categories are used, such as sàníbàad, bàheŋkhúd, lom sakun, and kìaw.

piˀ pàa

The diagnosis *piˀ pàa* (forest piˀ) is ascertained on the basis of a sudden appearance of yellow eyes and skin, without other prominent symptoms. The patient gets weak, but can usually still work.

Cause: The disease is caused by the intervention of a spirit from the forest.

Treatment: Magic.

Comments: It is different from *khǎj pàa* where there is a remittent fever and pale (not yellow) skin, though the causality is the same.

Diagnosis: Jaundice without fever.

pòoŋ

pòoŋ is a disease that attacks the joints and muscles. Several clinical pictures of pòoŋ were recorded:

> *lom píd pòoŋ*~pòoŋ dùug. The bones and muscles are eaten, giving pain and high fever. The legs shrink (khăa lìib) and become permanently useless. May result in paralysis (ʔammápâad).

Diagnosis:* Poliomyelitis. People in the village with sequelae of polio were given as examples of the condition. Another course of the disease is high fever, painful joints, staring eyes, and confabulation. Death follows within seven days.

pòoŋ may also attack the joints in arms, fingers, and lower limbs (especially the knees), leaving them stiff and flexed, painful and slightly swollen. May also be accompanied by pain in the loin. There is no fever.

Cause: People trample on holes or termite mounds where the pòoŋ-spirit lives. The spirit in revenge somehow injects a pòoŋ-poison into the victim's body, thus causing the disease. A serious wind appears, giving the characteristic symptoms and signs.

Diagnosis:* Chronic rheumatoid arthritis, arthrosis deformans.

Treatment: As the cause is magical, the cure is naturally magical too (pàw, céd hɛ̀ɛg), but medicines do exist. In fact, in three of the manuals we find altogether eight prescriptions against this disease, under headings like thùug phĭi pòoŋ phĭi ñam and kɛ̃ɛ píd pòoŋ píd ñam. Most of them are in the form of compressions (jaa kɔ̂ɔb).

Comments: Some people called it phaj pòoŋ, but the majority strongly objected to its having anything to do with phaj.

pòoŋ may also attack cows and buffalo, and is then called pòoŋ ŋua pòoŋ khwaaj.

lom sakun

lom sakun (family-wind)~kìaw lom sakun~piʔ sakun~piʔ tanuu sĭŋ. The main symptoms of this disease are as follows: A person suddenly gets a stroke, falls over, and loses consciousness. Some people become stiff and die within minutes or hours without regaining consciousness. Others wake up, but their minds are absent. They do not understand what you say and they cannot talk; they just mumble. They cannot move, because their limbs have become paralyzed (ʔammápâad).

Cause: A lom lŷad appears and ascends to the head, and is responsible for the sudden stroke. May pass from parents to children.

Comments: One informant used the term *lom sakun* in a more restricted meaning, only covering the condition of losing consciousness followed by wake-up. In this respect *piʔ sakun* and *piʔ tanuu sǐŋ* are synonymous terms. The condition of unconsciousness and sudden death should, according to this informant, be termed piʔ fáa mɛ̂ɛb or piʔ sajob, which is caused by a more serious wind.

Diagnosis: Apoplexy (cerebral stroke).

ned

ned~nedsy̌ŋ. This term is used to describe the sensation of a sleeping limb—as in a leg after sitting on it for a long time—resulting in a numb feeling in the legs and loss of sensation for a short while. It may be regarded as a mild form of kìaw (muscle cramps), and is then called lom kìaw nedsaa.

Diagnosis:* Numbness, prickling, tingling (paresthesia).

Note: The Bangkok-Thai cognate *nèb* means "numbness, tingling."

nedsaa

nedsaa is an insidious disease with gradual loss of sensation in the legs. The legs feel heavy with a numb sensation as if mud were stuck to the foot, which one cannot brush off. It expands slowly upward, and the patient becomes weak and loses all strength in his legs. The patient may fall and not be able to get up. The legs are still mobile, however, and the flesh is normal (in contrast to the condition ʔammápâad, when the flesh becomes soft, like that of a baby). After several years the whole body may be affected, and the patient can no longer even move his legs. Then the disease has turned to ʔammápâad nedsaa (nedsaa paralysis). It is "the sibling of ʔammápâad." It is usually seen in patients aged fifteen years and older.

Cause: Comes from outside the body.[10]

Treatment: It is a cold disease that requires a hot medicine. It can be cured, but the medication is not really any good. Modern medicine gives injections, but the disease does not really disappear. Food prohibitions are part of the treatment.

Diagnosis:* Polyneuritis. In Thailand usually due to vitamin-B deficiency (dry beriberi).[11]

Comments: Two of the five manuscripts mention the terms ned and nedsaa in altogether nine prescription headings, often in connection with other diseases like kìaw, sàníbàad, bàheŋkhúd, and also wind (lom).

ˀammápâad

This term is used to describe the condition of a general paralysis or paresis of the limbs. Some persons are born ˀammápâad, others become ˀammápâad as a result of other diseases. A person may be ˀammapâad in the whole body or just in one or two of the limbs. One half of the body may be ˀammápâad, in which case it is called tǎaj phàag (hemiplegia). A person can live as ˀammápâad for months or years before he dies. Some victims are also unable to talk.

Cause: Bad blood. One informant mentioned that spirits could be responsible for bad blood.

Treatment: There exist oral and topical remedies, but none is regarded as really good.

Comments: The informants agreed that lom sakun, nedsaa, and pòoŋ are the diseases that most commonly result in ˀammápâad. According to one informant ˀammápâad was called ŋɔ̂ɔj in older times. One or two remedies for ˀammápâad were found in each of the manuscripts studied.

10. phag tamlyŋ—which is regarded as cold—may cause this disease (Yoddumnern 1976:9).

11. The Bangkok-Thai cognate *nèbchaa* is used for "an infective form of polyneurosis, resulting in anesthesia of the skin." The term *chaa* by itself means numb. (McFarland 1944:940, 289).

satog

satog is an archaic term meaning to "pull with a jerking movement" or the "jerking movement" itself. The term *cág* is a synonym commonly used today. Satog is usually a symptom of complex diseases, such as khãj satog and sàníbàad satog. However, if intermittent or chronic convulsions occur by themselves without other conspicuous symptoms, the diagnosis khǎaŋ satog, lom satog, or just satog is given. A child with fever and intermittent contractions of muscles may get the diagnosis khãj satog. The situation of generalized epileptiform convulsions is recognized as the disease phǐi bãa mǔu.

There are from one to three prescriptions in each manuscript against satog in general.

khãj satog

khãj satog~khãj lɛ́w saduang satog~lom satog. This is a disease usually seen among children. The skin and flesh get very hot and a wind ascending to the head (lom khỹn) makes the patient soporose and absentminded, the eyes turn up and the body gets stiff with uncontrolled contractions of the arms or legs (satog). These convulsions or jerks may come and go; if not adequately treated with medicines, the patient will usually remain stiff, with the eyes fixed in an upward position, until he finally dies.

Cause: Unknown.

Treatment: Oral remedies and magic.

Diagnosis: Fever cramps; infectious diseases with cerebral affection (e.g., encephalitis, meningitis, etc.).

sàníbàad

This long-term disease, which normally attacks adults, is described as taking many possible forms, which are given different descriptive names according to the most prevalent symptoms. A person usually has only one type of sàníbàad at a time, but one type may change to another. The disease comes suddenly, but is usually preceded by fever. Once the disease has been contracted, attacks occur at intervals ranging from minutes to days. The frequency of the attacks varies from one to three times during the whole life span to ever-recurring attacks, making the disease chronic. The disease may, however, culminate in convulsions and death. Some typical manifestations are:

sànibàad bà pàag~sànibàad dag—the patient is mute, but after a while he may start to talk profusely

sànibàad sǎaw máj—the patient lies down kicking and writhing

sànibàad sadũŋ~sànibàad phǐi pɛ̌ɛŋ—he tears things to pieces, grits his teeth violently, and may bite the tongue

sànibàad bãa—he looks mad, and may run away for no apparent reason

sànibàad ŋâaw lab—the patient is sleepy

sànibàad satog~sànibàad cág—this is the situation when an adult person has repeated attacks of uncontrolled jerks (fits) or convulsions of the limbs, head, neck, or just around the mouth or eyes. If small children get the same symptoms during or after a period of high fever, it is called sànibàad dib (raw sànibàad) or, more commonly, khãj cág (pulling fever) or khãj satog (jerking fever). If the symptoms remain after the children have reached adulthood, the diagnosis will change to sànibàad satog.

Cause: It is caused by a wind (lom sànibàad) coming from outside. The similarity to being possessed by spirits is mentioned, but spirits have actually nothing to do with these conditions.

Treatment: The various kinds of sànibàad are regarded as difficult to cure. Many of the medicines used to treat sànibàad are of the cág type, a "pull out" medicine. A liquid herbal mixture is made, into which some leaves are dipped, and the patient is rubbed from head to toe—with or without magical formulas being recited—thus the disease is "pulled out." There are also some oral remedies.

Diagnosis: The diverse symptomatology makes sànibàad a rather broad and variable concept. It certainly covers the clinical pictures of several mental and neurological disorders, but also points to more or less chronic fever diseases as a part of the concept. An old lady in our village with the clinical picture of Parkinson's disease was given the diagnosis sàníbaàad cág.

Comments: It was stressed by the informants that sàníbàad has nothing to do with madness (bãa), although a patient's behavior may be similar in some cases. In the manuscripts sàníbàad (sometimes spelled sănníbàad) is amply represented. We have noted over seventy prescriptions that treat—among other diseases—sàníbàad. sàníbáad occurs in the prescriptions together with a host of other disease terms such as khăaŋ, saaŋ, piʔ, lom tàaŋ tàaŋ, kìaw, bàheŋ-khúd, hâag sàag, and even tùm. Some manuscripts refer to "the ten kinds of sàníbàad' and 'the eight kinds of sàníbàad" without further specification.

In the Bangkok-Thai tradition, "there are several kinds of sannibãt, the disease which develops when all three of the tridosa are active. One form occurs as a tremor similar to Parkinsonism, another form produces symptoms of fever caused by mucus, with fainting, sweating and bleeding" (Mulholland 1979*b*). In a Burmese manuscript we find the term *tha-nee-bât* described as "long and protracted fever" (Macdonald 1879: 27).

lom phid dyan

Dizziness and fainting in connection with menstruation or childbirth is called *lom phid dyan.*

Cause: Wrong food, bad smells, spoiled blood, or loss of blood.

Treatment: There exist many prescriptions against this ailment in the manuscripts, and traditional medicines against it are on sale everywhere.

Comments: This syndrome is usually a result of postpartum anemia. M. A. Muecke (1979) translates the term *lom phid dyan* as "wrong menstrual wind illness; afflicting wind of the month," and gives the causality "breach of post partum custom by women."

bãa

bãa means madness or mental disorder. The traditional doctors regard this disease as incurable. One informant described the disease in the following way: "Mad (bãa) persons may be violent and can harm people, or they sing and cry without apparent reason, give irrelevant answers, and talk to themselves. Some are scared and believe people will hit them. It is most common with women, and they are particularly exposed to this disease after they deliver a baby, due to weakness and loss of blood. Unmarried women may turn mad, too, especially when their menses are irregular or fail to come."

Comments: Although bãa has some symptoms in common with certain wind diseases, and certain diseases caused by spirits, it is—in principle—regarded as something entirely different from these. It does not rightly belong to the wind group of diseases. There are no traditional medicines against it, and the term is not recorded in the medical manuscripts studied. Our team did not collect information about this disorder, but refer our readers to the thesis of Walter Irvine (1982) on this subject.

4.2.5. Blood diseases

kìaw

kìaw~kèw seems to cover "rigidity and painful, spastic cramps in muscles and joints." The term occurs frequently in names of diseases in which cramps and stiffness are prominent symptoms, most of which are located in the legs. kìaw is generally accompanied by a wind, thus the terms kìaw lom and lom kìaw are often met with.

> *kìaw kɔ̃ɔm* (small kìaw)~kìaw khɔ́n kɔ̃ɔm (cudgel, or truncheon kìaw)~kìaw had kìaw háaw (pulling kìaw)~kìaw nɔ̂ŋ (calf kìaw) is simply muscle cramps, usually in the legs, but may also appear in other parts of the body like waist, breast, and arms. Disappears after a while without treatment.
>
> *kìaw lûug nǔu* is painful, stiff legs with palpable small nodules in the flesh of the leg.
> *Diagnosis:* Varices?

kìaw faj~kìaw mãj (fire cramps)~kìaw khãj (fever cramps)~kìaw sàn (shivering cramps) is cramps and stiffness in connection with fever, ranging from temporary cramps to more serious conditions leading to unconsciousness and death. (Septicemia?)

kìaw dam (black kìaw)~kìaw dam kìaw dɛɛŋ (red and black kìaw)~ʔintákhǐn khỹn kìaw dam. This is a serious, often fatal disease recognized by all the practitioners. The patient suddenly becomes weak and stiff and cannot move his limbs. Cramps appear in the chest region and cause pressure on the heart and difficulties in breathing. The skin becomes cool and turns red or dark blue—as the name of the disease suggests—especially on the hands, feet, lips, and eyelids, but the patient is hot inside. The patient lies inanimate and is somnolent. He may lose conciousness and then die. It is common in the hot season, and is usually seen among adults.

Cause: kìaw dam is caused by "unwholesome or bad blood" (lŷad phíkaan, lŷad sǐa) or "black blood" (lŷad dam) or "warm blood" (lŷad hɔ̂ɔn) together with a warm wind. It may be induced by the intake of food that the patient is not used to.

Treatment: kìaw dam must be treated with a warm medicine taken orally "to get the fire out to the skin." A good piece of advice is to pour alcohol—which is considered hot—into the patient's mouth or apply it to the skin.

Diagnosis: The symptomatology points to the manifestations of anaphylactic shock, and may have its cosmopolitan counterpart in the clinical condition of severe anaphylaxis.

In the manuscripts we have found some thirty-seven prescriptions that cure kìaw in one of its many manifestations, together with other diseases like piʔ, sàníbàad, and khǎaŋ. The manuscripts also mention kìaw kǐn tɔ́ɔŋ mɛ̂ɛ maan (cramps eating the womb of a pregnant woman). (Pregnancy pangs?)

Other terms have been recorded, unfortunately without full documentation: kìaw myyn, kìaw mahǎamyyn lǔaŋ, kìaw cɔ̂ɔŋ, kìaw ʔɔ̀ɔn kìaw mɔ̂j.

kǎan

In its broadest sense *kǎan* is a term used for hemorrhages of spontaneous origin.

kǎan lŷad (blood kǎan)~kǎan dam kǎan dɛɛŋ (black and red kǎan)~khãj kǎan (fever kǎan). The cardinal symptoms are high fever and the appearance of characteristic eruptions within the skin (kǎan fóg, pěn kǎan). The skin eruptions are understood as the blood breaking out and trying to escape from the vessels through the flesh, then becoming visible in the skin. The patient may bleed from the mouth or nose, too. If the eruptions appear on the hollow parts of the body, that is, the stomach, chest, and around the throat and neck, they are considered particularly dangerous. After some days this stagnant blood becomes spoiled (lŷad sǐa), the poison permeates deep into the body (píd khãw naj) and results in a pressing pain in the chest, difficult breathing, and death within a few days. It is not always fatal, though, and sometimes it may heal by itself or with medical treatment (most cases are regarded as intractable). It is seen among both children and adults.

Cause: The disease is caused by the blood getting warm and trying to escape from the body. One informant pointed out that if the placenta and blood are left in the uterus after birth, it can give rise to kǎan lŷad of the mother in the period after birth, causing death.

Treatment: It is a warm disease that must be treated with a cold medicine, both orally and topically, together with magic incantations. The herbalists admit that their medicines are not very effective against this disease. It was also stressed that the name of the disease should not be mentioned to the patient because that would cause an abrupt exacerbation of the disease.

Comments: The term *kǎan lŷad* is also used by some herbalists to describe in general bleedings from the nose, mouth, or vagina. Another term in current use for these conditions is lídsaduaŋ lŷad. One informant said that kǎan lŷad was synonymous with kìaw dam. It is notable that some informants equate kǎan lŷad with the modern Thai medical term *khwaam dan sǔuŋ* (high blood pressure), though the disease probably has nothing to do with hypertension.

Diagnosis: From the variable symptomatology, including both mild, severe, and fatal attacks of the disease, it is evident that it covers elements of many different cosmopolitan disease units. However, the central symptom, kǎan fóg, certainly represents capillary hemorrhages, purpura, or ecchymoses of the skin. It is assumed that both clinical syndromes of anaphylactoid purpura (infections, drug sensitivity), trombocytopenic purpura, as well as secondary, symptomatic purpura (among others a symptom of leukemia, sepsis, and carcinomatosis) will be classified as kǎan lŷad. (as for fǐi kǎan, see tùm líi.)

4.2.6. Diseases with swellings (edema) and tumors as prominent signs

tɔ́ɔŋ kə̃əm

tɔ́ɔŋ *kə̃əm*~tɔ́ɔŋ kə̃əm tɔ́ɔŋ kãam (hard stomach). The abdomen becomes hard, first on the right side, and then all over. As noticed by the practitioners, there is a hard, palpable resistance or several hard lumps in the abdomen. If progressing, the eyes and skin will turn yellow. The patient loses appetite and gets thin (phɔ̆ɔm hɛ̃ɛŋ), while the abdomen gets bigger and bigger. There is a piercing pain in the abdomen and upwards. It may be accompanied by bouts of fever. Occurs only in adults.

Cause: According to one informant, tɔ́ɔŋ kə̃əm is due to an expanding or rotten liver, while another respondent thought it was due to an enlargement of the spleen. One informant had heard that excessive consumption of alcohol could cause this complaint, but he maintained that alcohol could not alone be responsible because some people who never drank had succumbed to it.

Treatment: There exist some traditional remedies taken orally, but tɔ́ɔŋ kə̃əm is regarded as difficult and often impossible to cure.

Comments: One informant said that if a generally hard stomach was accompanied by blood in the stools he would call it lídsaduaŋ tɔ́ɔŋ kə̃əm, and if the stools were followed by fat he would call it khǎaŋ tɔ́ɔŋ kə̃əm. A generally hard stomach could also be termed sǎan tɔ́ɔŋ kə̃əm. One informant maintained that a khǎaŋ might develop into a saaŋ, which would progress to tɔ̂ɔŋ kə̄əm if not cured.

Diagnosis:* tɔ̂ɔŋ kə̄əm is rather comprehensive if evaluated from a cosmopolitan medical point of view. In order to find the Western counterparts of this disease, one has to consider all conditions of expansive processes in the abdominal area. One patient given the diagnosis tɔ̂ɔŋ kə̄əm had, clinically, a large abdominal tumor with multiple metastatic processes of the liver. According to the patient, a doctor at the hospital had inserted a needle into his liver (liver biopsy), and afterward the doctor had told him that he suffered from máreŋ (cancer).

sǎan (tumors, nodules)

sǎan or fǐi sǎan is the name of a group of diseases with the common characteristic of tumors or hard nodules appearing somewhere in the body, usually within or just beneath the skin. A sǎan does not burst by itself (bà tɛ̀ɛg, bà nâw ʔeeŋ) and is often accompanied by a wind (lom sǎan). This wind is characteristic and, when it appears by itself without any visible tumor, it is often indicative of a sǎan hidden somewhere in the body. In most cases, however, the diagnosis rests on the presentation of some visible or palpable tumors.

Cause: The disease appears by itself (ʔɔ̀ɔg càag naj maa), and is caused by an unidentified etiological agent (mii mɛ̂ɛ). It has nothing to do with the elements, but is rather a result of individual fate (wâadthanǎa).

Treatment: sǎan is said to be a hot disease, but still requires a hot medicine. The treatment is often protracted, involving many steps and several kinds of medicines and magic. The basic idea behind the treatment is to "pull the tumor out" and to cure the accompanying wind. The wind is treated with a ground medicine taken orally (jaa lom sǎan). The tumor is "pulled out" with a topical medicine that literally "eats its way down around the tumor," leaving behind a deep wound, which is healed by another topical medicine. Food prohibitions are part of the treatment. However, a tumor may be located on a spot where it would be too dangerous to pull it out; for example, in the throat. The traditional doctors will then at first move the tumor (jáaj sǎan) to a less dangerous spot on the body, for example, the arm, and pull it out there. No one in Northern Thailand (whom we met) doubted that this could be done successfully. We have not ourselves seen a successful transference of a tumor, but we have seen attempts that did not look very promising. We are nevertheless inclined to believe that the traditional doctors actually may be able to accomplish this feat in certain cases.

Various kinds of sǎan

It seemed that the more data we got about the different sǎan diseases, the more contradictory the picture became, both as to number and content of the various types of sǎan. We ended up with some fifty different names for sǎan (of which many may be identical, although the informants did not agree as to which) and numerous ways of grouping these diseases. In despair we have had to create a system that largely is our own, not based on any general consensus among the practitioners, but on our own "educated guesses." Below follow some sǎan concepts: general, specific, and unidentified.

sǎan lŷad (blood sǎan). Our information on this is contradictory. It is probably an etiological concept referring to any kind of sǎan that originates in the blood. This kind of tumor is soft and movable. As time goes by, it may develop roots, changing into a stationary sǎan (sǎan hǐn).

sǎan hǐn~sǎan kɔ̃ɔn (stone sǎan) is a general term for tumors that are hard and stationary because they have developed deep roots. They appear normally on the fleshy areas of the body. The patient becomes weak and thin. It is usually not fatal, but may cause much intermittent pain, and may give rise to a wind.

lom sǎan~sǎan lom (wind sǎan) is a soft tumor that appears in the front of the throat. It is not painful, but the patient loses appetite and may vomit. When the patient eats or smells something wrong, he becomes dizzy.

Comments: According to one informant lom sǎan is different from khɔɔ fɔ̂ɔg where the "tumor" is harder and more tense (tyŋ), appears symmetrically on both sides on the throat, and does not affect the appetite.

*Diagnosis**:* Diffuse struma (goiter).

lom sǎan bàheŋkhúd is a more serious version of lom sǎan, above. The wind accompanying this disease causes severe headache, red and running eyes, dim sight, reduced hearing, and loss of sense of smell.

sǎan man mǔu (pig-fat sǎan)~sǎan nɔ̂ɔg ŋua (cow hump sǎan) is a rather soft and movable tumor that appears in the skin most commonly on the neck, around the joints, or other places where the skin is thick. It does not burst. The inside of the tumor is homogeneous in consistency and resembles pig fat, as the name suggests. There is normally no pain, and it is not dangerous. It can grow big, though, and if located in the neck may cause headache. Seen with all ages, but not common among children.

Treatment: Medicine is smeared on to make it retract (lɔ̀ɔd, júbloŋ). The hospitals just operate them away.

*Diagnosis**:* Lipoma, but probably also including other types of benign tumors of the skin.

sǎan bàkham hɔ́ɔj~fǐi bàkham hɔ́ɔj~sǎan lǎam khɔɔ~sǎan nám lǐaŋ. First an ascending wind causes aching in the body and joints; then several nodules, the size of peas, appear under the ear, spreading to the throat and to the chest. When mature, they will take the form of a fǐi, burst, and give off secretion and blood, leaving behind ulcers that dry up. The disease spreads around in the body following the blood. The patient loses appetite and becomes weak and may die. A person gets it only once. More common now than before. No fever, no itching, not contagious.

Cause: Some informants gave "spoiled lymph" (nám lǐaŋ sǐa) as the cause, others did not know the cause.

Treatment: Must be moved to the shoulder and pulled out there. Strict food prohibitions.

Comments: According to one informant it is identical to the modern Bangkok-Thai concept máreŋ méd khǎaw naj sên lŷad (leukemia). Others said that the modern terms for it were *tɔ̀m thɔnsin* (tonsillitis) or *tɔ̀m thajlɔj* (thyreo-adenitis).

sǎan dɔ̀ɔg bug~sǎan bua bug~sǎan dɔ̀ɔg bua. This "flowering" (baan) tumor is considered very dangerous and often leads to death. The patient feels hot, gets pain, and becomes weak. A tumor appears in the skin. After some time it will break open (tɛ̀ɛg, baan—"flower") and several tùm will appear on its surface, giving off pus and blood, and leaving behind holes. The flesh rots away, but the tumor keeps growing. If one tries to cut it off, it will grow out again. It has roots like those of the banana palm. It results in dizziness and swimming eyes. Appears mainly on the upper part of the body (both sides of the neck, upper back, the corner of the mouth, armpits, chest, cheeks, and the tongue), but it is also seen in the groin and on the heels. After the "flowering" phase has occurred, the patient gets fever, coughs blood (if it is located on the throat) and it is then fatal within two to four weeks.

Cause: Poisonous blood (lŷad pěn píd).

Treatment: Compress of a caustic medicine (jaa kad khɔ̂ɔb) (but do not pull, because some of the roots may be left behind), plus an oral medicine against the accompanying wind (jaa kǐn kan lom) together with magic. It must not be operated on, although one informant said the hospitals can operate on it successfully. Food prohibitions are an important part of the treatment.

Comments: When shown pictures of malignant melanoma, mycetoma, and spinocellular carcinoma, one herbalist called them all sǎan dɔ̀ɔg bug. The concept probably includes different malignant processes of the skin. The term *fǐi dɔ̀ɔg bug* is used for smaller tumors.

sǎan khanthámaalaa. One or more tumors appear on the outside of the throat under the ear. The patient gets pain in the throat, and may cough blood that is dark and sticky. Accompanied by a "poisonous wind" (lom píd khŷn), causing attacks of unconsciousness. The disease is fatal, but fortunately quite rare.

Cause: From poisonous blood (lŷad pĕn píd).

Treatment: Very difficult.

Comments: One informant equates this term with săan dɔ̀ɔg bug. It was pointed out that săan kanthámaalaa has several features in common with other diseases. It is accompanied by "an ascending poisonous wind" (lom píd khŷn) as is bàadphañág; the patient coughs blood, as with lídsaduaŋ naj khɔɔ; and it also resembles tùm píd.

săan khăw tɔ̀ɔg (puffed rice săan)~săan dɔ̀ɔg (flower săan). One informant, who also had been present at an obduction where he had seen white tumors in the esophagus and the gastrointestinal tract, attributed these conditions to săan khăw tɔ̀ɔg.

săan kɛ̀n făaj~săan méd făaj (cotton-seed săan). Many small oblong nodules—the size of cotton seeds—appear simultaneously in the skin on some part of the body. They burst open by themselves and the inside is cream-colored (but there is no fluid). Not serious, but it does not disappear by itself.

Treatment: Oral medicine is taken to "chase it out" (khab ʔɔ̀ɔg). Magic (céd hɛ̀ɛg) is also commonly made use of. No food prohibitions.

săan lûug nŭu (mice-children săan)~fĭi lûug nŭu. Some white nodules—the size of maize kernels—suddenly appear in the skin somewhere on the body. They do not burst open by themselves. One informant regarded it as very serious, saying that the skin became hot, the patient would swell up, and not be able to eat and consequently die (usually within two months). Another informant regarded the disease as completely harmless.

Comments: The similarity to bàheŋ khàj păa was noted.

săan lídsaduaŋ is a general term for nodules—the size of plums—with a soft substance ("like that of the brain"—ʔɔ̀ɔg

ʔɔɔ) which can be squeezed out. No medicine needed. It has a head, but is not painful (and can thus not be classified as a fĭi). It is not stationary and can appear anywhere on the body. *Diagnosis*:* Folliculitis (pimples).

sǎan lídsaduaŋ khɔɔ dya. White or reddish tùm appear in the throat around the uvula (dya, lûug kadya). They burst open and result in a stinking smell in the mouth. The patient then becomes hoarse, loses his voice, coughs, vomits, and dies. Nothing is seen on the exterior surface of the throat.

Treatment: Very difficult to cure, and impossible after the patient has lost his voice. Strict food prohibitions.

sǎan naj tɔ́ɔŋ~sǎan kãam lŷad naj tɔ́ɔŋ (sǎan in the stomach). A hard, palpable lump or resistance appears in the stomach, causing pain, and an ascending wind arises that results in pressure in the chest region, difficulties in breathing, and headache. At first one can feel the hard lump moving slightly when it is pressed with the fingers, but later it becomes stationary as roots develop. It is serious, and the patient may die.

Cause: Something to do with the food. It is said to develop from "a khǎaŋ that has descended into the stomach."

Treatment: Oral medicine with salty taste.

Comments: The distinction from fĭi sǎan naj tɔ́ɔŋ is made on the basis of the more piercing pain and the absence of a palpable tumor with the latter. In a cosmopolitan medical sense sǎan naj tɔ́ɔŋ and fĭi sǎan naj tɔ́ɔŋ may be manifestations of the same underlying processes, such as ulcerous and carcinomatous lesions of an abdominal organ.

sǎan jaŋ nom (sǎan in the breast)~sǎan nom ñuaŋ (hanging breast sǎan). A hard lump or tumor in the breast of women. This term seems to cover all types of mammary tumors of females. (See also bàheŋ nom ñuaŋ.)

The following names for sǎan diseases were mentioned by one informant only, but not accepted by the others: sǎan ŋuu hàw, sǎan bàbãa, sǎan dùug, sǎan sapaw, sǎan sɔ̃ɔŋ naaŋ nâŋ hãj, sǎan lûug sakhẽe, sǎan mɔɔn pǔu, sǎan sabaaj, sǎan sǎaj.

Disease names containing the morpheme sǎan, but classified as non-sǎan diseases: sǎan khɔɔ fɔ̂ɔg (see khɔɔ fɔ̂ɔg) and sǎan lammá-nâad (see khǎaŋ lammánâad).

As for the confusion between the bàheŋ and the sǎan concepts, see the section on bàheŋ.

A total of forty-two prescriptions against sǎan diseases were found in the manuscripts. Very often the term *fǐi sǎan* was used, and the wind (lom) and the blood (lŷad) were often referred to in the names, as in lom sǎan, sǎan lom lâa, and sǎan lŷad. Other diseases may co-occur with sǎan, like khǎaŋ, mahòog, and bàheŋkhúd. Specific sǎan disease names mentioned were: fǐi sǎan lûug nǔu, fǐi sǎan naj tɔ́ɔŋ, fǐi sǎan wian phǐi, sǎan mŷn, sǎan pãaŋ kâj, sǎan ʔaj, sǎan lǔaŋ, and sǎan khãw khɔ̂ɔ.

khɔɔ fɔ̂ɔg

khɔɔ fɔ̂ɔg~sǎan khɔɔ fɔ̂ɔg~khɔɔ nŷaŋ.

A tumor appears on the front of the throat. The patient eats well, but still gets thin. There are two types. A hard one, called khɔɔ nŷaŋ, is neither painful nor accompanied by any wind. It resembles a sǎan. The soft variety—khɔɔ fɔ̂ɔg—is, in contrast, both painful and accompanied by a wind that presses on the eyes, making them "big and protruding." Strict food prohibitions.

Treatment: Oral medicines (general sǎan-medicine). It is possible to move the tumor by means of magic and a topical medicine to another and less dangerous spot on the body (for details, see sǎan).

*Diagnosis**:* goiter (thyreotoxicosis). (See also lom sǎan.)

hâa wɔ̂ɔg

hâa wɔ̂ɔg~kaaŋ pɔɔŋ (monkey pest, swollen chin).

Thick, oblong swellings of the cheek and under the mandible appear, accompanied by pain when swallowing. Normally seen among children, but also in adults (see also khǎaŋ lammánâad).

Treatment: Magic and topical medicine (lime).
Diagnosis: Mumps (parotitis).

maan nám

maan nám~maan hung (archaic)~maan nám maan hung~maan hung maan nám (pregnant with water).

maan nám is a disease in which the abdomen swells in the same way it does in a pregnant woman, but the patient does not eat more than normally. When the abdomen becomes large the patient has difficulty in breathing, and his heart starts to palpitate. It is very serious, and the patient will usually die. It is seen among adults, usually female.

Cause: The practitioners all gave modern explanations of the etiology, such as the uterus being out of order (mód lûug phíkaan) or cancer of the uterus (máreng mód lûug) or the liver being out of order (tab phíkaan), knowledge obtained by feedback from patients who had been in the hospital.

Treatment: There exist some traditional remedies, but according to the herbalists themselves they are not good. It was also emphasized that modern medical doctors could not cure the patients either. One informant had heard that the patients were punctured in the abdomen in the hospital, causing fluid to come out.

Comments: The close relationship to the condition pɔɔŋ was pointed out by some informants. One informant pointed out that a person with maan nám could have pɔɔŋ of the legs at the same time.

Diagnosis:* Ascites. The verbalization of the accompanying symptoms and course reflects some characteristics of the basic disorders underlying this condition (carcinomatosis, cardiac failure, hepatic failure).

pɔɔŋ

This is a disease in which the skin and flesh are swollen on various parts of the body, usually on the lower legs. When the skin is pressed, finger pits appear, but disappear after awhile.

Treatment: Both topical and oral remedies.

Diagnosis:* Pitting edema (localized lymphedema).

hăm ʔòod

hăm ʔòod (swollen scrotum)—sãj loŋ hăm (intestines falling down in scrotum).

A new, borrowed concept not clearly understood, but applied for the conditions of inguinal and scrotal hernia as well as scrotal edema of different origin.

khăa maan (pregnant leg)

The leg is swollen from the ankle to the groin. It is usually seen in children over ten years old and in young adults. There is nɔ̌ɔŋ (pus) inside the leg. Usually not painful. Finally the patient may die.

Diagnosis:* Lymphedema (localized to the leg), commonly an expression of filariasis.

loŋ săw~loŋ săw khỹn săw
(down into the legs or, literally, "poles")

This is an expression or attribute used when a disease spreads down in the legs and causes aching and/or swollen limbs and joints. It may be a result of different conditions: bàhòog loŋ săw, bàheŋ-khúd loŋ săw, módtakhyd loŋ săw, kìaw loŋ săw, lídsaduaŋ loŋ săw. Among others, generalized lymphedema (elephantiasis) is covered by this concept.

4.2.7. Infections and fever diseases

khãj means fever, but is also used in a more general sense for "being sick," as in khon khãj (a patient) and pĕn khãj (be sick, have a fever). The term *khãj* may or may not be prefixed to the many disease terms that have fever as a prominent symptom.

The traditional doctors recognize degrees of fever, but have no way to measure it, beyond feeling the skin of the patient. On a verbal level, they differentiate between:

–khãj ˀob (low, constant fever)

–khãj hɔ́ɔn~hɔ́ɔn nýa hɔ́ɔn khiŋ (fever)

–khãj hɔ́ɔn nág~khãj sǔuŋ (high fever)

–khãj kǔm~khãj bà lòb~khãj hýa~khãj sỳam~khãj sỳm (high, constant fever)

–khãj bà húu swàaŋ~khãj bà húu wan bà húu khyyn (high, constant fever with patient in a soporose condition)

There are also expressions for the frequency of the fever attacks:

–ñŷag hɔ́ɔn ñŷag nǎaw~cŷyd nýa cŷyd tǔa~khân nýa khân tǔa (now hot now cold)

–khãj wén wan~sǎam wan dii sìi wan khãj (fever every second day)

–khãj háan khãj hýa (repeated, sudden attacks of fever)

Distinction is also made between:

–fevers without sweat (khãj hỳa bà ˀɔ̀ɔg), which are considered particularly dangerous, and fevers with sweat (khãj hỳa ˀɔ̀ɔg)

–fevers when the patient feels hot (tǔa hɔ́ɔn nýa hɔ́ɔn khiŋ, khãj bà nǎaw), and fevers when the patient feels cold and shivers (khãj nǎaw sàn)[12]

The aim of the remedies used in treating diseases with a mounting fever (khãj khỹn) is naturally to bring it down (hãam

12. Similar types of fevers in Laos are mentioned in Spire 1907:19.

khãj, dab khãj). There are special remedies for babies with fever (lûug ʔɔ̀ɔn khãj). The fever remedies as a rule contain a mixture of bitter and warm ingredients.

The traditional doctors admit willingly that "fever diseases are both difficult to diagnose and difficult to cure" and that the Western medicines are superior to the traditional ones in the treatment of these diseases. (Some of them do use Western medicines to bring the fever down.) This is also the general attitude of the villagers.

The traditional doctors only vaguely hinted at the blood or the wind as being the cause of fever. Only one prescription—out of a total of some sixty—mentions the fire element as the ultimate cause of fever.

khãj hâag sàag

khãj hâag sàag~khãj hâag sàad~hâag sàag~phĭi lâad sàad.

The symptoms are weakness, spells of fever going a little up and down in peaks, but usually high and increasing and accompanied by loss of appetite, headache, pains in the body, and difficulties in sleeping. The skin turns pale, and the soles of the feet and the palms of the hands become glossy red, black, or yellowish. The patient may confabulate and becomes thin. After a week or two the feces turn red and then black, but are not particularly loose in consistency. If not successfully treated the patient may die within twenty days. (One informant, however, claimed he had had this disease several times.) The disease is seen with all age groups, and is more serious than pãaŋ. Previously common, now rare.

Treatment: Oral remedies. Eight prescriptions have been recorded from the manuscripts.

Comments: In modern Bangkok Thai, the term *khâj râag sàad* means typhoid. Some of the Northern Thai informants also identified khãj hâag sàag with thajfɔɔj (typhoid) and málɛɛlia (malaria), although when we asked the informants on other occasions what thajfɔɔj was called in Northern Thai they would say khãj luʔ (fever and diarrhea). One informant also called this disease lûud dam lûud dɛɛŋ lûud lÿaŋ (black, red, or yellow lûud).

Diagnosis: khãj hâag sàag is, from the description, assumed to represent a common clinical picture of typhoid.

khãj pàa (forest fever)

The patient feels tired, followed by a sudden onset of fever that goes up and down every day and may be accompanied by uncontrolled jerks of the limbs. The patient gets weak and pale. The disease can last for weeks. It is serious and the patient may die, but usually it is not fatal.

Cause: May be caused by a forest spirit. One informant had heard that bites from a particular insect might be the cause.

Treatment: Oral medicine, together with incantations.

Diagnosis: Our inquiries revealed no other symptoms beyond the unspecific fever symptoms mentioned above. These symptoms may be applicable to a number of infectious diseases of different etiologies. A cosmopolitan counterpart in medical practice might be *febris causae ignotae.* However, the pattern of an intermittent and/or remittent, long-lasting fever disease void of other specific symptoms is a common clinical manifestation of malaria in the area, making it highly probable that some cases of malaria are given this traditional diagnosis.

pãaŋ

pãaŋ~khãj pãaŋ~khĩi pãaŋ~pãaŋ kãam~mɛ́m kâj~mám kâj.

The patient gets fever, but feels cool and starts to shiver. The fever goes up and down for days. The patient may vomit, his skin turns pale, and he starts to confabulate. The abdomen becomes inflated and painful, typically on the left side due to the spleen that is enlarged (one informant believed due to the liver).[13] The fever then disappears for days or weeks, only to reappear if not successfully treated. The fever attacks can last for years. It may be fatal, and is mainly seen among children.

Cause: Generally unknown, but the fever is said to be caused by the enlargement of the spleen.

Treatment: One informant would use a hot medicine to "set fire to the spleen and thus make it shrink." Another informant had

---

13. Laotian traditional medicine uses the term *khipang* for "enlarged spleen" (Spire 1907:12, 19).

heard that modern doctors treated the disease with nám kinin (quinine water). Food prohibitions are part of the treatment.

Diagnosis: Malaria (see discussion under khãj málɛɛlia).

khãj sàníbàad lýa (chronic sàníbàad fever)

This disease was not familiar to all the respondents, but in some manuscripts it was listed as a specific kind of sàníbàad, and some short descriptions were also provided: one or two years of fever and heavy headache; two to three years of fever, easily angered, never get things finished, short of breath; fever on and off, completely exhausted.

One informant gave the following description: the patient gets a moderate fever that lasts for some hours, but then disappears. It comes back, however, usually the next day or at intervals of up to three days. The disease may last weeks, months, or even years. Usually the patient can walk and work with this fever, but if it continues for a long period, the patient loses his appetite and gets weak. It is called sàníbàad because of its long-term nature.

Diagnosis:* The verbalization of the concept as a chronic fever disease with a recurrent fever points to different disorders, but most cases are likely a result of malaria (see khãj málɛɛlia).

khãj málɛɛlia

This is a modern term for the disease malaria. The variable clinical manifestations of malaria have up to now probably been encountered in diseases and diagnostic entities such as khãj pàa (forest fever), khãj sàníbàad lýa (chronic recurrent fever), khãj wén wan (fever every second day), khãj háaŋ khãj hýa (repeated, sudden attacks of fever), khãj nǎaw sàn (cold and shivering fever), khãj cab sàn (shivering fever), and pãaŋ (fever with an inflated abdomen—now recognized as due to an enlargement of the spleen).

Other clinical manifestations of malaria, however, such as fever followed by stupor and/or convulsions (cerebral affection, especially in children), liver enlargement and jaundice (hepato-biliar affection), diarrhea and abdominal pains (a dysenteric picture)—and still there are others—make a considerable extension of the possible traditional counterparts (see khãj cág, khãj bàhúu swàaŋ, piˀ pàa, ŋúan tǎa lɯ̌aŋ, bàhòog lɯ̂ad).

ŋúan tǎa lɯ̌aŋ

ŋúan tǎa lɯ̌aŋ~ŋúan tǔa lɯ̌aŋ~khãj tǎa lɯ̌aŋ.

This disease is found in many manuals, but is not recognized by all the informants. Furthermore it is conceptualized in quite different ways by some respondents. According to one informant it is characterized by yellow discoloration of the skin and eyes, fever, weakness, and difficult urination. No one noticed any changes in the feces or the urine.

Treatment: The therapy is a combination of an oral remedy and magic incantations.

*Diagnosis**:* "Jaundice" of variable etiology.

khãj wad

khãj wad~khãj phid dɛ́ɛd phid nám—have a cold.

This disease is caused by changes in the weather or sudden changes in body temperature, as when bathing at the wrong time of the day. We have recorded no specific medicines for this ailment.

khãj wad jàj

khãj wad jàj (a big cold)—influenza and possibly also pneumonia.

khãj nóg naaŋ ˀɛ̀n

khãj nóg naaŋ ˀɛ̀n is an archaic term for a disease with high, constant fever and frequent spastic cramps, under which the body is stretched in an arch (opistotonus). One informant called this disease a kind of sàníbàad.

Diagnosis: Meningo-encephalitis.

tăa lyang (yellow eyes)

Yellow eyes and yellow skin are important symptoms of many traditional disease entities. As this symptom usually requires its own specific medicine, the diagnosis lôog tăa ly̌aŋ (yellow-eye disease) is used. However, the practitioners are fully aware that yellow skin (icterus) is a result of diseases of different etiology and the diagnosis lôog tăa ly̌aŋ is rarely made in actual medical practice but used as a supplementary diagnosis to diseases such as ŋúan tăa ly̌aŋ, piʔ pàa, saaŋ, and tɔ́ɔŋ kə̄əm.

tăa dɛɛŋ (red eyes)

The patient gets red and itching eyelids, followed by a smarting pain and secretion. The disease will easily spread to both eyes, and it is regarded as very contagious. Common among children.

Cause: Outside agents (maa càag nɔ̂ɔg).

Treatment: Magic and topical medicine.

*Diagnosis**:* Conjunctivitis and other inflammatory diseases of the eye, including trachoma.

Comments: One informant maintained that tăa dɛɛŋ might be a development of módtakhyd. The development of the disease then starts as above, but by and by the eye sockets turn red and finally black, and the patient becomes blind. This development of the disease is not regarded as contagious.

Other eye diseases: The common sty (hordeolum) is known as tɔ̌ɔn or tăa pĕn kũŋ. With the impact of Western medicine, new eye diseases are now recognized, and terms borrowed from Bangkok Thai are used for them: for example, glaucoma = tɔ̃ɔ hĭn, cataract = tɔ̃ɔ kacog.

laduu khăaw (white discharge)

This is the term for white discharge from the vagina (leukorrhea). It occurs especially in the postpartum weeks if women do not keep their food prohibitions, or if they are exposed to strange, strong smells in that period. The prevention is to eat only vegetables, keep inside the house, and avoid bad smells.

Treatment: Medicines, used in the bath and taken orally.

Comments: It may also be a development of khǎaŋ naj mód lûug or khǎaŋ naj puŋ ñîaw.

píd lɔ́ʔ

píd lɔ́ʔ~píd paj. This disease is above all circumscribed in etiological terms. It has its origin in a wound, such as from a rusty nail, a wooden splinter, bites from insects and animals. A poison enters the body through this lesion and, when it ascends, it results in a painful, stiff, and swollen limb, high fever and, in serious cases, unconsciousness, sometimes convulsions and, finally, death. The area around the wound turns greenish black. Sometimes several papules appear in the skin, thus the name tùm píd lɔ́ʔ is commonly applied.

Treatment: Incantations commonly used, but nowadays the herbalists usually send the patients to the hospital for injections.

Comments: Several informants equated this disease with the Bangkok term *bàadthǎjág* used for the disease tetanus, and some clinical features of tetanus are likely to be encountered in the traditional concept of píd lɔ́ʔ. However, the central part of the concept with a stiff, painful limb following a skin lesion on hands or feet, equates the condition with lymphangitis. The more serious course with unconsciousness and convulsions indicates the inclusion of toxemia and septicemia as a part of the concept, too.

Some informants maintained that if the disease culminated in convulsions, they would call this condition sàníbàad cág. (See also bàheŋ faj laammɔ̂ɔn.)

4.2.8. Skin diseases

4.2.8.1. Vocabulary related to skin diseases

Before the skin diseases are surveyed in detail, a presentation of the vocabulary used to describe the symptoms and signs in this group of diseases is given.

A. ***Skin lesions and efflorescences***

phɛ̆ɛ	Wound.
lŷad khɔ̄n	Extravasation of blood (ecchymosis, suggulations).
máan lŷad = cám lŷad	Dark patch in the skin, as after being hit.
máan dɛ̀ɛd = cám dɛ̀ɛd	Dark patch in the skin, as after being sunburned.
hɔɔj phɛ̆ɛ	Scar (general term).
pãw	Scar (following an eruption).
thə̀əg	Excoriation.
tùm	An isolated macule, papule, vesicle, pustule, or bulla. Vesicles and bullae are also referred to as tùm nám lɣ̌aŋ (with watery secretion), while pustules may be specified as tùm nɔ̆ɔŋ (with pus).
méd	Small red macule, papule, or tiny vesicle (smaller than tùm).
phỳn	A patch of primary efflorescences in a dense cluster; a plaque.
bə̃ə	Thick, keratotic plaque.
ked	Crust, scale.
dãan	Flat nodule or granuloma within the skin; sharply demarcated keratotic plaques (callus).
dàad	Thick white (hypochrome) plaque or macule; a patch (as of a rash). (See pĕn dàad, below.)

pǎan	Red, black, or yellow macule; birthmark.
fãa	Large, dark patch in the face (nevus, angioma).
pǎan dam pǎan dɛɛŋ	Freckles.
fǎj = fǎj dam fǎj dɛɛŋ	Slightly elevated black or red mole; senile wart.
tǎj	Small papule (itching).
fóg = dan	Tumid lymph node or gland beneath the skin.
mɛɛŋ ŋon	A flat mole.
hùud~hud	Wart (verruca). (Also used as a disease term; see hùud~khĩi hùud.)
mỹn	Wheal (urtica). (Also used as a disease term.)
kǎan	Dark macules appearing by themselves; purpura. (Also used as a disease term.)
fĩi	Abscess (painful tùm with pus). (Also used as a disease term.)
sǐw	Follicular papule, pimple in the face. (Also used as a disease term.)
sǎan	Tumor. (Also used as a disease term.)

B. *Quantitative and qualitative appearance of efflorescences*

One by one

–*Small units:* pěn méd pěn méd, pěn tîi pěn tîi, pěn cud pěn cud, pěn tɔ̀m pěn tɔ̀m (arch.), pěn tùm pěn tùm, pěn tùm pěn tǎa

–*Larger units:* pěn lûug, pěn nùaj, pěn kɔ̃ɔn, pěn kə̃əm

In patches, in groups: pěn ñùm pěn ñùm , pěn ñɔ̀m pěn ñɔ̀m
Eruptions, rashes: pěn phὲn, pěn phỳn, pěn dàad, pěn bə̃ə, pěn thỳm

Depressions: pěn khŭm pěn mɔ̃ɔŋ, pěn wέεm

C. *Discharge from the skin*

khĩi hãŋ kεε = kàag hãŋ kεε = khĩi haŋ kεε = khĩi hâag kεε	Dandruff.
khâab = thə̀əb	Skin peeling.
khĩi khaj	Desquamation.
khĩi khŭj	Refuse matter from vesicle (yellow crust).
ked	Squamous discharge, scale, crust.
hỳa	Sweat.
hỳa khaj kháaw	Big sweat pearls, which appear on the body of a dying person.

D. *Occurrence and progression of skin eruptions*

D.1. *To swell*

pɔɔŋ = buam	To swell (general) (as the cheek when having a quinsy or alveolar abscess; or scalds from boiling water).
pûud	To swell, expand (locally) (as tumors), to protrude (as eyes).
byn	Soft swelling around the edge or border (as swollen lips; or the concomitant swelling around the edge of a wound).

kâj	Tense swelling (like a flatulent corpse that has been in water for some days; or like an advanced expanded tumor in the abdominal area).

D.2. *To retract*

pɛ̂ɛb	Shrink, deflate (of swellings).
tɛb	Flatten out and disappear (of wounds).
wâab = wɛ̂ɛb	Disappear (of wounds).
ñúb	Diminish, subside (of vesicles).
lɔ̀ɔd	Diminish, subside (of carbuncles); miscarriage, spontaneous abortion.
hód	Shrink, contract.
hɛ̃ɛŋ	Dry up.
múd	Disappear.
hǎaj	Recover, be healed.

D.3. *To spread*

laam	Spread (on the body).
phɛ̂ɛ	Spread (in general).
cɔɔn	Spread, in the case of vesicles appearing close to the original ones.
sod = phod	Spread, in the case of vesicles appearing far from and independent of the original ones.

wyyn	Flare up, to get worse (as, for instance, vesicles that get worse with wrong diet).
tûan = tôon	Spread (of an epidemic).

D.4. *To rot and decompose*

phə́ˀ	Stained excoriations (e.g., tùm phə́ˀ, pàag phə́ˀ).
hŏm	Inflamed (e.g., tùm hŏm).
ˀagsèeb	Inflamed (e.g., phɛ̆ɛ ˀagsèeb).
phúaˀ	Decay, ooze.
nâw	Putrefy (general).
lwâan = lâan = pỳaj	Decompose and disintegrate, be in a state of putrefaction.

4.2.8.2. Groups of traditional skin diseases

There are four large groups of skin diseases primarily circumscribed on the morphological picture of the skin eruptions: the tùm group, the fĭi group, the săan group, and the bàheŋ group.

tùm group

A tùm has a head (hŭa), but no root (hâag), and is not painful (bàceb)—(papules, vesicles, pustules). The eruptions are isolated, scattered, and usually widespread and itching (khan). Typical diseases of this group are children's diseases such as measles (tùm had), German measles (tùm dɛɛŋ), and chicken pox (tùm săj). The conditions of smallpox (tùm sug), prickly heat (tùm hỳa), and other conditions of papular and vesicular skin eruptions also have their natural position here.

fĭi group

A fĭi has a head (at least in its initial stage), normally no root, but is painful. As a disease term it covers different pyodermal lesions such as furuncles (fĭi khĩi kàj), carbuncles (see fĭi hỳm hăj), and echtyma (see fĭi laˀàag, fĭi bɔ̀ɔ jìan).

săan group

A săan has both head and root, and is normally not painful. It may be hard or soft, movable or stationary. It appears as a tumor or large nodule of the skin or the underlying tissue, or it may be localized inside the body. Some of the săan are regarded as skin diseases, like lipomas (săan lûug nŭu), skin carcinomatosis (săan bua bug), and lymphadenoma (săan nám lŷaŋ), while there are others that have nothing to do with the skin. We have chosen to keep the săan diseases as one group, and avoided applying the localization criteria, which would have split the group up. All the săan diseases are thus treated together in section 4.2.6. Diseases with Swellings and Tumors as Prominent Signs.

bàheŋ group

Here the eruptions take the form of a mixture of phỳn and tùm affecting the "surface" of the skin only. The tùm eruptions are partly wet, but without pus, at least in the initial stage of the disease (vesicles and/or bullae). The lesions generally itch and may burn (ceb hɔ́ɔn hɔ́ɔn).

The bàheŋ group certainly includes a very wide variety of skin diseases of the cosmopolitan medical system. Skin diseases with a picture of erythema and vesiculobullous eruptions of both infectious and noninfectious origin are parts of the bàheŋ concept.

The diagnostic criteria for a delimitation of the four main groups of skin diseases are summarized in table 3, below.

A fifth group, made up of *cɔ̃ɔ*, *khĩi tûud, khĩi kɔɔ*, and *khúdtálâad* also constitutes a natural entity due to the morphology of the lesions and the serious course. The lesions are described as thick, demarcated plaques and nodules (granulomas) (pĕn dãn pĕn bə̃ə), and it is assumed that leprosy and yaws make up central parts of these concepts.

The subtypes of *lídsaduaŋ*, which affect the skin, are also primarily circumscribed by morphological characteristics: the eruptions take the form of thickened, indurated lesions or plaques, and "eat the bottom of the skin."

In contrast, the diseases *hŷan* and *hɔ̃ɔ* show a broad variation of eruptions, while they have a common localization; namely, on

TABLE 3

DIAGNOSTIC CRITERIA OF tùm, fĭi, sǎan, AND bàheŋ DISEASES

Disease	Head (hǔa)	Root (hâag)	Pain (ceb)	Eruptions
tùm	+	÷	÷	papules, vesicles, pustules
fĭi	+ (÷)	÷	+	papules, pustules
sǎan	+	+	÷ (+)	tumors, nodules
bàheŋ	÷	÷	(+)	papules, vesicles, bullae, partly in confluent, superficial patches

the distal parts of the limbs. In this group the localization is given heavier weight than the morphological picture. hýan and hɔ̌ɔ border on both eczematous and mycotic conditions with, however, infective eczemas and trichophytosis of forearms, hands, lower legs, and feet, having the greatest importance in the concepts.

4.2.8.3. Cosmopolitan versus traditional skin diseases

In table 4 the correspondence of cosmopolitan and traditional diagnoses in cases of acne, psoriasis, eczemas, and dermatophytoses are summarized.

In cosmopolitan medicine the condition of *acne vulgaris* has a broad content and includes inflammatory processes of the sebaceous glands and hair follicles in general. At least five corresponding traditional entities have been recorded, each having a restricted meaning both to the morphological picture and to location. The situation is similar for *psoriasis,* for which the traditional diagnoses are primarily based on the size, color, and degree of dissemination of the eruptions, while in cosmopolitan medicine the diagnosis is based on morphological characteristics of the skin lesions.

In the *allergic dermatitis* group, the two cases of hýan were both localized to the hand, taking the form of erythema with fissurating, scaling skin, although one case showed somewhat swollen indurated patches justifying the use of the term *lídsaduaŋ*. In both cases dirty water was given as the etiological agent. The two cases

TABLE 4

DIAGNOSTIC CONSIDERATIONS OF ACNE, PSORIASIS, ECZEMAS, AND DERMATOPHYTOSES
(The number of observed cases is given in parenthesis)

Acne vulgaris	sǐw (1) sǐw cáaŋ (1) lídsaduaŋ lŷad (1) khǎaŋ lídsaduaŋ (1) sǎan lídsaduaŋ (1)
Psoriasis vulgaris	phadoŋ lŷad (1) lídsaduaŋ khǎaŋ lŷad (2) lídsaduaŋ dàad (1)
Eczemas	
Allergic dermatitis	
Dermatitis medicamentosa	bàheŋ khan (1)
Contact eczema	bàheŋ mǎa ñŷaŋ (1) bàheŋ lŷad (1) hýan nám (1) hýan lídsaduaŋ (1) lídsaduaŋ fáa máan (1)
Unspecified	bàheŋ mǎa ñŷaŋ (2) khǎaŋ khan (1) lídsaduaŋ khan (1)
Seborrheic eczema	lídsaduaŋ khan (4) lídsaduaŋ tēn (1)
Nummular eczema	bàheŋ tēn (1) lídsaduaŋ tēn (1)
Asteatotic eczema	hýan nám (1)
Infective (microbial) eczema	hýan nám (3)
Tropical eczema	hýan cáaŋ (1) phaj nám (1)
Lichen simplex (circumscribed neurodermatitis)	lídsaduaŋ khan (2) lídsaduaŋ dàad (1) hýan nám (1)
Infantile eczema (atopic dermatitis)	khǎaŋ nám nom (1) khǎaŋ lŷad (1)
Dermatophytoses	
Tinea capitis (ringworm of the head)	lídsaduaŋ nám lǐaŋ (1)

TABLE 4 (*continued*)

DIAGNOSTIC CONSIDERATIONS OF ACNE, PSORIASIS, ECZEMAS, AND DERMATOPHYTOSES
(The number of observed cases is given in parenthesis)

Tinea corporis (ringworm of the trunk and limbs)	hýan nám (1), khĩi khàag (1)
Tinea cruris (ringworm of intertriginous areas)	khĩi khàag (1)
Tinea manuum (ringworm of the hands)	mõo lŷad (1), hɔ̃ɔ faj (1)
Tinea pedis (ringworm of the feet)	mõo lŷad (1), hýan nám (1)
Tinea (pityriasis) versicolor	khǎaŋ lŷad (khĩi sĩan) (1)
Cutaneous candidiasis (intertrigo)	hýan wíd (1), bàheŋ lŷad (1) khǎaŋ lŷad (1)

of lídsaduaŋ both demonstrated chronic eczematous lesions with thickened, somewhat lichenified skin. In one case the eruptions were on the neck (lichenified plaques due to allergy to a metallic chain—lídsaduaŋ fáa máan), in the other on the arms and neck. Although the lesions should qualify for hýan as well, the localization does not, thus making lídsaduaŋ the appropriate term. The more widespread eruptions were recognized either as bàheŋ or khǎaŋ. The case of bàheŋ had isolated, itching papulovesicular eruptions, being subdivided into bàheŋ khan (itching bàheŋ) and bàheŋ mǎa ñÿaŋ (bàheŋ with itching like that produced by touching the hairs of the plant mǎa ñÿaŋ [Mucuna pruriens DC-Fabaceae]). khǎaŋ was reserved for a case of disseminated papules of the skin.

For *seborrheic eczema,* the diagnosis lídsaduaŋ khan was used in four cases, all representing typical erythematous, scaling patches with itching seborrhea. In one case in which the lesions were more scattered, the diagnosis lídsaduaŋ tẽn (dancing lídsaduaŋ—eruptions) was given.

The typical coin-shaped, secreting lesions of *nummular eczema* had their counterparts in bàheŋ tẽn and lídsaduaŋ tẽn, the attribute tẽn stressing the typical "dancing" behavior of the lesions appearing in one place and then gradually healing, only to reappear in another place. *Asteatotic eczema, infective eczema, and tropical eczema* were diagnosed as hŷan or phaj, as they all occurred on the legs and wrists. The clinical picture of tropical eczema with thick, secreting granulomatous or verrucose plaques was kept distinct, being recorded as hŷan cáaŋ or phaj nám.

The *lichen simplex* group has been identified in three traditional diagnoses, each emphasizing different morphological or distributional characteristics. In two cases the itching aspect of the lesions was stressed (lídsaduaŋ khan), in one case the well-circumscribed hypochrome plaques (lídsaduaŋ dàad), and in one case the predominating localization on the legs (hŷan nám).

Infantile eczema with eruptions, also affecting the face, was placed in the khǎaŋ group: khǎaŋ nám nom was used for an eight-month-old boy where the cause of the disease was assumed to come from the mother's milk, and khǎaŋ lŷad in a six-year-old girl, for which the diagnostician emphasized the blood (lŷad) as the probable causative agent.

Among the *dermatophytoses,* one case of *tinea capitis* with oozing and itching circular lesions of the scalp was given the diagnosis lídsaduaŋ nám lỹaŋ owing to the deep lesions (lídsaduaŋ) with secretion (nám lỹaŋ). A superficial, itching lesion without secretion would have justified the diagnosis khĩi khòog.

Tinea corporis was diagnosed as khĩi khàag in a case with two single, isolated mycotic plaques of the trunk, while hŷan nám was applied to a case of widespread gyrate and coalescent plaques all over the body. According to the latter informant the condition represented a severe, progressed stage of hŷan nám caused by dirty water.

Tinea cruris with a picture of some isolated itching and tineiform lesions of the groin also qualified for the diagnosis khĩi khàag.

Two patients with two clinical varieties of *tinea manuum* were recorded as quite different skin diseases. mõo lŷad was recorded in a case of thick, scaling plaques with circinate borders of small vesicles and pustules on both palms, whereas hɔ̌ɔ faj was reserved for a case with a prevailing intertriginous form with redness, scaling, and fissures of the palms and interdigital spaces.

Tinea pedis was observed in two cases; one case with the typical picture of an acute pustular form—with a single patch on one of the foot-soles—was given the diagnosis mõo lŷad, whereas hŷan nám was diagnosed in a case of red, itching, and somewhat vesiculating patches in between the toes.

An unambiguous picture of *tinea versicolor* was tentatively given the diagnosis khǎaŋ lŷad by the diagnostician, whereas the patient maintained that it was undoubtedly khĭi sĭan.

Three cases considered to be *candidal intertrigo* were given different diagnostic designations mainly owing to different localization. hýan wíd was used in a case of dry, red, itching patches of the skin in the groin; khǎaŋ lŷad for similar lesions localized to the axillas; and bàheŋ lŷad was recorded in a female with red, itchy, scaling patches of both the axillas and the groin. The latter condition was attributed to the menstrual blood.

Comments

As evident from our studies, the main diagnostic criteria used in the circumscription of skin diseases by the practitioners are the *morphological picture* of the lesions and the *localization of the eruptions,* that is, the same criteria that are the basis for disease recognition in Western dermatology. In traditional Northern Thai medicine, the bàheŋ group is defined mainly on the basis of the morphological picture of the eruptions, while in hɔ̌ɔ and hýan the localization is regarded as the most important criterion. Such parallel situations are also found in cosmopolitan medicine where, for example, the morphological picture of the lesions is decisive in the eczema group (also embracing some types of bàheŋ), while the dermatophytoses (including hɔ̌ɔ and hýan) are defined mainly by localization.

4.2.8.4. Traditional diseases primarily affecting the skin

tùm dɛɛŋ

tùm dɛɛŋ~ˀɔ̀ɔg dɛɛŋ (red tùm).

This is a common, well-known disease. The child gets tùm (i.e., macules, papules, and vesicles) all over the body, sometimes also in the mouth, accompanied by a slight fever. The child recovers within three to five days. It is not serious.

Treatment: Oral medicine (of the "expelling" type (jaa thìib)). See section 5.1. Omnipotent Remedies.

Diagnosis: German measles (rubeola).

tùm sug

tùm sug~ʔɔ̀ɔg sug~tùm lŭaŋ~khāw māj ked lɛ̂ɛd~fĭi sug~fĭi dàad~fĭi pùag.

The patient gets fever and pustules that are black on the top. The pustules burst open and discharge the pus. Dark crusts appear, which leave scars when they heal. The disease attacks all age groups, and previously quite a few died. Nowadays not seen, because of vaccination. It is considered a very contagious and a rather dangerous disease.

Cause: The sug-spirit.

Treatment: Magic and medicine.[14]

Diagnosis: Smallpox (variola).

Comments: When there were cases of tùm sug in a village, the dogs would bark at night because they could see the sug-spirit. The disease is called fĭi dàad or khâj thɔɔráphíd in Bangkok Thai. Smallpox—which was previously very common—is called mak souk in Laotian (Sassady 1962:41, citing Macey 1910), or kok mak-souk (Spire 1907:24). Spire gives an interesting example of how the Meos treated this disease. (See also tùm líi.)

tùm săj

tùm săj~ʔɔ̀ɔg săj (transparent tùm).

A children's disease in which the patient gets scattered vesicles that spread over the body. The vesicles dry up leaving crusts that eventually fall off. Not serious.

14. One informant said that it is common to make an offering to the spirits as a part of the treatment of tùm sug, tùm săj, tùm had, and tùm dɛɛŋ and that salĭi-muun medicine is commonly used.

Treatment: Oral medicine of the "expelling" type (jaa thìib).

Diagnosis: Chicken pox (varicella).

Comments: The similarity to tùm sug was pointed out by some practitioners, but eruptions of tùm sug have black heads and are more serious.

tùm hỳa (sweat-tùm)

The patient gets tùm (macules and papules predominating) on the trunk and arms.

Cause: Appears when sweating.

Treatment: None. It disappears by itself after two or three days.

Diagnosis: Prickly heat.

tùm had

tùm had~ˀɔ̀ɔg had.

A skin disease among children, rare among adults. The child gets fever and coughs for a while, then macules and papules appear all over the body. The child loses appetite, but usually recovers after some days, although it may be fatal in a few cases.

Treatment: Decoction of leaves from the had-tree for the patient to bathe in to relieve the itching.[15]

Diagnosis:* Measles (morbilli). One patient with papular urticaria due to insect bites (strophulus) was also given this diagnosis.

Comments: Also called "the younger brother of tùm dɛɛŋ."

tùm píd

tùm píd (poisonous vesicles)~bàheŋ tùm píd~phaj píd (poisonous phaj). Other terms that are part of the concept: phaj cáaŋ, phaj hɛ̂ɛd, phaj mɔ̌j, phaj ŋua, phaj khwaaj.

---

15. had—two species of the genus *Celtis* (Ulmaceae) have been collected under this name—*C. tetrandra* Roxb. and *C. cf. timorensis* Spanoghe (see Appendix).

tùm píd is a general term for certain types of vesicles appearing after the patient has eaten the meat from (or just touched) the corpses of diseased or plague-ridden animals. The flesh of these animals has a phaj-agent that enters the body giving rise to a poison (píd) responsible for the following symptoms: After two or three days the patient gets fever and begins to shiver, his sight becomes dim, his hearing dull, and he may lose his voice. Then one or more vesicles (the size of maize kernels) appear, shaped like volcanoes, the bases of which are white and the hollow parts black. They may be localized anywhere on the body, but normally they are found on the hands, arms, chest, or back. They are neither painful nor itching, but rather dangerous. When the vesicles are mature, the tops shoot up and a poisonous wind (lom píd) ascends to the chest giving a pressing pain around the heart. There are difficulties in breathing, the heart gets weak, and unconsciousness and death may follow. The stools turn black and the urine becomes hot. Previously common, now rare.

Treatment: Magic (blowing on the head) and a poison-expelling medicine (jaa thàaj píd) taken orally. None of our informants had ever treated this disease. All of them stressed the importance of food prohibitions, alcohol being regarded as particularly dangerous. Injections must be avoided at all costs, as they are the shortest way to death!

Comments: One informant operated with four subtypes of tùm píd: a white one, a creamy yellow one, a red one, and a black one, the two latter being particularly dangerous. Some informants asserted that tùm píd was not always dangerous and could disappear by itself, unless the patient smelled something bad or ate unwholesome food (kǐn khɔ̌ɔŋ salɛ̌ɛŋ), which would cause the poisonous wind to ascend, resulting in unconsciousness and death.

Some informants regarded tùm líi as a kind of tùm píd. One informant said that if a tùm píd occurred in the face it should be termed sǐw cáaŋ.

Diagnosis: The explication of the disease varies, but the condition of septicemia is probably responsible for the more serious clinical pictures; namely, the primary skin lesions and/or secondary skin manifestations that often accompany this disease.

tùm líi

tùm líi (hidden cyst)~kǎan tùm líi~fǐi kǎan.

This disease is verbalized as a tùm with blood inside appearing somewhere on the body, usually on the fingers or just around the anus; in the latter case often preceded by diarrhea and headache. One informant distinguished between a red, harmless variety and a black, dangerous variety.

Cause: Unknown. A spirit was suggested as a possible causative agent.

Treatment: Puncture and squeeze the blood out. Magic may also be required.

*Diagnosis**:* Hemorrhagic cyst.

Comments: kǎan tùm líi is usually not dangerous, but according to one informant it may be accompanied by fever and then cause headache, pains in the loins, and even unconsciousness due to a poisonous wind that arises. The condition is then recognized as khǎj tùm líi. One informant equated khǎj tùm líi with phǐi dàad and khǎj thɔɔláphíd, which are both translated as "smallpox" in modern Bangkok Thai. (See tùm sug.)

fǐi

fǐi is a group of diseases, most of which are suppurative skin diseases with lesions like carbuncles, furuncles, and so forth. They are characterized by having a head (hǔa) with pus (nɔ̌ɔŋ), being painful and causing a "poison" (píd) to arise. Food prohibitions are part of the treatment. Several kinds of fǐi do not fit these general characteristics; for example, fǐi bɔ̀ɔ jìan and fǐi laʔàag. Some types of fǐi may also be alternatively classified; for example, fǐi mûaŋ is here arranged as a subtype of módtakhyd, whereas fǐi sǎan has been classified as a separate entity. fǐi kǎan is another name for tùm líi. Some of the informants subdivide the fǐi into those occurring on the left side of the body (female fǐi) and those occurring on the right (male fǐi). (See section 3.8.7. Left-right and female-male.)

The data we collected on the fǐi diseases are rather inconsistent. None of the informants knew all the subtypes mentioned below, they disagreed as to what names where identical, and often on what the content of the concepts were. The reason is partly that the herbalists differ in degree of splitting—some operate with three kinds of fĭi, others with ten—but mainly because there is confusion and overlapping with other major groups of diseases, especially tùm and săan. We have the impression that the herbalists chose one of these groups as the major one at the expense of the other groups, that is, some operate with many kinds of fĭi, but relatively fewer kinds of tùm and săan, while others use săan as a lump group, and therefore operate with fewer tùm and fĭi. The most common recorded fĭi are:

> *fĭi hŭa khwăm* (head-down fĭi). Small heads (hŭa) appear with red borders and white centers. When opening they will discharge greyish-white pus. The fĭi will then take the form of a volcano with a depressed center, because the head now turns inward. It becomes painful and is often accompanied by fever. May be localized anywhere on the body except the face. Dietary restrictions are a necessary part of the treatment. If one eats wrong food, it may result in death, according to the manuscripts, although the informant had never seen this actually happen.[16]
> *Diagnosis*:* Furunculosis, pyodermia.

> *fĭi khɔɔ sɔ̂ɔj*~fĭi sɔ̂ɔj~fĭi săan khɔɔ sɔ̂ɔj (necklace fĭi) appears first as small, hard, and swollen tùm in strings on the neck—usually on one side only. The tùm contain some pus, and result in a stinging pain and slight itching. They have no root or head, as a fĭi normally should have, but the informant still classified it as a fĭi owing to the pain and itching symptoms. It can take two to three years to disappear. It is not as uncomfortable or serious as a bàheŋ.
> *Cause:* Perhaps from the blood.

16. The Laotian term *fi houa kouam* is translated as "abscess of the liver" by Sassady (1962:74).

fĭi laʔàag~fĭi maʔàag~fĭi wɔ̂ŋ laʔàag. A round, itching, red or brownish spot (without a head [hŭa]) appears on the skin, gradually growing bigger and eating its way through the flesh until it finally may reach the bone (which is not attacked), resulting in a hole in the flesh. The edges swell and become red and hard. The wound gives off a little secretion or pus. It is painful and is accompanied by fever. Usually only one lesion. It may occur anywhere, but is normally seen below the elbows and on the legs.

Cause: Unknown. Appears by itself, not from outside (of the body).

Treatment: Topical medicine. Difficult to cure.

Comments: One informant insisted that this is not a fĭi as it has no head or root, but is rather a kind of tùm.

Diagnosis:* Echtyma.

fĭi hy̆m hăj~fĭi thy̆m hăj~fĭi hŭa bua~fĭi fag bua~fĭi bua~fĭi khya (lotus-head fĭi [i.e., fruit] or fĭi bunch). First a warm, pale circle appears on the skin. After two or three days it turns red and painful. A big fĭi shoots up with several small yellow heads that discharge pus. It appears as a cluster of about ten confluent fĭi. It is accompanied by a slight fever and headache, and surrounding lymph nodes may swell. There is only one, usually occurring on the buttocks and around the waist and the back (soft places). After some days (max. 30 days) the fĭi bursts and discharges pus and blood leaving behind a scar. Usually not dangerous.

Cause: Unknown.

Treatment: Pull the head out with a thread, or squeeze it out.

Comments: One informant regarded fĭi hy̆m hăj as synonymous with fĭi cĭm cîi.

Diagnosis:* Carbuncles.

fĭi bɔ̀ɔ jìan~bɔ̀ɔ jìan~fĭi bɔ̀ɔj jìan~fĭi bùag jìan (eel-well fĭi) starts as a tùm with a head containing secretion. Then it eats its way through the skin and flesh to the bone, continually giving off secretion, resulting in a big, deep hole—as wide as a finger—with a swollen, sharp border. There is usually only one at a time. There is no (or hardly any) pain. It may appear anywhere on the body.

Cause: The following etiological agents were recorded: (a) from the "sap of eels" (jaaŋ pǎa lǎj); (b) from a thin and hardly visible insect (with an eel-like shape); and (c) unknown, but from outside (of the body).

Treatment: It is regarded as difficult or impossible to cure, but some topical medicines are available. One informant treated the diseases fǐi hỹm hǎj, fǐi la?àag, fǐi dàad, and fǐi bɔ̀ɔ jìan with the same topical medicine.

Diagnosis: Echtyma. (Cutaneous Leischmaniasis?)

Comments: The description of fǐi bɔ̀ɔ jìan is very similar to that of fǐi la?àag. One informant lumped these two concepts together, whereas other informants kept them apart.

fǐi khĩi kàj~fǐi kõn kàj~fǐi khĩi cîi~fǐi cǐm cîi~fǐi hǔa ŋǎaj (chicken shit fǐi, chicken ass fǐi, head-up fǐi). The eruption starts as a head with a broad, flat, hard red base. When this fǐi is mature, there is a broad red zone with a small head containing pus in the center. It is painful and itches. It finally bursts giving off pus and blood. It smells like chicken feces (as the name indicates). One to several eruptions appear anywhere on the body, most often on the buttocks, knees, stomach, and waist. It is not serious. It may develop into tùm píd if one eats the wrong food.

Cause: Unknown.

Treatment: The head can be squeezed out. A topical medicine can be applied (see Notes, under "Treatment of fǐi—general aspects," below).

Diagnosis: Furuncle, abscess.

fǐi dàad~fǐi sug~fǐi pùag (see tùm sug).

Treatment of fǐi—general aspects

The common kinds of fǐi do not need therapy, but should be left to mature by themselves. After they have opened and discharged the pus, they will heal by themselves. There are medicines applied topically to stop them from growing big. If the fĭi grows big and becomes painful, it may cause a poison (píd) and a wind (lom) to arise in the body. It is then considered serious, and needs treatment, which consists of both magic and topically applied warm medicine; for example, the root of Plumbago indica (píd piw dɛɛŋ) ground in water and mixed with alcohol may be used to treat fĭi mûaŋ and fĭi khĭi kàj, and the sap of Streblus asper (khɔ̀ɔj) is used against fĭi hŷm hăj and fĭi khĭi kàj. Lime is smeared on in some cases.

Notes: We have also recorded some descriptive fĭi names: fĭi lŭaŋ (big fĭi); fĭi dam (black fĭi); fóg fĭi (swollen fĭi) occurring in the groin and in the armpits, probably representative of lymphadenitis.

Manuscripts: fĭi is represented in all the manuscripts, with altogether some sixty prescriptions. There is no elaboration following the names of the various fĭi types. The names themselves are thus our only source of information.

a. Color-descriptive:

–fĭi him khăaw/dam (white/black-rimmed fĭi)

–fĭi hŭa khăaw/dam (white/black-headed fĭi)

–fĭi pàag dɛɛŋ (red-mouthed fĭi)

–fĭi khya khăaw/dam (bunches of white/black fĭi)

–fĭi khăaw (white fĭi)

–fĭi cám lom phĭi ñíaʔ (dark fĭi with wind caused by spirits)

b. Other visual impressions:

–fĭi hŭa khûab~fĭi hŭa khwăm (fĭi with the head turned inward)

–fĭi pŷaj nâw (rotten fĭi)

–fĭi sug paj taŋ khiŋ (mature fĭi all over the body) (see tùm sug)

–fĭi fóg (swollen fĭi)

c. Places of occurrence:

–fĭi naj tɔ́ɔŋ~fĭi săan naj tɔ́ɔŋ (fĭi in the stomach) very common; eight prescriptions (see fĭi săan)

–fĭi ŋúan săan naj tɔ́ɔŋ~fĭi hâa ŋúan

–fĭi naj sãj~fĭi lăam sãj (fĭi in the intestines) = fĭi maleŋ lom; four prescriptions

–fĭi jaŋ nom (fĭi in the breast) = maleŋ nom ñuaŋ

–fĭi jaŋ khɔɔ (fĭi on the throat)

–fĭi naj kaaŋ (fĭi in the jaws) = maleŋ taŋ

–fĭi naj hŭu (fĭi in the ear)

–fĭi lŭaŋ tîi lăŋ/tɔ́ɔŋ (big fĭi on stomach or back)

–fĭi lŭaŋ tîi ʔɛɛw loŋ tĭin (big fĭi from waist downward)

–fĭi lŭaŋ tîi pɔ̃ɔŋ khêŋ pɔ̃ɔŋ khăa (big fĭi on the legs)

d. Other:

–fĭi bua tŭa mia /tŭa pûu (male/female lotus fĭi)

–fĭi khanthámaalaa

e. Compound names with other disease terms: fĭi maleŋkhúd (occurs on throat and between the eyebrows), fĭi săan, fĭi lammánâad, fĭi khăaŋ cáaŋ, fĭi kăan, fĭi khăaŋ lom púʔ

f. fĭi diseases not mentioned in the manuscripts: fĭi hỹm hăj, fĭi khĩi kàj, fĭi khĩi cîi, fĭi khɔɔ sɔ̂ɔj, fĭi bɔ̀ɔ jìan, fĭi laʔàag, fĭi mûaŋ, fĭi pùag.

In some prescriptions the functional properties of the medicines are given as:

–hãam píd fĭi (stop [literally, forbid] the poison of the fĭi)

–dab píd fĭi (extinguish the poison of the fĭi)

–cũu píd fĭi (press [on] medicine [to stop] the poison of the fĭi)

–thìib píd fĭi (drive out the poison of the fĭi)

–kad fĭi (bite the fĭi)

–sáʔ hŭa fĭi (cleanse the head of the fĭi)

–hɔ̀ɔ hŭa fĭi (envelop the head of the fĭi)

bàheŋ

There is a lot of confusion concerning the concept of bàheŋ, partly because of the lack of standardization of terminology and partly because the bàheŋ concept seems to have been in a continual state of flux during the last few decades.

When talking about bàheŋ the traditional doctors describe certain ideal types of this disease, which probably do exist, but we have not had the opportunity to see examples (see group A). In clinical situations, however, diseases that are not part of these ideal types are still referred to as bàheŋ (group B).[17] Furthermore, in the manuscripts the bàheŋ concept is used in a very general sense, and many of the various bàheŋ types mentioned there are now classified under the headings fĭi, săan, and lídsaduaŋ. To make the confusion complete the Bangkok-Thai cognate of this word—*máreŋ*—has been adopted by modern medicine for the cosmopolitan disease entity cancer. This new concept is well known in Northern Thailand, and is gradually eroding the traditional concept of bàheŋ, and also that of săan.[18] Still we feel it is possible to summarize the general characteristics of the traditional bàheŋ diseases as follows: a group of skin diseases with itching, superficial, and wet eruptions (vesicles and bullae) localized anywhere on the body.[19] The unspecific causa-

17. As only one of our informants was confronted with many different cases of skin diseases, we cannot exclude the possibility that his use of the bàheŋ concept in these situations is idiosyncratic.

18. When an herbalist says he can cure bàheŋ, it has been misunderstood to mean that he can cure cancer. We would therefore emphasize that the remedies in common use against bàheŋ in Northern Thailand have no actual reputation as remedies to treat cancer.

19. P. Macey recorded a disease in Laos called pha nhat khi ma hèng, which he equates with shingles—*zona* in French. (Sassady 1962:41, citing Macey 1910:87).

tive agent (mɛ̂ɛ—"mother") makes the blood poisonous (lŷad pěn píd) and causes severe itching. bàheŋ is considered to be a hot disease, and it requires magical treatment together with food prohibitions. Oral medicines, acting as purgatives, may also be given to "expel the poison" (jaa thàaj píd), together with a medicine to "kill the mother" (jaa khãa mɛ̂ɛ), which is applied topically as an antipruritic remedy.

A. *Theoretical or ideal types of bàheŋ.*

A-1. *bàheŋ types familiar to all practitioners.*

A-1.1. *bàheŋ fáa máan*~bàheŋ faj mãj (dark sky bàheŋ, burning bàheŋ).

Rather big patches (the size of a hand) composed of small papules in dense clusters appear on the skin, normally on the upper trunk, but also on the legs and arms. These patches (phŷn) are at first reddish, later on turning dark brown or blackish. The skin lesions are painful and burning, itch slightly, and are accompanied by fever and weakness. A poison (píd) has entered the patient's body resulting in a wind (lom) that causes a pressing pain in the lower chest and back, making it difficult to breathe. Fatal within two to four weeks if not treated.

Cause: The blood has turned poisonous (lŷad pěn píd) for unknown reasons. According to one informant it may appear as a result of too long exposure to the sun. Most informants maintain the cause as external.

Treatment: In addition to magic and jaa thàaj píd, a topical cold medicine is applied on the burning lesions.

Comments: Although everyone agrees that the disease is fatal if not treated ("the manuals say so"), nobody has actually seen anybody die from it. On the contrary, some say they have been able to cure many cases with their powerful incantations. When incantations are blown on, the dark patches stop spreading and gradually turn paler and disappear after some two weeks of treatment. Some informants equate bàheŋ fáa máan with bàheŋ ʔɔ̃ɔm, but usually the latter is kept apart on the basis of its peculiar way of spreading and its dreaded course.

A-1.2. ***bàheŋ khàj pǎa*** (fish egg bàheŋ).

Groups of five to ten tùm with nám lŷaŋ (vesicles) resembling fish eggs appear and spread on the upper trunk, buttocks, arms, and legs, that is, the "soft parts" (but not the mouth, lips, tongue, nose, or fingers). The eruptions vesiculate or just dry up without opening, and heal with formation of crusts. The lesions are somewhat itchy and burning, and a slight fever may appear. It is seen in all ages, but most often among children from five to fifteen years of age. It is not contagious and a person may get it several times. The informants maintained that the disease might be serious and even fatal if it spread all over the body, but as the treatment is effective, no one has seen such a course.

Cause: Unknown. One informant ventured the possibility of getting it after eating the fruit sõm bàfyaŋ (Averrhoa carambola—Oxalidaceae). The blood turns poisonous and a lom lŷad appears, which is responsible for the symptoms.

Treatment: The therapy is magical (incantations and lustral water). In addition, a jaa thàaj píd (poison-expelling medicine) is given.

A-1.3. ***bàheŋ tẽn*** (dancing bàheŋ).

A few isolated eruptions, usually not more than two or three, appear on some part of the body. At first they are red (papules), then they turn paler and wet (vesicles), and finally burst, giving off secretion. The size is from that of maize kernels to one centimeter in diameter. After a week the skin is healed, but new eruptions appear on another part of the body. The lesions itch, and burn slightly, and the patient usually scratches until crusts are formed. It is not regarded as serious.

Cause: The blood has turned "poisonous" for unknown reasons.

Treatment: Magic and jaa thàaj píd (poison-expelling medicine).

Comments: Not all informants recognized bàheŋ tẽn as a specific disease, but regarded it as a descriptive term for any kind of bàheŋ "dancing" on the skin, a general characteristic for several of the bàheŋ types; for example, bàheŋ khàj pǎa and bàheŋ jɔɔm tĩin mǎa.

A-1.4. *bàheŋ ʔɔ̄ɔm* (encirling bàheŋ).

On the lower part of the abdomen and the back, small, burning eruptions arise in well-circumscribed patches, forming a continuous stripe and gradually spreading around the circumference of the abdominal and lumbal region. The patient gets fever. When the circle is complete—which will take about thirty days—the patient dies in a matter of hours, crying out at the moment of death. It is regarded as extremely serious, but as it is very rare, none of the informants had ever seen it.

Cause: The blood has turned "poisonous" for unknown reasons.

Treatment: Magic and jaa thàaj píd.

Comments on familiar bàheŋ types (A-1): During our investigation we met fourteen patients who were given the diagnosis bàheŋ, of whom only one was diagnosed as having one of the four main types of bàheŋ, that is, bàheŋ tẽn, a condition that turned out to be a nummular eczema. Theoretical knowledge of the main types of bàheŋ thus seems to be of little help in medical practice.

Diagnosis: Concluding remarks about the possible conditions in Western dermatology that underlie the traditional diseases bàheŋ fáa máan, bàheŋ khàj pǎa, bàheŋ tẽn, and bàheŋ ʔɔ̄ɔm must be postponed until some controlled observations and casuistics are available. It is assumed, however, that several groups of skin diseases such as allergic dermatitis, eczemas, different types of vesiculobullous and herpetiform eruptions are partly covered by these indigenous disease entities. bàheŋ khàj pǎa, centered around the characteristic of vesicles more or less in dense clusters, points to diseases such as herpes simplex, herpes zoster, and dermatitis herpetiformis as possible Western counterparts. bàheŋ tẽn, which is shown to cover at least a clinical manifestation of nummular eczema, might fit some pictures of impetigo (scrumpox) as well.

A-2. *Some bàheŋ entities known only to some of the practitioners.*

A-2.1. *bàheŋ jɔɔm tǐin mǎa* (dog footprint bàheŋ).

The patient gets groups of three or four tùm, which look like the footprint of a dog, and vesiculate and dry up after a while. They may spread to all parts of the body and may be accompanied by fever. Usually, this disease clears up by itself, but severe cases need treatment. Seen in all ages.

Cause: It comes from lom lŷad, due to poisonous blood.

Treatment: Magic.

A-2.2. *bàheŋ faj laam mɔ̂n.*

This concept was clearly expressed by one informant: The patient gets a tùm on the foot or hand. It develops by itself. Then long red stripes develop beneath the skin ascending to the knee or shoulder, respectively. The patient gets terrible pain, and the affected limb gets stiff. The patient gets hard, painful nodules called bàdan hɛ́ɛ in the groin or armpits. He gets warm, and a fever arises. If it progresses, the patient may lose consciousness and die.

Cause: From lom lŷad (blood-wind), due to poisonous blood.

Treatment: Magic.

Diagnosis:* The clinical picture equates with the Western medical entity truncular lymphangitis, and has the appearance of a regional lymphadenitis (bàdan hɛ́ɛ). The severe course of this type of infection, with the possibility of spreading to the blood bringing on sepsis and death, is also conceptualized by the informant.

A-2.3. *bàheŋ nom ñuaŋ* (hanging breast bàheŋ).

This disease is well circumscribed by its localization on the nipples of the breasts of women during the suckling period. The woman gets tùm or phŷn around the nipple, usually on one breast only, and the breast becomes painful and red, sometimes giving off pus.

Diagnosis:* This disease corresponds to the Western entity mastitis with or without an intramammary abscess.

The condition of an intramammary abscess was kept apart as a specific disease called fĭi jaŋ nom by another informant. This informant distinguished among the diseases bàheŋ nom ñuaŋ, fĭi jaŋ nom, and săan jaŋ nom, a division that has its cosmopolitan medical counterpart in mastitis, intramammary abscess (phlegmone), and intramammary tumor, respectively. A third respondent put all these conditions into the single concept of săan nom luan.

B. ***The pedestrian types of bàheŋ used in clinical situations by one of our informants, illustrated by some selected casuistics.***

B-1. ***bàheŋ khan*** (itching bàheŋ).

A twenty-three-year-old woman had for seven days suffered from an itching exanthema of the trunk and limbs. Inspection revealed partly confluent papules and macules with excoriations and scaling. She had during the previous few weeks been taking some unidentified tablets bought at the local pharmacy to make her gain weight. The condition, interpreted as a manifestation of an allergy (dermatitis medicamentosa), was maintained as bàheŋ khan on the basis of its severe itching and superficial, scattered eruptions not making the skin thick (indurated). Another patient given this diagnosis had no primary eruptions at all, only excoriations and scars due to itching for several years. (Essential prurigo? Allergic manifestation of a chronic intestinal infestation?)

Treatment: Steam-bath made from a decoction of herbal ingredients boiled in a pot (jaa ʔàab).

B-2. ***bàheŋ mǎa ñÿaŋ*** (mǎa ñÿaŋ is the name of the plant Mucuna pruriens (Fabaceae) which has hairs that can produce severe itching if touched).

A twenty-four-year-old woman had been suffering for eighteen months from an itching, well-circumscribed exanthema of the forearms, upper chest, and neck, taking the form of vesiculopapular eruptions on an erythematous base. The itching was especially aggravated in the sun. She had been in the habit of wearing metallic ornaments on the affected places.

A forty-nine-year-old man had had erythema and large itching urticarial efflorescences of the face and neck for a month.

A seventy-one-year-old man revealed a generalized papulous dermatitis with scaling and excoriations affecting the whole body except the head.

Comments: All these cases were interpreted as different manifestations of an allergic dermatitis due to metallic allergy, photoallergy and, in the last case, with no obvious allergic agent. According to the traditional doctor the diagnosis bàheŋ mǎa ñÿaŋ was assessed on the basis of superficial lesions of the skin not making the skin thick and hard, the papulo-urticarial lesions with erythema around them, together with the severe itching (as if the patient had touched the pruritic plant mǎa ñŷaŋ). A successful treatment was reported to rest on food prohibitions in addition to a topical medicine that was smeared on.

B-3. *baheŋ lŷad* (blood bàheŋ).

A forty-five-year-old woman presented patches of vesiculopapular eruptions and secondary scaling and atrophic skin of hands and feet, which had lasted for some months. Periodic itching.

A forty-five-year-old woman had suffered from an itching dermatitis in the groin and armpits for one month. The rash consisted of small papules and well-circumscribed red and dry patches.

The first case was taken as a manifestation of an eczema (toxic) due to contact with some allergens, the latter case as an intertriginous Candida-dermatitis.

Comments: The informant pointed out the similarity between the last case and the disease hŷan, but as he was sure that this condition had its origin in the blood and had not come from the outside (as is the case with hŷan), it was classified as bàheŋ lŷad. The diagnosis was used for a localized, superficial, itching dermatitis where there was no information indicating any specific releasing factors, and the conditions were consequently attributed to the blood.

bàheŋ diseases in the manuscripts

Three of the manuscripts did not mention the term *bàheŋ* at all, two manuscripts had one prescription each against this disease, while one manuscript contained twenty-seven prescriptions against *maleŋ*.[20] The following kinds were recorded (the parentheses contain the practitioners' understanding of the terms):

---

20. The spelling maleŋ was standard in the manuscripts, suggesting that at least the spelling of this word is influenced by that of Bangkok Thai (although the spelling bàheŋ was met with in two instances).

maleŋ phag bua (fĭi fag bua)

maleŋ pàag nâw (lídsaduaŋ lammánâad)

maleŋ nom ñuaŋ (fĭi jaŋ nom, săan jaŋ nom)

maleŋ pĕn khŭm (a kind of săan?)

maleŋ fáa fâad (bàheŋ fáa máan?)

maleŋ taŋ (fĭi naj kaaŋ)

maleŋ cɔɔn (bàheŋ tẽn?)

maleŋ laam (bàheŋ laam mɔ̂n?)

bàheŋ khãw mãj (tùm sug)

maleŋ khan (?)

maleŋ ñwâad (?)

maleŋ cáaŋ (?)

maleŋ dan (?)

maleŋ laa (?)

maleŋ kɔ̃ɔn (?)

maleŋ lom (?)

fĭi maleŋ lom (?)

bàheŋ mòn (?).

The use of the bàheŋ concept in the manuscripts indicates the possibility that bàheŋ was once a very general term including other subgroups like fĭi and săan, a possibility that is supported by the fact that none of the theoretical types of bàheŋ (group A-1), which were well known to all practitioners, is mentioned in the manuscripts at all. The spelling of the word, however, plus the general confusion surrounding this term may indicate that the concept of bàheŋ corresponds in fact to the theoretical types outlined above, and that the confusion—which is also apparent in the manuscripts—is rather recent.[21] At any rate, conclusions regarding the development of this term must be postponed until more evidence has been gathered.

mẙn

The patient suddenly gets swollen red wheals up to three or four fingers broad, without secretion inside. The eruptions are very itchy, but disappear without treatment after some days. Usually they come back at intervals. The wheals may occur all over the body, but they are not serious.

Cause: Given variously as wrong food, insect bites, and changes in weather. A wind arises in the body causing the eruptions.

Treatment: Usually none, but some prescriptions are found in the manuscripts.

Diagnosis:* This disease entity is reserved for the condition of large wheals on the skin, and it corresponds to urticaria (nettle rash). (One patient observed.)

hùud

hùud~khĩi hùud~hud is verbalized as a hard, rough tùm. It corresponds to the English term wart. hùud is also a disease in which the patient has disseminated warts (verrucae vulgaris).

Cause: Warts are said to come from touching the blood of eels (lŷad pǎa lǎj) or from the sap of toads (jaaŋ khaaŋ khóg).

Treatment: Topical medicines.

phadoŋ lŷad (blood phadoŋ)

This disease was not known to the practitioners interviewed,

21. One might object that the manuscripts are old and should be taken as better evidence than the oral tradition. This is not always true. The manuscript that contained the many bàheŋ (maleŋ) prescriptions referred to above is said to have been written by the uncle of the present owner. He was Burmese and had traveled widely. There could easily be a heavy influence from Burmese traditional medicine, as well as that of Central Thai, in this manuscript.

except for one who used this diagnosis in a case of guttate-nummulate psoriasis.

Cause: From the blood.

Comments: The term phadoŋ lŷad is not found in the manuscripts. Probably it is a recent borrowing from the Bangkok-Thai term pràdoŋ where it is used for "a rash or skin disease characterized by excessive itching and burning, a form of eczema" (McFarland 1944:499). This description did not fit the case diagnosed as phadoŋ lŷad.

pɛ́ɛ ˀaakàad

The term *pɛ́ɛ* is used in modern medicine for allergy, and the disease pɛ́ɛ ˀaakàad was described by one informant as sneezing, coughing, and difficulties in breathing. Two patients, both suffering from an allergic dermatitis, were also given this diagnosis. It is generally said to be caused by hairs from insects and animals, or from dust, as from trees or flowers (pollen), and is therefore also called pɛ́ɛ fùn láˀɔɔŋ (be defeated by dust and particles). pɛ́ɛ ˀaakàad may develop into khǎaŋ khañyy.

ɓág

This is the name of a tree, but also the name of a disease one may get when passing under such a tree, resulting in a swollen, red, and itching face.

Diagnosis: Allergic dermatitis?

ɓǎan

This is the name of an insect, but also the name of a disease one gets when the caterpillar of this insect, living on the banana palm, touches the skin, causing a smarting, burning, and itching pain.

Treatment: Rub the affected spots with locks of human hair.

Diagnosis: Contact dermatitis.

mɛɛŋ khian

This disease is named after an insect that "eats up the head," causing the hair to fall out in clumps.

Treatment: Topical medicine. The traditional doctors maintain that the disease can be cured.

Diagnosis: Alopecia areolata.

Comments: This disease is distinguished from khĩi khòog by the lack of lesions on the scalp: the hair just falls out without other signs. It is different from hǔa láan (bald-headed), which cannot be cured.

khĩi khòog

This is a disease that primarily attacks the scalp, but also the forehead, neck, and cheeks. It appears as round plaques, each with a light brown center and with red or white spots on the circumference. The central part then turns darker, gives off secretion, and crusts develop. The crust cracks, the secretion dries up, and the scales fall off, leaving a light-red lesion. It itches and burns. The hair may or may not fall out. It is regarded as contagious, and previously the disease was especially common among the novices in the temples.

Cause: It comes from the outside. The disease has a "mother" that enters the skin.

Treatment: Topical medicine.

*Diagnosis**:* Tinea capitis (favus), seborrheic eczema of the scalp, psoriasis of the scalp.

Comments: The entity probably includes different diseases attacking the scalp, resulting in ulcers and secretion with or without heavy dandruff. One informant had a deviating opinion concerning this disease and maintained that with khĩi khòog there are only plaques and scaling, but no secretion. According to him the disease lídsaduaŋ khan (itching lídsaduaŋ) represents the pictures of secreting lesions of the scalp. This comes from the blood and is not contagious. khĩi khòog is not recorded in the manuscripts studied.

khĩi khàag

The disease appears as round, sharply demarcated plaques, each with a slightly swollen and red border and brown scales in the center. They gradually expand and itch, and may be localized all over the body except the head.[22]

Cause: It comes from the outside.

Treatment: There are many topical medicines in common use.

*Diagnosis**:* Trichophytosis (ringworm).

Comments: khĩi khàag seems to equate with the cosmopolitan entity trichophytosis when affecting the trunk and limbs except for the feet, hands, and head. Two patients were observed with what looked like tinea corporis and tinea cruris. Trichophytosis with a restricted distribution to the head or the hands and feet is classified as khĩi khòog, hýan, hɔ̌ɔ, or khĩi móo. One informant classified khĩi khàag as a subgroup of hýan, another grouped the diseases khĩi khòog, khĩi kɔɔ, and khĩi khàag together.

khĩi khàag nám nom (khĩi khàag due to mother's milk)

Superficial, scaling red plaques appear on the face or neck of babies and small children. The lesions are dry and red and spread along the circumference. After scaling the skin turns white.

Cause: Said to be caused by mother's milk that spills over the baby when it is sucking.

Treatment: Topical medicine. It is emphasized that remedies against khĩi khàag cannot be used.

Diagnosis: Pityriasis alba. (Candida intertrigo?)

Comments: The description seems to fit the clinical manifestation of pityriasis alba, but perhaps also cutaneous candidiasis of the face of small children. It is distinguished from khĩi khàag by the more superficial lesions leaving white, depigmentated patches, whereas khĩi khàag produces redness and eats deeper into the skin.

22. In Laotian the term *khikak* means ringworm (Sassady 1962:41, citing Macey 1910). The Bangkok-Thai cognate is *khîi klàag*.

hɔ̌ɔ

1. *hɔ̌ɔ cwáʔ*~hɔ̌ɔ nám~hɔ̌ɔ phə́ʔ~hɔ̌ɔ ñāa nâw~hɔ̌ɔ tǐin~hɔ̌ɔ. It appears between the toes, but may spread to the rest of the foot. Round, sharply dermarcated, red itching plaques composed of vesicles appear, giving off a malodorous secretion. The vesicles do not eat deep into the skin, but they may produce a burning sensation. The nails are not affected. Common in rainy season.

Cause: From dirty water or rotten grass.

Treatment: There are a lot of alternative topical medicines. Can disappear by itself. Food prohibitions are sometimes part of the treatment.

Comments: Most informants emphasized that the lesions look like hýan and, if they spread further up on the wrists and lower legs, the disease would be classified as hýan. One informant said it could develop into phaj.

Diagnosis:* Tinea pedis (intertriginous and vesicular form).

2. *hɔ̌ɔ dān* is characterized by yellowish-white tùm appearing in patches within the skin on the foot-soles and between the toes, but also sometimes on the lower legs, wrists, and hands. The eruptions have dirty content (pustules). They usually do not burst open, but remain within the skin, which then turns hard (pěn dān). Some eruptions may open, however, giving off a little secretion. They eat deep into the skin, and are very itchy.

Cause: From dirty water. One informant said it comes from bad nám lýaŋ (lymph).

Treatment: We have recorded six different prescriptions based on topical treatment. It is said to be easily cured by pressing salt on the affected skin. Some say it may disappear by itself.

Diagnosis:* Tinea pedis (hyperkeratotic and pustular form), tinea manuum.

Comments: The description also leads us to assume that hɔ̌ɔ dān represents a form of trichophytosis of the feet (and hands). It is distinguished from hɔ̌ɔ cwáʔ by the hard, flat nodules (pěn dān) in the skin that eat deep into the flesh, and minimal vesiculation. Some informants say it resembles hýan, except for the localization. One informant had heard the English term Hongkong-foot (= tinea interdigitalis) used for this condition. One patient, given the diagnosis hɔ̌ɔ faj, owing to the burning sensations (faj) of the affected skin of the hands, suffered from tinea manuum.

3. *hɔ̌ɔ dyan* appears as painful, red, swollen skin around the nails of fingers and toes. The nails may finally fall off.
   Diagnosis: Paronychia. (See phãm.)

phaj

phaj is a term that covers two groups of diseases, both labeled phaj. One group, called phaj píd, is accompanied by poison (pǐd) and is potentially dangerous. It is classified as a subtype of tùm píd.

The other group contains certain skin diseases that belong to the phaj concept proper. One informant regarded burns as a kind of phaj. The demarcations of the concept of hýan are unclear. Some informants use phaj and hýan as synonyms, others maintain that hýan may develop into phaj, while still others keep these two concepts strictly apart.

phaj nám (water phaj) is localized on the feet, lower legs, and hands. It starts as small, reddish, itchy papules that turn into darker, burning, and painful patches that finally form thick, confluent plaques of the affected skin. The lesions ooze and may spread from the original locations. Fever may arise.

Cause: Dirty water, such as water where grass has been rotting.

Treatment: Topical medicine (same as for hýan nám). In addition, magic and food prohibitions are required. It is regarded as difficult to cure.

Comments: Some informants equated phaj nám with hýan nám, while others kept them apart mainly on account of the symptoms of fever, painful oozing lesions, and the more serious course typical of phaj nám. One informant said that phaj nám was the same as the Central Thai term pràdoŋ nám. Only one of the manuscripts mentions phaj nám, providing two prescriptions.

Diagnosis:* Infected eczema (of the legs), tropical eczema. One patient was observed with an infected chronic eczema of the lower legs with deep fissures and verrucose thickening of the skin.

phaj bõoŋ (caterpillar phaj) is an itching skin eruption caused by irritation from hairs as, for example, from the bõoŋ (caterpillar), from hairs of mǎa ñy̌aŋ (Mucuna pruriens-Fabaceae), from thùa ly̌aŋ (the yellow beans), from molds (haa hed), and from rotten wood (haa máj phúaʔ). The more one sweats, the more it itches.

Treatment: Blow incantations into sticky rice and roll the rice over the skin. The hairs will then adhere to the rice.

Diagnosis: Contact dermatitis.

hýan

hýan~khĩi hýan is the name of a group of skin diseases. The most common members of this group are:

hýan nám~hýan mə̌j~hýan (water hýan, dew hýan). The characteristics of this disease are red-white, elevated, slightly secreting, itchy plaques, surrounded by a red border. They appear normally on the skin of the wrists, the anterior part of the legs, the knee folds, or on the hands, but may finally spread all over the body. Most common in the cold season.

Cause: From dirty water, rotting grass, or molds of rotting trees (haa).

Treatment: It is difficult to cure, but some prescriptions (topicals) together with magic incantations can be effective.

Comments: Some informants equate the disease with phaj nám, while others keep the two apart. Some say it resembles khĩi khàag, others hɔ̃ɔ. Of the nine patients observed and given this diagnosis, three turned out to have microbial eczema (infective eczema) of the legs, one had lichen simplex chronicus (of the legs), one had asteatotic eczema (feet and hands), one toxic contact dermatitis (of the hands), one tinea corporis, and two tinea pedis. As will be seen from this list, hýan nám concerns chronic eczematous lesions and dermatomycosis primarily localized in the lower legs, feet, and hands.

hýan cáaŋ~hýan kwǎaŋ (elephant hýan, deer hýan). The skin of the lower legs, wrists, and feet gets thick and grayish with fissures and secretion. The skin burns and itches. The name indicates that the skin looks like that of an elephant. It does not spread to other parts of the body.

Cause: From outside, especially from dirty water.

Treatment: Topical medicine, magic, and food prohibitions.

Comments: Some informants maintain this to be a specific disease with no connection with hýan nám, while others treat it as a progressed, final stage of the latter disease. A variant mentioned by one informant is hýan kwǎaŋ (deer hýan), in which the skin looks like the skin of a deer. The patient gets white-grayish plaques on the lower legs and wrists. One patient given the diagnosis hýan cáaŋ actually had a verrucose, secreting and crusted eczema of the legs, a condition commonly referred to as tropical eczema in cosmopolitan dermatological textbooks. A similar clinical picture of tropical eczema was diagnosed as phaj nám by another informant.

hýan wíd~hýan sũam~hýan sǎŋkhaŋ (toilet hýan). Patches of dry, red, itching lesions appear in the groin, on the scrotum, and around the anus; slightly scaling.

Cause: Contagion from toilet.

Treatment: It may disappear by itself, but there are some topical medicines against it, too.

Diagnosis:* Intertriginous dermatitis (Candidiasis). (One patient seen.)

Comments: hýan can be summarized as diseases primarily affecting the distal parts of the limbs and the groin. They all cause itching, and the skin lesions are in patches or plaques, usually with thickening of the skin.[23] The etiological agent comes from outside the body and settles down in the skin. Dirty water is the most common causative agent. In Western dermatology the various hýan represent certain pictures of eczema and dermatomycosis.

23. The cognate for hýan in Bangkok Thai is *rýan,* now meaning "leprosy." Macey identifies the Laotian term *khi huan* with dry eczema (Sassady 1962:41, citing Macey 1910).

There are cases in which a patient's symptoms do not fit any one of the existing local disease concepts. This results often in a "mixed diagnosis," as in the following example: The patient had itching, red, fissurated, and vesiculating patches on the hands. The skin was inflamed and swollen, and the patient reported that she had got it after using a special kind of washing powder. The traditional diagnosis of hýan lídsaduaŋ was given, which rested on the localization to qualify it for hýan, but the indurated, swollen skin, and the lesions going deep in the skin, qualified it for lídsaduaŋ. The patient revealed a typical contact dermatitis of the hands.

khĩi sĩan

This is a skin disease composed of white-yellow, scaly patches that spread all over the upper trunk, neck and face. When scratched, small scales fall off. The patches are very itchy, especially when exposed to the sun or when the patient sweats.

Cause: Unknown, but it comes from outside, as can be seen when a person wears a shirt borrowed from someone suffering from it and gets it, too.

Treatment: It will not heal by itself, and it is difficult to cure. We have recorded three different prescriptions against it.

Diagnosis:* Pityriasis versicolor.

Comments: One patient given this diagnosis had a typical picture of pityriasis versicolor. One informant called the disease "the younger sibling of khĩi khàag." Another respondent divided the disease into khĩi sĩan khǎaw (white) and khĩi sĩan lýaŋ (yellow) with predominately white or yellow scales and patches, respectively. The disease was not found in the manuscripts studied.

khĩi móo

khĩi móo~móo. Thick, hard, red or dark plaques and nodules (ked dam dɛɛŋ khɛ̌ŋ nǎa) appear in the skin somewhere on the body, usually on the feet, legs, and around the knees. The lesions are painful, the thick plaques crack, and oozing wounds appear. It finally may spread all over the body. Some lesions disappear, but new ones appear somewhere else. The disease is contagious and will not heal by itself. It normally attacks adults.[24]

Cause: The cause was alternatively given as bad blood, dirty water, or bites from insects leaving their urine within the skin. This disease may also be transferred from the parents (through the blood).

Treatment: Oral and topical remedies and, in addition, food prohibitions. It is regarded as difficult to cure.

Comments: This skin disease was unfamiliar to most of our respondents, and the provided descriptions are rather divergent. One informant divided the disease into two subtypes: (a) móo thammádaa (common móo) = móo khǎaw (white móo) = móo nám lỳaŋ (secreting móo) with the symptoms above, and (b) móo lŷad (blood móo) = móo dɛɛŋ (red móo) that gives off bloody secretion and never attacks the nose. This subdivision was unknown to the other informants. Several informants mentioned the similarity with khĩi tûud. One informant called it "the younger sibling of khĩi tûud," but maintained that it could not develop into khĩi tûud. Another informant said that it was identical with khĩi tûud. One remarked that it resembled hýan cáaŋ.

khĩi móo is not recorded in the manuscripts studied, but we have collected one prescription.

Diagnosis:* The diagnosis móo was used by one of our informants in four cases of skin diseases. Three patients given the diagnosis móo lŷad turned out to have trichophytoses of the hands and feet (tinea pedis [1], tinea manuum [1]) and a possible secondary stage framboesia of the leg (1), taking the form of several granulomatous, ulcerating lesions and edema of the lower leg. The diagnosis móo faj was applied to a patient with a group of discoid, scaling plaques of the limbs compatible with psoriasis (see also khĩi tûud).

---

24. In one Northern Thai dictionary ***khĩi móo*** is translated with the Central-Thai term ***khúdtháråad*** (framboesia, yaws) (mêed 1965:44). Spire has recorded a disease in Laos referred to as khi mo, which he identifies as "le pian" (framboesia) (Spire 1907:12, 22).

khĩi móo nɔ̀ɔ

khĩi móo nɔ̀ɔ~móo nɔ̀ɔ~khĩi nɔ̀ɔ~tǎa pǎa~pěn cán. Nodules of hard skin appear on the soles of the feet and hands. The nodules have a deep root, and pressure on them causes pain.

Diagnosis:* Clavus, verrucae plantaris.

Comments: One patient with clavus of the foot soles was observed. The attribute nɔ̀ɔ (bamboo shoot) points to a seasonal aspect of the disease; namely, that the disease is commonly seen in the rainy season when the bamboo shoots appear.

khúdtálâad

khúdtálâad appears as red or dark red nodules and plaques (pěn dãn pěn bɔ̃ə) that ooze along the rinds. The skin turns thick and white with scales and crusts. "The skin is eaten from inside." It may affect all parts of the body, but is usually found in the skin of the arms, hands, and feet. The fingertips and toes turn black. It may be fatal.

Cause: Unknown. One informant mentioned "bad blood."

Treatment: Both oral and topical remedies (jaa salǐimuun), and food prohibitions. Difficult or impossible to cure.

Comments: One informant called the disease "the younger sibling of leprosy," and the other informants all maintained that the disease was similar to khĩi tûud, or just a variety of it. One respondent distinguished it from khĩi kɔɔ by the incurability of khúdtálâad, whereas khĩi kɔɔ can be cured. Another equated khúdtálâad and khĩi kɔɔ. We have found one prescription for khúdtálâad in the manuals. It is possible that the term khúdtálâad is a recent borrowing from Bangkok Thai, where it has now been adopted for "framboesia, yaws."

Diagnosis: See khĩi tûud.

cɔ̃ɔ

cɔ̃ɔ is a serious disease with many manifestations. It generally starts with fever. Then some parts of the body swell and become painful, usually the feet or hands. The fingers may become gnarled. The flesh of the body, including the face, gets red and swollen. Dark, thick skin lesions appear, some taking the form of nodules (pĕn dãn). The patient may lose skin (the skin is eroded away). It may also affect the nose. It resembles khĩi tûud but, unlike this disease, the lesions itch and are painful, and there is no loss of sensation.

Cause: May come from water, but normally caused by spirits (phĭi sàj) or black magic (thùug sidpakhun khɔ̆ɔŋ pə̂n, thùug cɔ̃ɔ, thùug sàj wãan).

Treatment: Sweat-baths and oral remedies (purgatives).

Diagnosis: See khĩi tûud.

khĩi kɔɔ

This disease is maintained to be a contagious, dry, itchy skin disease taking the form of thick, hard lesions (năŋ dãn dãn năa năa [granulomas, nodules]) that may be scattered all over the body. The lesions clear up with heavy loss of scales, giving a repugnant impression.

Cause: Unknown.

Treatment: The remedy is taken both by mouth and applied topically at the same time.

Comments: The disease was not recorded in the manuscripts studied. Two informants said they had seen it once, but they had never tried to cure it. Some said it resembled khĩi tûud and one suggested that it was another word for khĩi tûud in an early stage when there are no ulcerations and no secretion. One informant put khĩi kɔɔ and khĩi hid in synonymy. Another said it was a Northeastern Thai word for khúdtálâad, while yet another maintained that it was different from this, as khúdtálâad could not be cured.

Diagnosis: See khĩi tûud.

khĩi tûud

khĩi tûud~tûud~pháñâad lŭaŋ (the great disease)~lôog lýan (Bangkok Thai). The herbalists recognize several stages in the development of khĩi tûud, and there are several clinical manifestations. The disease may start in between the first and second finger, where the muscle is eaten away (kĭn mɔ̆ɔn myy). Then swellings occur, followed by loss of fingers. It commonly attacks the toes and the nose, too. The eyeballs and teeth are not affected, but aside from this it may appear anywhere on the body. khĩi tûud may also appear as dry, scaling plaques with partial or complete loss of sensation in the affected area, often preceded by itching and pain. Sometimes the skin is just insensitive and the color of the skin changes. Certain types of lídsaduaŋ—the incurable ones—may develop into khĩi tûud. There may be long intervals when the disease seems to stop developing, but in the long run the patient will become crippled.[25]

Cause: khĩi tûud is generally considered to be caused by "germs" (mii cýa mii mɛ̂ɛ), which are found encapsulated in the earth. If, while digging, one hits one of these lumps containing "germs" and breaks it and the contents touch the body, one will get contaminated, although it may take years before the disease actually appears. Contamination through direct contact with a khĩi tûud-affected person is also possible, although people have observed that in a married couple where one person is attacked by this disease the other person does not necessarily get it. The same is the case with children of khĩi tûud patients: they may or may not get the disease of their parents. If they do, it does not normally appear before the age of seven. It is commonly believed that a person with khĩi tûud may cause others to get the disease by cursing them. Finally, it is said that eating the púdsaa-fruit (Chinese date; Ziziphus jujuba-Rhamnaceae) may be a cause of this disease.

Treatment: A combined treatment of sweat-bath and oral medicines, some acting as purgatives, is tried. The treatment is only effective in the very first stages of skin lesions. If fingers and toes have started to fall off, cure is impossible. Food prohibitions are included.

Diagnosis:* Three patients given the diagnosis khĩi tûud all had manifestations of the early stage of tuberculoid leprosy, with anesthetic, infiltrated macules and patches localized on the lower legs.

---

25. According to Spire, the Laotians distinguish between three kinds of leprosy: ki-hueum (= khĩi hýan?), "lèpre au début," tout thao (= tûud . . . ?) "lèpre avec ulcérations," and ki-tout (= khĩi tûud?) "lèpre avec nodosités" (Spire 1907:24).

The delimitation of the diseases cɔ̃ɔ, khĩi tûud, khĩi kɔɔ, khúdtálâad, and khĩi móo is not clear, and probably these diseases are variably applied by the practitioners. While the four first-mentioned diseases mainly put emphasis on the appearance and characteristics of the lesions, khĩi móo is also to a large degree determined by the localization of the skin lesions. From the descriptions provided, it is assumed that cɔ̃ɔ, khĩi tûud, khĩi kɔɔ, khúdtálâad, and khĩi móo cover certain manifestations of leprosy and yaws, including some of their complications. While khĩi tûud more specifically points to an affinity with tuberculoid leprosy, also verified by the observed casuistics, the other four with the descriptions of thick skin lesions (nodules, granulomas) probably border on both lepromatous leprosy and secondary and tertiary stages of yaws. The more localized picture of yaws, when hands, feet, and lower legs are typical sites of predilection, will probably be recognized as a part of the khĩi móo concept. A widespread lepromatous leprosy with nodular lesions (lepromas) and the similar and often clinical indistinguishable picture of a secondary stage yaws probably recur in the concepts of cɔ̃ɔ, khúdtálâad, and khĩi kɔɔ. As already pointed out, the two latter diseases are commonly intermixed, and the verbalization is similar. This may indicate that they represent alternative terms for the same concept, possibly having their origin in different geographical areas.

Comments: None of the terms khĩi tûud, tûud, pháñâad lŭaŋ were found in the manuscripts.

khĩi hid

> Patches of tiny papules and vesicles appear between fingers or toes, on arms and head, and may sometimes, though rarely, spread all over the body. The patches itch, and the skin turns red when scratched. The itching increases when the skin is exposed to sunshine.[26]

Cause: Generally unknown, however, one informant said that it appears when haj-insects or meen-insects (from chickens) enter the skin through the pores, leaving a white residue around the entrance.

26. khĩi hid has also been recorded as a common disease in Laos under the name khi it, "la gale" (scabies) (Spire 1907:21).

Treatment: Different therapeutic methods were recorded, such as lying down in a mud-hole, or drinking and bathing in a specific decoction. The informant who referred the disease to the existence of insects in the skin said that an effective cure was to expose the body to the sun and afterward spray the skin with a solution of insect-killer. If no treatment is applied, the patient will suffer from it for months.

Diagnosis: Scabies.

Comments: One informant compared the disease with khı̌i sı̌an, another with khı̌i kɔɔ. Five prescriptions were collected; one prescription was found in a manuscript, and four prescriptions were obtained directly from the practitioners.

sı̌w

sı̌w is the condition of scattered follicular papules (pimples) of the face and neck (Acne vulgaris).

sı̌w cáaŋ

sı̌w cáaŋ (elephant pimple) is a sı̌w (pimple) on the face or the forehead that turns red and dark and starts to grow. If it bursts, the pus inside comes out and it disappears. If it does not burst, a serious poisonous wind will arise and ascend to the face causing it to swell around the sı̌w. The poisonous wind presses the heart and may result in unconsciousness and death in a few hours. A sı̌w cáaŋ must not be touched, and the patient must avoid bad smells or unwholesome food; if he does not, the wind will ascend and cause attacks.

Cause: Unknown.

*Diagnosis**:* Furuncle, cystic acne. (One patient observed.)

Comments: This disease concept seems to cover the condition of a cystic acne that may be infected, giving an abscess formation (furuncle). The dreaded course of a furuncle of the face, which can extend to and infect the central nervous system, causing unconsciousness followed by death, has also been observed in connection with this "disease."

lídsaduaŋ of the skin

lídsaduaŋ dàad (lídsaduaŋ with dàad-lesions) is the name used to describe thick, sharply demarcated, pale skin lesions that have heavy scales or are hypochrome. When the affected skin is completely white, the diagnosis kõoŋ is used. In the medical practice the diagnosis lídsaduaŋ dàad was given to a patient with a localized scleroderma and sclerodactyli (morphea) of the forearm, including some patches of vitiligo; to a patient with a guttate psoriasis with thick scaling of the well-circumscribed lesions; and to a patient with a dry, scaling, and well-circumscribed chronic eczema.

lídsaduaŋ khǎaŋ lŷad (blood-khǎaŋ lídsaduaŋ). Two patients given this diagnosis both had a widespread nummulate-discoid psoriasis with heavy scales. A delimitation against phadoŋ lŷad was made on the basis of a less generalized distribution of the latter.

lídsaduaŋ lŷad (blood-lídsaduaŋ). This diagnosis was assessed in a case of cystic acne all over the face.

lídsaduaŋ nám lǐaŋ (lymph-lídsaduaŋ). One case seen with tinea capitis taking the form of favus.

lídsaduaŋ tẽn (dancing lídsaduaŋ) is the name used to describe the condition of sharply demarcated, predominantly coin-shaped lesions with a little scaling, which are scattered and "dancing" on the body, that is, the lesions disappear in one place, but will reappear in another. Two patients observed. One had a typical nummular eczema of the legs and trunk, the other probably seborrheic eczema with coin-shaped lesions predominating.

lídsaduaŋ fáa máan (dark sky lídsaduaŋ). One patient given this diagnosis had two dry, bluish, lichenified and scaling plaques of the neck, interpreted as chronic contact dermatitis due to allergy to a metallic chain, which is widely used as an ornament.

lídsaduaŋ khan (itching lídsaduaŋ). This diagnosis was commonly made use of to describe itching, scaling plaques somewhere on the body. Seven patients given this diagnosis had different manifestations of eczemas, such as lichen simplex chronicus (2), seborrheic dermatitis (eczema) (4), and acute eczema with lichenification, probably on an allergic base (1).

phãm

This is a painful disease that attacks the tips of the fingers or toes. The finger or toe swells up, the distal joint turns stiff, and the disease starts eating its way through the skin and flesh around the nail, which turns black. It may also destroy the bone. It is extremely painful, but the pain can be diminished by holding the hand up, thus preventing the blood from reaching the finger.

Cause: Some informants say that it starts as a small wound as a result of being pricked by a thorn, or that a wound appears by itself. Others say that it comes from a kind of luminous black caterpillar, which causes itching if touched, with the same name as the disease, namely, bõoŋ phãm.

Treatment: It is regarded as difficult to cure, but magic or medicine may be effective. We have seen no prescriptions against phãm.

Diagnosis: Pyogenic paronychia.

Comments: One informant compared this condition to hɔ̌ɔ dyan, another to bàadphañág.

kõoŋ

kõoŋ~tûud kõoŋ (leprosy kõoŋ)~tûud phỳag (albino leprosy)~dàad khǎaw (white patches)~bàheŋ khĩi dàad (bàheŋ patches). This name is used for the condition of white patches of the skin. It is commonly applied to the condition of vitiligo. Some say it can develop into leprosy, others that it cannot. It is regarded as difficult to cure, but a lídsaduaŋ dàad medicine may be used. Some equate this condition with lídsaduaŋ dàad, but most practitioners keep them apart. Food prohibitions are normally part of the treatment.

4.2.9. Modern concepts

baw wǎan—diabetes mellitus. This disease was not known earlier, but the new term—borrowed from Bangkok Thai—has been widely accepted and is fairly well understood. The complication of gangrene is also mentioned. One informant meant that patients with diabetes mellitus probably were given the diagnosis khǎaŋ loŋ liŋ in older times. We have come across one newly created prescription against baw wǎan.

bãa mǔu~phǐi bãa mǔu—epilepsy.

khwaam dan sǔuŋ—high blood pressure (hypertension). The concept has been recently introduced and is frequently heard. However, there is no deeper understanding of the concept. We have come across one prescription.

khɔɔ thìib—diphtheria. (See also under khǎaŋ.)

khãj lŷad ʔɔ̀ɔg is a modern concept borrowed from Bangkok Thai for hemorrhagic fever. Previously the disease was not known, but both the disease term and its content are now widely used and understood.

khãj dam dɛɛŋ is a modern concept borrowed from Bangkok Thai for scarlet fever. Not yet generally known.

lôog lýaŋ—a modern, borrowed term for jaundice (icterus).

ʔaj dãn—whooping cough, pertussis. (See also under khǎaŋ.)

sãj tiŋ—appendicitis.

5

Drugs and Diseases

5.1. OMNIPOTENT REMEDIES

It is not uncommon to find that more than one medical preparation in the therapeutic arsenal—irrespective of its taste and quality (hot, cold, indifferent)—is used to treat one and the same disease. A first assault may be made using a medicine against the disease group in general; for example, a general remedy against khăaŋ. A second assault may be made using other medicines aimed at eliminating or diminishing some specific or disabling symptoms of the disease, such as itching, vomiting, or headache. A third assault on the disease may be made using a drug against the presumed etiologic agent or the process held responsible for the symptoms. For example, when a disease is due to the intervention of a poisonous agent (píd), this agent has to be killed or dispelled; or when the symptoms are attributed to a serious wind (lom), the wind must be kept in check by a wind medicine. But there also exist some omnipotent remedies—both preventives and curatives—prescribed for a wide range of diseases, either to induce strength and vigor in the patient when he feels weak and disabled, or to expel and combat the fundamental causes of the disease. In theory, these remedies are given credit for many and variable actions and effects, but in current practice they are regarded as alternative remedies in the treatment. The more common of these are briefly described below.

jaa thâad (medicine for the elements)

This remedy is given to a person suffering from general fatigue, or to one who is weak and disabled, whether due to disease or not. It is commonly made use of to give children an appetite and to restore their strength. Nowadays, there is a tendency to give these remedies a value as appetite stimulators, though originally, as the name indicates, they were believed to strengthen the elements, which are thought necessary for recovery. jaa kǐn khãw lam (medicine [which makes] the rice taste nice) is another traditional remedy that points more specifically to the desired result of stimulating appetite. A jaa thâad is prepared either as a decoction or as a powder, in the latter case usually mixed with honey before it is taken orally.

jaa bamluŋ kǎmlaŋ (strength-enhancing medicine)

This is the principal restorative remedy, giving strength to the body in general. It is usually taken as a preventive. These remedies are also used as heart tonics and as sexual stimulants, promoting both sexual desire (aphrodisiac) and endurance.

jaa ʔaajúʔ wádthánáʔ (medicine to prolong life)

This preventive remedy acts along the same lines as the two above: to strengthen the body with the purpose of prolonging life.

jaa salǐimuun (omnipotent salǐimuun medicine)

This remedy is given the ability to combat the fundamental processes of disease independent of what the disease may be. It is prescribed in addition to other more specific remedies. Another procedure is to use the salǐimuun medicine as a base and then add some specific ingredients directed against the actual disease, rendering the medicines according to their applications; for example, "jaa salĭimuun lom kìaw" against kìaw, "jaa salĭimuun lom bàheŋkhúd" against bàheŋkhúd, and so forth.

jaa kɛ̃ɛ (medicine to relieve . . .)

This is also a general remedy used as a basis for the treatment of a variety of diseases and complaints. A jaa kɛ̃ɛ sapaʔ (medicine relieving all kinds [of disease]) is a remedy for every variety of human disorder, but usually a jaa kɛ̃ɛ is given a more specific application—for groups of diseases or just a single disease or symptom. For example, jaa kɛ̃ɛ lom (medicine to relieve the wind) is used for all diseases in which wind is prominent; jaa kɛ̃ɛ sǎan (medicine to relieve the sǎan) or jaa kɛ̃ɛ ceb tɔ́ɔŋ (medicine to relieve stomachache) for sǎan and ceb tɔ́ɔŋ, respectively. It is again the combination of ingredients which decides the medical application.

jaa thìib (expelling medicine)

The purpose of this remedy is to expel certain symptoms or diseases from the body. The desired effect is to get rid of the causal agent of the complaints. Some thìib remedies have a general application, whereas others are more specific; for example, jaa thìib khãj (medicine to expel fever) and jaa thìib píd (medicine to expel poison).

A jaa kɛ̃ɛ and a jaa thìib have the same domain of application, but are, in theory, regarded as different. The former is ascribed the property of minimizing the effects (symptoms) of the disease agent, and the latter is given the ability to expel the causal agent from the body.

jaa thàaj (expelling-through-intestine medicine)

jaa thàaj medicines, which may be regarded as a subgroup of jaa thìib, expel the causal agent of the disease through the anus. They are applied when the causal agent has entered the body with food. A jaa thàaj is almost without exception a purgative, thus provoking diarrhea. Some remedies are of a more general nature, being able to expel all kinds of agents, whereas others have a more restricted use; for example, jaa thàaj pháñâad (medicine to expel worms [vermifuge]) and jaa thàaj píd (medicine to expel poison).

In the next section we will deal with medicines of a more specific kind than the omnipotent ones cited above. Before we do this, we will make some observations about ingredients in general:

First, it is our impression that the herbalists normally have no clear opinion on why each ingredient actually is included in a prescription.

Second, the pharmacy textbook of Wat Pho mentions the existence of subsets of ingredients in the prescriptions; that is, groups of ingredients which, for various reasons, are frequently lumped together. The herbalists in Northern Thailand did not mention such subsets; still we assume that they may exist there as well, especially symptom-specific subsets with properties like "beat down fever," "check the wind," and so forth. The existence of such subsets could be explained historically as a merger of two or more prescriptions.

And third, not all ingredients in a prescription have a claimed curative effect. Ingredients may be included intentionally for cosmetic (taste, flavor, color) or other noncurative purposes; for example, to conceal the real content of the medicine, or just to make it easier to form it into pills, to swallow, to apply to the skin, and so on.

5.2. THE RELATIONSHIP BETWEEN DRUGS AND DISEASES[1]

We now turn to the crucial questions concerned with the relationship between diseases and drugs because, obviously, the curing process consists of identifying or diagnosing the condition of a sick person, and then selecting a number of materia medica to be used to treat that condition. In other words, the focal point of the curing process is the establishment of specific links between one particular disease and one particular selection of materia medica in

1. Sections 5.2, 5.3, 5.5, and 5.6 constitute a revised and enlarged version of "The Relationship between Drugs and Diseases in Northern Thai Traditional Medicine," a paper presented by Viggo Brun at ASOMPS IV, Bangkok, 15–20 September 1980.

each concrete case of the disease. The problem is, how are these links established? How clear and unambiguous are they? How many are there? In brief, what is the nature of these links?

There are two specific sources in the tradition where concrete links between diseases and plants are established; namely, in the prescriptions, and in the statements concerning the curing properties of single plants. In the following section we will discuss the nature and implications of the information in these two sources.

5.3. THE PRESCRIPTIONS

An overall description of the prescriptions has already been given in sections 3.5.3 and 3.5.4. The tradition has developed three standard units of information presented in a fixed sequence. The curing range is given in the "head" of the prescription. Then follows the "corpus" of the prescription, which contains an enumeration of the ingredients used in the prescription and, finally, the "tail," which contains the directions for treating, mixing, and prescribing the ingredients.

It must be kept in mind that:

1. A prescription may be used against more than one disease.
2. A prescription may be composed of many ingredients, from one to about a hundred, but normally four to ten.

TABLE 5

STANDARD FORMULA OF NORTHERN THAI PRESCRIPTIONS

Subunit	Information
"Head": curing range	In case of disease A (B . . . N) and symptoms a (b . . . n)
"Corpus": ingredients	take ingredients 1, 2, 3 . . . n
"Tail": directions	and mix them in the following way . . . and give it to the patient in the following portions and frequency . . .

3. There are many ways in which ingredients can be prepared and mixed. The relative weight of each ingredient may be indicated; the ingredients may be boiled, crushed, mixed raw, and so on, and they may be eaten, inhaled, applied to the skin, and so forth.

This is illustrated in table 6.

In our example, prescription P_1 is given medical properties against diseases D_1 and D_2 by means of the ingredients I_1 and I_2, which should be boiled, and the decoction then drunk.

Several plants *together* account for the claimed medical property of a prescription. If we take into consideration that there are, let us say, some one hundred local disease concepts, some two thousand different ingredients, plus twenty ways of treating and mixing these ingredients, then we arrive—theoretically—at a virtually unlimited number of possible combinations or, in other words, chaos! The virtue of any medical tradition must be that it somehow has enabled its practitioners to reduce a theoretically unlimited number of combinations to a limited number; that experience has reduced chaos into some kind of system. But how systematic are the various medical traditions in this respect? Or, in other words, if one seeks within a tradition for the answers to such specific questions as, How can one cure disease A? or, What are the characteristics of disease B? how many different answers will one find, and how various are these answers?

In the case of the Northern Thai medical tradition, we can safely say that it has moved away from chaos, but at the same time it still is far from having a system: From the tradition, one can still come up with many different answers to the same question. There are, for example, many prescriptions against the same disease, and descriptions of the content of the specific disease terms vary considerably.

How many prescriptions are there in the medical tradition in Northern Thailand? The prescriptions are found in medical manuscripts and there are hundreds and hundreds of these manuscripts lying around in temples and private homes. The manuscripts consist mainly of sequences of prescriptions (and incantations and related magical information) and, taken together, they must contain a very

TABLE 6

THE CURING RANGE, INGREDIENTS, AND THE PREPARATION AND ADMINISTRATION OF THE INGREDIENTS IN FIVE (HYPOTHETICAL) PRESCRIPTIONS

Prescription (P)		P_1	P_2	P_3	P_4	P_5
Curing range	D_1	x	x		x	
(D = Disease)	D_2	x		x		
	D_3		x			
	D_4		x			x
	D_5			x		x
	D_6			x		
	⋮					
	D_n				x	
Ingredients (I)	I_1	x			x	x
	I_2	x		x		
	I_3		x			
	I_4		x	x		
	I_5		x		x	
	I_6		x		x	x
	I_7		x	x		x
	⋮					
	I_n			x		x
Preparation and administration		Boiled, per os	Dried, ground, per os	Dried, ground, mixed with oil, topically	Crushed raw and taken per os, + incantations	Boiled, per os

large number of prescriptions—our estimate is tens of thousands. Focusing on a few prescriptions or even on all the prescriptions of a single herbalist thus gives a simplistic and distorted picture of the tradition as a whole. The experience making up the tradition cannot be gleaned from the knowledge of one informant only. In fact, the body of knowledge is so vast that one person cannot possibly manage to carry the whole tradition in his head. Furthermore, the secrecy surrounding the prescriptions favors a bits-and-pieces transfer of the knowledge. The secrecy functions, in fact, as a centrifugal and disconnecting force scattering the knowledge about randomly to the different curers. Therefore it becomes of utmost importance to search for the *sum of knowledge* contained in the *tradition as a whole.* A close look at the standard units of information in the prescriptions will demonstrate this.

5.3.1. The curing range

The curing ranges, found in the headings of the prescriptions, vary considerably. They may be limited to one disease only—sometimes enlarged with a few symptoms—or they may contain several, or a large variety of, diseases and symptoms. In other words, the curing ranges of the prescriptions are *more or less extensive* and they *more or less overlap* one another. This immensely complicates not only a comparison of the prescriptions but also a comparison of the medical applications of the plants within the prescriptions. One would, for example, like to compare the various prescriptions against the same disease. In the case of disease D, one may find ten different prescriptions that cure disease D alone. These can easily be compared as to ingredients. There are many prescriptions, however, that cure disease D plus a variety of other diseases and symptoms. How should we analyze this type of information?

The prescription headings mention many disease concepts, but give little information about the content of these concepts. The focus of the prescriptions is on the ingredients, and the diseases are just mentioned by name, evidently assuming that the reader already knows the content. The contents of the diseases are transferred orally, and a proper understanding of them can only be arrived at through direct interviews with local doctors and, preferably, through direct observations of specific cases of diseases together with an herbalist.

But besides these complications, the prescription headings can also be considered as a blessing in disguise because, within the entire tradition, it is only in the headings that diseases are in any way classified. Because of the overlapping, however, this classification turns out not as a clear-cut one but as patterns or tendencies to classification. Still, these patterns can be used to form the basis for a more systematic and detailed classification.

A brief look at what can be gained from a disease classification based on the prescription headings may be useful at this point. In section 3.8.12 we pointed out that we could plot the diseases on a "map" and then encircle those cured by each prescription. If a prescription had a narrower, specific application, the circle would be accordingly small, whereas a prescription with a wide or general curing range would encompass many diseases. If more and more prescriptions were treated in this manner, more and more diseases would need to be plotted, and clearer and clearer concentrations (patterns) of circles would—presumably—emerge (although there would undoubtedly be many vague or uncertain edges). These patterns obviously group the diseases together because they have certain medical properties in common. What these properties are must await further investigation in each concrete case, of course.

Prescriptions are a part of practice, thus a classification of the diseases based on a large number of prescriptions is a classification based on the practice of the tradition. To the individual herbalist, however, the whole body of prescriptions is irrelevant. He bases his disease classification—however incomplete—on his own limited experience and knowledge, together with whatever theory has been crystallized within the tradition; thus his cognitive view of the diseases is likely to turn out to be both a partial and an idealized version of practice. The two classifications—based on parts of the knowledge and the whole of the knowledge, respectively—are not necessarily congruent, but they can be compared. The degree of difference between them would reflect the degree of distance between practice and theory in the tradition.

If we take the prescription headings as our only source of information, we can conclude that a number of medical concepts have developed within the tradition, but that practitioners are still in the process of stabilizing and classifying them.

5.3.2. The ingredients

We will next analyze the second standard unit in the prescriptions: the materia medica. An important question is which of the ingredients in a prescription are essential, that is, which of them contain bio-active principles that may cure the disease?

On a purely logical level we would assume that ingredients with a high recurrency rate in prescriptions against one specific disease are promising in terms of possible therapeutic effects. However, the ingredients with a high frequency score in prescriptions against many other and quite different diseases as well are not likely to be the most essential parts of a prescription. The promising ingredients are especially those with a high frequency score in prescriptions against one disease and no other, or those which are restricted to prescriptions against diseases with a common or similar pathogenesis (in a biomedical sense).

At first glance it also looks reasonable to assume that *the shorter the prescriptions, the more likely they are to contain the most effective ingredients.* The logic behind this assumption is plain enough: centuries of trial and error should have resulted in the effective ingredients being retained in the prescriptions and the ineffective ones being gradually dropped out. As will be demonstrated later, the evidence we have does not support this assumption.

At this point in our exposition it is natural to raise the fundamental question: *To what degree do the ingredients actually recur in prescriptions against the same disease?* A tentative investigation shows ingredient-overlapping to be low indeed.

From a corpus of some thirteen hundred randomly collected prescriptions, we have picked out all the prescriptions against two diseases and analyzed them (for details, see below).

We found a total of twenty-one prescriptions against nĩw, with an average of four ingredients per prescription. None of these prescriptions had identical ingredients! Six short prescriptions had no ingredient in common with any other prescription, and the rest had one or two ingredients in common with one or two other prescriptions.[2]

2. The traditional medicines against nĩw are widely reputed to be effective. One would therefore have expected few and clear links between this disease and the materia medica used against it. The actual heterogeneity of the ingredients is therefore particularly surprising.

In the case of bàheŋkhúd, we found thirty-seven prescriptions with an average of eight ingredients per prescription. None of these prescriptions had identical ingredients, and there was a low degree of ingredient-overlapping. As much as 90 percent of the ingredients occurred in only three prescriptions or less out of the total of thirty-seven.

This preliminary statistical survey clearly demonstrates that identical prescriptions are rare—nonexistent in our survey—and that in spite of some recurring ingredients, the prescriptions against these two selected diseases are characterized by a high degree of heterogeneity.

At first glance these results are surprising because, in spite of the bits-and-pieces transfer of the knowledge, one would expect the prescriptions to be a stable part of the tradition. This assumption is strengthened when we take into account the fundamental rule regarding transfer. "The prescriptions have been passed on from time immemorial and should not be tampered with, therefore: do not omit any of the original ingredients." With this rule in mind it becomes a paradox to discover the diversity and heterogeneity of the prescriptions.

Before we try to explain this paradox, let us for a minute ponder the ideology behind this rule: "Today's variety and fragmentation goes back to an original unity. In the beginning everything was one: there was *one* original Teacher who had *the* answer." Apparently he had found *the* cure (prescription) for each disease. The idea is that the past was glorious (and, implicitly, the present less so) and one should respect and cling to it. Therefore: do not omit anything![3] This goes for all aspects of the tradition, but we suspect particularly for the superstructure—the practitioners' own understanding of the tradition.

This is obviously an idealized vision of history, and the ultimate consequence of such a view is stagnation. In spite of this reverent and conservative attitude, the medical tradition has not been

3. Another reason for not wanting omissions of ingredients in the prescriptions could be that a certain combination of drugs has been proven to have medical effects that might disappear if some of the ingredients were left out.

stagnating, but has on the contrary been continually changing. So much so that heterogeneity has become a fundamental characteristic of the practice of the tradition today. The reason is that besides the above-mentioned rule, which aims at stability and homogeneity, there also exist three other implicit rules for transmission, which secure change and development of the practice of the tradition; namely, addition, replacement, and creation of new prescriptions.

Additions. The rule of adding allows for new experiences (i.e., curative properties of plants) to be added to existing prescriptions. One might suspect that, in cases of diseases that have turned out difficult to cure, the rule "if a prescription doesn't work, experiment by adding" has been applied, causing a continual increase in the number of ingredients in certain prescriptions. Another reason for the multi-ingredient prescriptions could be a general tendency in the tradition to incorporate rather than to exclude. Regarding drugs, practitioners of cosmopolitan medicine are prone to adopt the attitude: The less the better—in other words, isolate the active components and purify them, according to the rule. In the Northern Thai tradition practitioners seem to take the opposite position: The more the better.

Replacement. A practical reason for allowing the substitution of one ingredient for another is the situation herbalists commonly find themselves in when they cannot get hold of one or more ingredients they need right away. But replacements must have been restricted in one way or another for one cannot, of course, replace an ingredient with any other random ingredient. Obviously, the exchangeable ingredients must have some qualities in common. In the "Pharmaceutical Manual of Wat Pho" there is a list of some twenty plants that can replace one another, mostly imported plants to be replaced by local ones. Unfortunately, we did not pay sufficient attention to this problem of replacement during our data collecting, thus we do not know to what extent replacement of individual ingredients is practiced. But the problem is important and deserves to be investigated further.

Generally speaking, we assume that experimenting with additions and substitutions has taken place. These experiences, however, have not normally been passed on to other curers. The same experiments may thus have taken place over and over again, resulting in an ineffective and slow accumulation of knowledge.

Creating new prescriptions. We have come across examples of new prescriptions against entirely new disease concepts, like baw wǎan (diabetes), for example. Beyond that we cannot confirm that new prescriptions are being created. We cannot accept, however, that the rules of addition and replacement are sufficient to explain the heterogeneity of the prescriptions. The only way to explain this is to postulate that creation of new prescriptions (including loans from neighboring medical traditions) simply *must* have taken place, and still takes place, on a considerable scale.

We note, en passant, that the transition from adding and replacing ingredients and merging already existing prescriptions on one hand, and creating new ones on the other, is a relative and gradual one.

5.4. MEDICAL USE OF SINGLE PLANTS: RESULTS OF THE MEDICO-BOTANICAL INVESTIGATION

The core of the Northern Thai medical tradition is the curative aspect, and above all the utilization, of plants as medicinal drugs. In fact, the tradition as a whole is built on and around the practitioners' knowledge of plants and their experiences with them. Or as one of our informants put it: "The important thing is not what you call a disease, or from where it comes, but rather to know which preparation must be used to get rid of it." In the villagers' minds a good doctor is one who has effective medicines at his disposal.

An important part of our studies has been to record and collect medicinal plants from the area. The results of the ethnobotanical investigations are presented elsewhere (Bjørnland and Schumacher, in preparation). In this context we would like to extract and analyze the medico-botanical information obtained from the botanical informants (presented in toto in the column "Medical use[s]" in the List of Medicinal Plants in the Appendix). In the following section these data are compared to the information from our analysis of the prescriptions.

When we found plants on our botanical expeditions, our botanical informants readily offered answers to the question, What is this plant used against? The answers came in the form: This plant is used against disease A, B . . . N and symptoms a, b . . . n. In the botanical list we have taken great care to record the diseases and symptoms in the local vernaculars, because we believe easy translations on the spot by some interpreter are often more misleading than correct. [The content of the medical terms can be found elsewhere in the text via the index].

At first glance, it might appear that the Appendix contains the most concentrated and precise information about the medical properties of the plants. That is not the case.

First, this information cannot be based on experience with the plants in isolation because it is hardly ever true that plant A *alone* cures disease D. As already pointed out above, plant A is part of some prescriptions against disease D, but may at the same time also be part of prescriptions against quite different diseases. The information in the Appendix must thus be interpreted to mean that the plant is but one of the ingredients in prescriptions used to treat the mentioned disease or symptom.

Second, our medical data in the Appendix are incomplete, because we did not have the opportunity to discuss the medical use of the plants with more than a few informants from a few selected areas. More thorough interviews with more informants would certainly have extended the ranges of medical application of many of the plants.

Nevertheless, we have rearranged our present information on the medical use of single plants in table 7. In this table the medicinal plants have been assigned to eighteen subgroups of diseases/symptoms/remedies arranged into four major categories. As can be seen, diseases of the digestive system are treated with far the greatest variety of plants (237 species). A large proportion is also devoted to the group of omnipotent restorative and curative remedies (140 species). Fever (83 species), skin diseases—mucocutaneous lesions (56 species) and urogenitalial complaints, with some obstet-

TABLE 7

NUMBER OF COLLECTED MEDICINAL PLANTS ASSIGNED TO THE VARIOUS REMEDY GROUPS

Remedy group (to treat)		
Organ-Related Diseases	Digestive system	237
	Skin	56
	Urogenital system	53
	Nervous system	33
	Cardiovascular system	18
	Ophthalmic system	8
	Respiratory system	7
	Endocrinologic system	5
		Subtotal 417
Classified symptoms and signs	Fevers (khǎj)	83
	Body pains (ceb . . .)	20
	Bites (. . . khob)	14
	Dizziness (vertigo) (maw hǔa)	14
	Tumors (sǎan)	10
	Others	6
		Subtotal 147
Miscellaneous indigenous symptoms and complaints	kǐn phid/kǐn sàlɛ̌ɛŋ	42
	lom bàheŋkhúd	10
	lom (afflicting winds)	39
		Subtotal 91
Omnipotent remedies	jaa thâad, jaa bamluŋ kǎmlaŋ, jaa ʔaajúʔ wádthánáʔ, jaa salǐimuun, jaa kɛ̃ɛ, jaa thìib, jaa thàaj	140

ric conditions included (53 species) put claim to more than 10 percent of the plants each, while the remaining groups account for 1 to 8 percent of the material.

If we compare these data on the medical use of single plants (listed in the Appendix) with our preliminary analysis of the prescriptions, we find not only that certain diseases or complaints—for example khǎaŋ and bàhòog—account for the use of a great number of the single plants we collected but also that there are many different prescriptions for these diseases.

Many of these remedies are also complex with a lot of ingredients. An exception is prescriptions used to treat skin diseases, which consist of just a few (usually two or three) ingredients. An obvious reason for the great number of plants and the many prescriptions used to treat gastrointestinal disturbances, fever diseases, and skin lesions is the high prevalence of such conditions in the population. Furthermore, in these groups the diseases are many—both from an indigenous point of view and even more so in a biomedical sense. Consequently, a great variety of plants and remedies is needed.

Another plausible explanation may be a desperate search for effective remedies/cures within these disease groups. When no obviously effective remedy exists, a natural course would be to enlarge the existing prescriptions with new ingredients. Prescriptions against mucocutaneous lesions, however, which are treated with simple, topical medicines, whose effectiveness is easier to observe objectively, still include a large proportion of the plants. This should indicate that, at least for the skin diseases, ineffective therapy cannot be the only reason why there are so many plants in common use.

Many of the plants in the botanical list appear to have a restricted medical use in that they are recorded with one disease or symptom only, or with some closely related diseases (see the appendix). This assumption of restricted use may rest on the scantiness of our information on the medical uses of these plants. In any case, we are not in a position to identify the true single-use plants in the tradition—if they do exist. Nevertheless, it should be noted that the apparently high proportion of single-use species used to treat mucocutaneous lesions or bites may be real, because many of these plants are poisonous when taken orally and consequently have to be reserved for external use as topicals in skin diseases and related conditions. We assume, however, that the number of multiple-use species in the tradition far exceeds the number of single-use species.

5.5. THE MEDICAL USE OF PLANTS IN THE PRESCRIPTIONS

It would be natural to assume that, when a single plant in isolation is believed to have specific and desirable effects against a particular disease, that plant will: (a) be found in the prescriptions against that disease, (b) be among the most frequently recurring ingredients in these prescriptions, and (c) be found especially in the very short prescriptions with only a few ingredients.

But what seems natural to assume is not always correct, and in this case our assumptions were certainly not supported by facts. One of the greatest surprises the analysis of the prescriptions (see below) gave us was that only a few of the plants which, in isolation, were said to cure disease D were actually included in the recorded prescriptions against that disease.

In the case of nĩw, we found fifteen plants in the botanical lists which were said to cure this disease, but as many as nine of these plants were not found in any of the prescriptions against nĩw *at all.* Of the six species which occurred, only four recurred in several prescriptions, but not one of them was found in the very short prescriptions (see fig. 28). In the case of bàheŋkhúd, only one out of ten plants in the botanical list (see the appendix) was found in any of the thirty-seven recorded prescriptions against it! (see fig. 29).

An explanation of this almost incredible fact could be that there are synonyms among the vernacular plant names both in the botanical list and in the prescriptions. A plant may thus occur in both places, but under different names. We have not been able to weed out all possible synonyms—although a fair number of them have been picked up; still we believe that even if they occur, they must be rather few. Another explanation could be that our material is statistically unrepresentative. We cannot reject this objection entirely, although we will remind the reader that we have information about some five hundred plants from some thirteen hundred prescriptions. These numbers are relatively large and should at least show us a tendency.

We believe that neither of the two objections above invalidates our conclusion, namely, that the *information about medical properties of plants in isolation should be regarded with utmost skepticism,* as the information usually gives only a simplified, incomplete, and distorted picture of the reality. We will, on the contrary, argue that it is the prescriptions that reflect the complex reality of praxis, and that they are the important source of information regarding the relationship between drugs and diseases.

5.6. ANALYSIS OF PRESCRIPTIONS

It is now time to present the results of our analysis of prescriptions against two indigenous diseases, nĩw and bàheŋkhúd, in detail. The prescriptions analyzed are taken from a corpus of 1,300 prescriptions—1,200 coming from five medical manuscripts collected in various parts of the Chiangmai plain, and 100 having been obtained by way of mouth from our informants.

5.6.1. nĩw (Calculus pro parte)

As our first example we have chosen prescriptions against nĩw because (1) the symptomatology of this disease is clear and not easily confused with other indigenous disease concepts, (2) the traditional nĩw remedies in use have a reputation for being very effective, and (3) calculus is a common condition in Northern Thailand.

We have collected twenty-two prescriptions[4] specifically against nĩw, five of which we got orally from our informants, and seventeen of which we found in the manuscripts.[5] The twenty-one

4. One of the prescriptions stands out as exceptionally long (48 ingredients) compared with the others, and is also used against other major disease groups. In our discussion we will disregard this prescription.

5. Two of the manuscripts did not contain any prescriptions against this disease, and the three others contained ten, five, and two, respectively. We have not included prescriptions against symptoms or signs that may be connected with calculus; for example, prescriptions against symptoms like "muddy urine," "blood in the urine," and "pain in the back and loin." Neither have we included any of the numerous khǎaŋ prescriptions, some of which may also be used against calculus-related symptoms.

TABLE 8

FREQUENCY OF INGREDIENTS IN nĩw PRESCRIPTIONS

51	ingredients occur in	1	prescription
9	" " "	2	prescriptions
6	" " "	3	"
1	" " "	4	"
(67	in total)	(21	in total)

prescriptions analyzed contain a total of ninety ingredients, giving an average of a little more than four ingredients per prescription. The number of different ingredients is sixty-seven, and a summary of the frequency of the ingredients in the prescriptions is shown in table 8.[6]

The figures in table 8 show a surprisingly low frequency of recurrence of single plants in the prescriptions, and we must conclude that there is a low degree of homogeneity in the nĩw prescriptions. Behind these types of frequency lists—as we have already pointed out—lies the general assumption that the more frequently a plant recurs in prescriptions against a certain disease the more likely it is that it has specific medical effects against that disease. This assumption is limited by another assumption, however: If an ingredient has a high *general* frequency score—that is, if it often occurs in prescriptions against other and even quite different diseases—its "curing effect," if any, is assumed to be of such a "general nature" that it can be safely eliminated. If, however, an ingredient occurs only in prescriptions against diseases with a common or similar etiology or pathogenesis (in a biomedical sense), it should be considered promising in relation to some specific pharmacological property. In our example, we are neither in a position to eliminate or specify ingredients with a high general frequency score nor to single out the promising ingredients with a high specific frequency

6. The list is tentative, as we have not been able to check whether there are any synonyms among the local botanical names. If there are, the frequency of some plants would increase.

TABLE 9

NAMES OF INGREDIENTS OCCURRING IN TWO OR MORE nĩw PRESCRIPTIONS

Two prescriptions	Three prescriptions	Four prescriptions
bàfyaŋ	hǐn sõm	mánád = bàkhànád
bàpin	bàdəəj	
fãaŋ	bàdùug	
khácaaw	càkhaj*	
khwɛ́ɛŋ khǎaw	khãw mĩn*	
lom lɛ́ɛŋ	puuləəj*	
sõm hed		
máliw		
hɔ̌ɔm*		

score, as such complete frequency lists—based on all available prescriptions—have not been worked out. Still, our experience points at càkhaj (lemongrass), khãw mĩn (ginger), puuləəj (another ginger), and hɔ̌ɔm (onion) as belonging to the group with a high general frequency score and with a "curing effect of a general nature," which, consequently, could be eliminated. These are marked with an asterisk in table 9.

From the results shown in tables 8 and 9 we observe that:

1. Fifty-one ingredients (that is, 76 percent of the total) occur in only one prescription.
2. The plant with the highest frequency score—mánád, or bàkhànád (pineapple)—occurs in only four out of a total of twenty-one prescriptions, that is, in less than one-fifth, which is a surprisingly low score.

In figure 27 we have arranged the prescriptions so that those with common components are placed together. Each prescription has been given a number for identification. The fifty-one different ingredients occurring only once have not been named, but are indicated by a dash; the others have been written out in full.

As can be seen, the prescriptions against nĩw fall neatly into four groups, among which there are no common members (except for two minor instances). If we look closer at figure 27 we observe that:

1. Group IV (the "remainder" group) consists of six short prescriptions, of which four are single-ingredient prescriptions. One would have expected that the very short prescriptions would contain the "essence" of the tradition, that is, the specifically nĩw-active plants. It is therefore surprising to find that these prescriptions have no ingredients in common, nor have they ingredients in common with any of the other nĩw prescriptions. There is thus no statistical evidence to indicate that they are promising as nĩw-curing plants.

   The single-ingredient prescriptions ("If you have disease D, cure it with plant P") postulate the same one-to-one relationship between disease and plant as the statements about the curing properties of plants in isolation ("Plant P cures disease D"). Again we meet with the paradox: the more precisely the tradition attempts to answer, the more various the answers become. We are thus forced to look beyond these one-to-one statements to the more complicated and less precise prescriptions, and use their confusion and overlappings to arrive at a system—a system based on likelihood and tendencies—just as we had to do when we classified the diseases!

2. Group III consists of three prescriptions with several common components. But as these ingredients are of a "general curing kind," these prescriptions do not look very promising either.

3. Group II is centered around prescriptions 8 and 17 with the common ingredients bàdùug, khwɛ́ɛŋ khǎaw, and sõm hed. Loosely attached to them are five other prescriptions, each with one ingredient in common.

4. The statistically most promising prescription, number 2, is found in Group I, where five prescriptions are interwoven by means of the components mánád, hǐn sõm, bàfyaŋ, and bàdəəj hǐn.

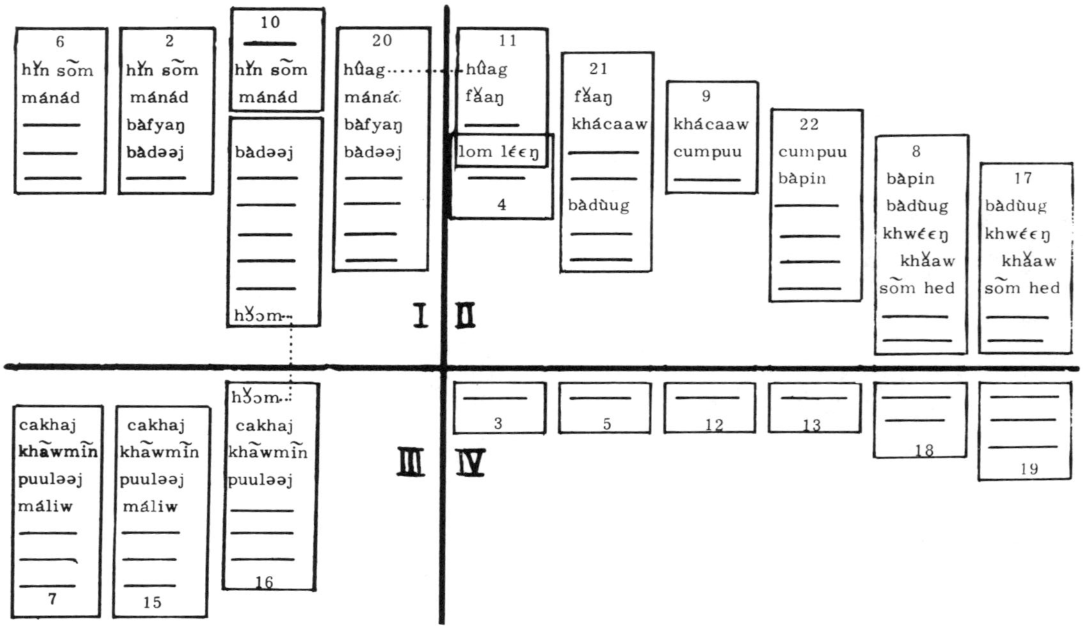

Fig. 27. Prescriptions against nĩw grouped according to common components.

In spite of the great diversity in the prescriptions against nĩw, a statistical approach thus yields in this case a slight indication of the likely prescriptions (and components) to be investigated.

Our next step is to go to our list of collected medicinal plants and extract from it the plants said to be used against nĩw, and then compare them with the results of our frequency study of the prescriptions. Fifteen plant taxa representing nineteen species in table 10 are prescribed against nĩw.

Of these fifteen taxa only six turned up in the prescriptions. The prescriptions against nĩw contain sixty-seven different ingredients. Our botanical list gives fifteen native plant taxa said to cure nĩw. A comparison of these sources gives an overlapping of only six taxa. That is, more than half of the collected plants said to cure nĩw do not occur in the investigated prescriptions against this disease at all! This is schematically shown in figure 28.

We note that all the plant taxa in table 10 (except the last) are refound in the prescriptions belonging to Group I and that prescriptions 2 and 20 again are singled out as the most promising. Unexpectedly none of the plant taxa in table 15 occurs in the prescriptions with only one ingredient. In fact, the single-ingredient prescriptions could simply be regarded as new additions to the botanical list.

5.6.2 bàheŋkhúd (painful conditions; among others, headache, migraine)

bàheŋkhúd is a disease term that covers, among others, the symptoms wind (lom) and pain (ceb), especially pains in the head, like headache and migraine, but bàheŋkhúd may also affect the eyes and ears, the muscles in general, the bones and joints, and it may result in general edema (see pp. 121–123).

In the medical manuscripts checked, we found thirty-seven prescriptions claiming curing properties against this disease. The prescriptions contain from 1 to 27 ingredients, with an average of 8 ingredients per prescription, and with altogether 174 different ingredients. The recurrence frequencies of the ingredients in the prescriptions are listed in table 11.

TABLE 10

SINGLE PLANTS FROM THE LIST OF MEDICINAL PLANTS ASSIGNED CURING PROPERTIES AGAINST THE DISEASES nĩw AND bàheŋkhúd

Disease	Plant taxon	Scientific species	Family	Occur in prescriptions (prescription numbers)
	ñãa thɔ̀ɔd pɔ̂ŋ	*Equisetum debile*	Equisetaceae	+ (20)
	ñãa khuaj ŋuu	*Achyranthes aspera* *Achyranthes bidentata*	Amaranthaceae Amaranthaceae	–
	ñãa khuaj ŋuu nɔ́ɔj	*Cyathula prostrata*	Amaranthaceae	–
	sɛ̀ɛ sǎalaa	*Thevetia peruviana*	Apocynaceae	–
	mánád~bàkhànád	*Ananas comosus*	Bromeliaceae	+ (2, 6, 10, 20)
nĩw	pùag nám	*Buddleja asiatica*	Buddlejaceae	–
	phɛ̂ɛŋ~sàkɛɛ	*Combretum quadrangulare*	Combretaceae	+ (19)
	bàfaj, bàfaj pàa, bàfaj dyan hãa	*Baccaurea sapida*	Euphorbiaceae	–
	khĩi mɔ̂ɔd, khàj mɔ̂ɔd	*Glochidion lanceolarium* *Glochidion sphaerogynum*	Euphorbiaceae Euphorbiaceae	–
	bàhǐŋ mẽn	*Flemingia macrophylla* *Flemingia sp.*	Fabaceae Fabaceae	–
	bàfyaŋ	*Averrhoa carambola*	Oxalidaceae	+ (2, 20)
	máj pḥàj cɛ̃ɛ	*Bambusa cf. blumeana*	Poaceae	–

TABLE 10 (*continued*)

SINGLE PLANTS FROM THE LIST OF MEDICINAL PLANTS ASSIGNED CURING PROPERTIES AGAINST THE DISEASES nĩw AND bàheŋkhúd

Disease	Plant taxon	Scientific species	Family	Occur in prescriptions (prescription numbers)
	bàdəəj hǐn	*Coix lacryma-jobi*	Poaceae	+ (2, 14, 20)
nĩw	ñãa phàag khwaaj	*Dactyloctenium aegypticum* *Eleusine indica*	Poaceae Poaceae	–
	máj hûag	*Thyrsostachys siamensis*	Poaceae	+ (11, 20)
	léb khúd, bàkhúd	*Polyscias fruticosa*	Araliaceae	–
	phag wǎan tõn	*Sauropus cf. amoebiflorus*	Euphorbiaceae	–
	phag wǎan bãan	*Sauropus androgynus*	Euphorbiaceae	+
bàheŋkhúd~ lom bàheŋkhúd	dɔ̀ɔg dãaj pàa	*Lobelia nicotianaefolia*	Lobeliaceae	–
	cáa phag wǎan, cĩi jɔ́ɔj	*Micromelum minutum*	Rutaceae	–
	phag pɛɛm pàa	*Toddalia asiatica*	Rutaceae	–
	pɔ̌ɔ tɛ̌ɛŋ	*Colona floribunda*	Tiliaceae	–
	pàan sǎa	*Boehmeria nivea*	Urticaceae	–
	sàg	*Tectona grandis*	Verbenaceae	–
	phag pɛɛm	*?*		–

TABLE 11

Frequency of Ingredients in bàheŋkhúd Prescriptions

120	ingredients occur in		1	prescription
30	"	" "	2	prescriptions
7	"	" "	3	"
6	"	" "	4	"
4	"	" "	5	"
1	"	" "	8	"
3	"	" "	9	"
1	"	" "	10	"
1	"	" "	12	"
1	"	" "	14	"
(174	in total)		(37	in total)

TABLE 12

Names of Ingredients Occurring in Eight or More bàheŋkhúd Prescriptions

Name of ingredient	Number of prescriptions in which the ingredient occurs
dìid	14
phag wǎan bãan	12
ŋaa cáaŋ (elephant's tusk)[7]	10
thùa puu	9
raaŋ jen	9
ñyaŋ	9
cɔɔj naaŋ	8

7. In the bàheŋkhúd prescriptions we find that "bones of animals" are very common ingredients—elephants' tusks, hooves, horns, and teeth of rhinoceros, bones of eagles, bones of black dogs, shells of turtles, shellfish, and even the jaws of the slow loris. If these "bones" were statistically lumped together they would receive the highest frequency score. This may have something to do with the fact that bones are regarded as cool, and that coolness is needed to calm down the roaming wind, which is the immediate cause of the pains accompanying this disease. In addition, some plants whose names contain the words for horn (khǎw) and cool (jen) may have been included because of sympathetic magic.

TABLE 13

NUMBER OF INGREDIENTS OCCURRING IN FOUR OR MORE PRESCRIPTIONS DISTRIBUTED AMONG SPECIFIC PRESCRIPTIONS

Prescription no.	Number of ingredients occurring in four prescriptions or more
11	9
15	8
36	8
4	6
20	6
37	6

We found that the main bulk of the ingredients, some 90 percent, occur in three prescriptions or fewer. But—in contrast with nĩw—we also found some ingredients with a high frequency of recurrence. In fact, seven ingredients occur in eight prescriptions or more, and the ingredient with the highest score occurs in nearly one-third of all the prescriptions. The seven most frequently used ingredients are listed in table 12.

Next, we singled out the prescriptions with the highest number of frequently occurring plants (table 13).

We have thus so far concluded that the plants and prescriptions against bàheŋkhúd listed in tables 12 and 13 are—from a statistical point of view—the most promising for further investigations.[8]

If we turn to our botanical list and extract from it the plant taxa used against bàheŋkhúd, we find the surprisingly low number of ten. Nine of these do not occur in the prescriptions against bàheŋkhúd at all! Only one does; namely, phag wǎan bãan,[9] which occurs in twelve prescriptions.

---

8. We are not—as has been mentioned above—in a position to identify and eliminate plants with an overall high frequency score. Nor have we been able to weed out possible synonyms among the local botanical names.

9. Two other species with similar names occur in the botanical lists (see the Appendix), namely, phag wǎan tõn and cáa phag wǎan. They are counted as not occurring in the prescriptions.

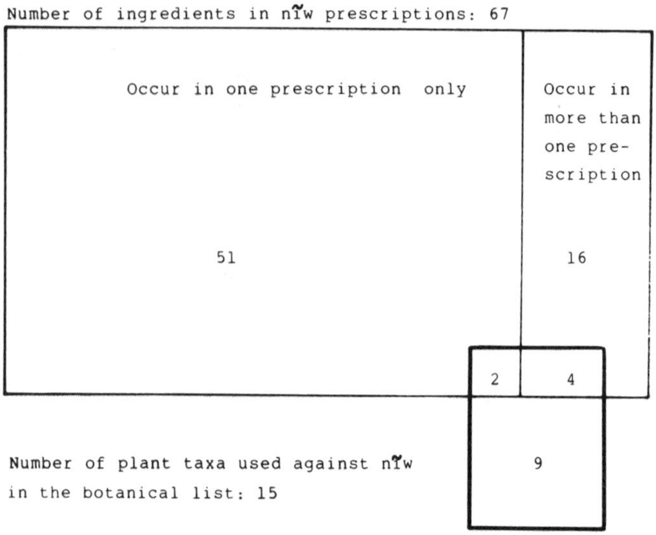

Fig. 28. Overlapping between ingredients in nĩw prescriptions and collected native plant taxa said to cure nĩw.

The relationship between the ingredients in the prescriptions and the plant taxa said to cure bàheŋkhúd is illustrated in figure 29.

5.7. CONCLUSIONS AND RECOMMENDATIONS

We are of the opinion that the most reliable information about the relationships between plants and diseases are to be found in the prescriptions, which are also regarded by the herbalists themselves as the essence of the tradition. Due to the many nonstandardized variables in the prescriptions, and their general heterogeneity, we propose a statistical study of a representative number of prescriptions as a rational way to extract information from the tradition.

Frequency lists of the ingredients should be worked out; one list with the score of all ingredients in all prescriptions should be compared with another list of all the ingredients in the prescriptions against each specific disease (or group of diseases). Then we

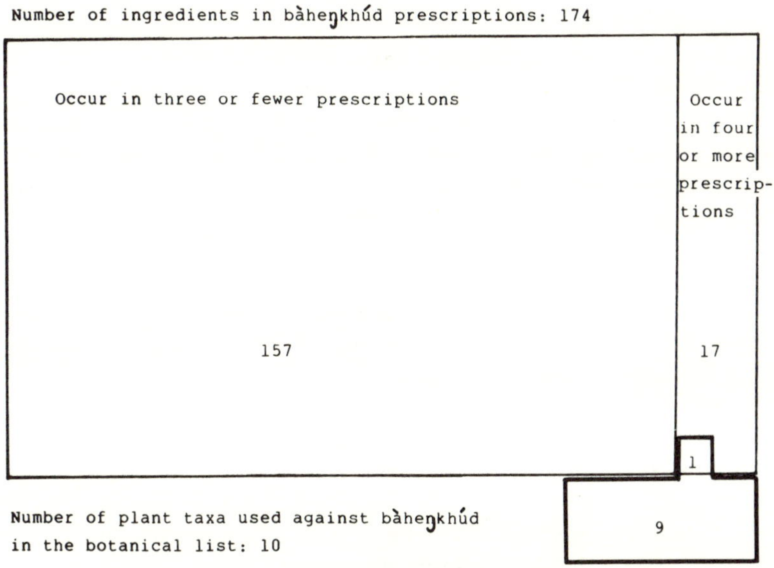

Fig. 29. Overlapping between ingredients in bàheŋkhúd prescriptions and collected native plant taxa said to cure bàheŋkhúd.

could perhaps single out the ingredients that are most likely to be the effective ones in each and every disease. At the same time, these lists would reveal: (a) the degree of homogeneity of the prescriptions against a given disease; (b) the whole range of applications of each ingredient; and (c) the names of the ingredients (plant taxa) that are made use of within the tradition.

A statistical analysis of the curing ranges in the headings of the prescriptions would also give us more information on how the diseases are perceived, organized, and classified, and put us in a better position to uncover and understand the theory and structure of the tradition as well.

One of the obstacles such a statistical study of a large amount of data will encounter is the problem of synonymy (one concept having more than one designation) and homonymy (one name used for more than one concept). A cognitive study of the kind presented in this volume forms a sound basis for solving this type of problem.

It is self-evident that statistics and computerization are not the final answers to structural and theoretical problems in general. It is, however, a natural and necessary step at this stage and should be followed by other steps; for example, focusing on the curers' own understanding and use of their tradition. We should alternate between a specific level, where a cognitive approach should be stressed, and a general level, where some objective criteria and methods of natural sciences should be applied.

The results of such an extensive statistical investigation would be a rational point of departure for further studies of many aspects of the tradition, but it would especially furnish representative data for a rational choice of the most promising medicinal plants suitable for further pharmacological and phytochemical investigations and screening programs. Far too often in the past the selection of plants for this purpose has been based on heresay or incomplete information.

Finally we would add that the historical dimension—the internal development of the tradition, the external influences on the tradition, and the relationship of the tradition with the development of Thai society in general—is not less important than the relationship between curing and prevention, especially regarding the dietary practices.

6

Will Herbalism Survive?

The survival of traditional Thai medicine, and the quality of such a survival, depends on many factors: the attitude of the government, the competition from Western medicine, the attitude of the patients, the recruitment to the tradition and, finally, the internal vitality of the tradition itself.

6.1. THE TRADITIONAL MEDICAL SCHOOLS

For about fifty years the traditional medicine was apparently only practiced actively in the countryside. Then in 1957 the royal tradition was reorganized with the establishment of the School of Traditional Medicine at Wat Pho in Bangkok. The old manuals used at Siriraj around the turn of the century were reprinted, and teaching commenced. Later, the school formed regional branches. There now exist—as far as we know—the following traditional medical schools using the Wat Pho manuals, or revised or abridged editions: Wat Pho, Wat Mahathat, and Wat Parinajok (all in Bangkok); Wat Jaj Sisuphan and Wat Phichaj (both in Thonburi); Wat Anatharam (Chiangmai), Wat Nong Nakhon (Lampang); and schools in the provincial towns of Udorn, Kon Kaen, Korat, Ubol, and Roi Et.)[1]

1. Personal interview with sèeg sɔ̌ɔnlam, Wat Mahathat, 18 November 1978.

These schools, which all are located in temples and thus closely connected with the Buddhist monks, are the most important centers for spreading the traditional medicine of the royal branch.

There is, furthermore, the Āyurvedic Society of Thailand (samaakhom pheesàd lέʔ ʔàjúráwêed booraan hὲεŋ pràthêedthaj), established in 1952, and since 1960 located in Wat Sam Phaya, Bangkok. The society treats patients (about 2,000 in 1974), and conducts classes in both traditional pharmacy and medicine, using the textbook *ʔajúráwêedsỳgsǎa* by Khun Nídthêedsùgkìd (1899–1953). The society has, since 1968, given courses in traditional medicine for commune medics (phε̂εd pràcam tambon) in cooperation with the Health Department and the Livestock Department. In the period 1968–1974, thirty-eight courses of this kind were given, with about one hundred participants attending each session. The president of the society up to 1974 was Khun Sophitbannalak, and his daughter Sajsanom Kittikacorn was vice-president.[2]

Lately, institutions have appeared which teach traditional medicine by mail. An example of this type of school is the institution under the rather pompous name of International Institute of Pharmacological Research Extension (sàthǎaban sòŋsə̌əm kaankhónkhwáa sàmǔnphraj ràwàaŋ pràthêed), which was established in 1977. The headquarters of this institute is located at Sam Phran, Nakhorn Pathom, but it also has contact persons throughout the country. The institute teaches traditional medicine by post at two levels. The first level, which takes about two months to complete, teaches the medical properties of plants, animals, and minerals, in addition to the method of mixing drugs. The second level takes another three to six months to complete, and the curriculum appears to be very much like the first level, only more detailed. (The medical properties of *1,000* plants are taught, as well as drugs to cure *every* disease.) The institute provides textbooks, and the curriculum stresses the importance of Western scientific methods. In fact, Western medicine is introduced at several levels in the curriculum.[3]

2. Summary from the society's journal, *nítajásǎan pheesàd-ʔajúráwêed,* nos. 18–38 (Jan. 1969–Jan. 1974).

3. Summary from the institute's journal, *sàmǔn phraj,* nos. 1–3 (June 1978–August 1979).

6.2. THE RECRUITMENT

The Ministry of Public Health has kept records of the number of people who have received a license from the ministry to practice in the three branches of traditional medicine. Unfortunately, we do not know from what year the statistics begin, but in tables 14 and 15 the figures for the period 1957–1978 are given.[4]

The total numbers for 1978 do not, of course, indicate the actual number of herbalists practicing with a license in that year. These figures are cumulative and include people who were then dead or too old to practice.

We note that the number of candidates passing the pharmacy examination is very large in comparison with those for the two other groups. The most interesting thing, though, is the trend in the figures. The number of traditional pharmacists is steadily increasing and should be quite sufficient to ensure the continuity of this branch of the tradition. In contrast, the numbers of midwives and general practitioners are dwindling rapidly, and in the six year period 1972–1978 came down to the surprisingly low numbers of three and five, respectively! These figures may give a slightly more pessimistic picture of the situation than is actually the case because some of those having a pharmacy license will in actual practice also

TABLE 14

TOTAL NUMBER OF LICENSES, 1957–1978

	Pharmacy	Midwifery	Medicine
1957	12,275	8,506	34,270
1962	12,663	8,518	34,317
1968	14,997	8,551	34,441
1972	15,681	8,576	34,492
1978	19,518	8,579	34,497

4. The figures were obtained from Mr. Woraphod Narakhorn, Ministry of Public Health, June 1978.

TABLE 15

INCREASE IN NUMBER OF LICENSES, 1957–1978

	Pharmacy	Midwifery	Medicine
1957–1962	388	12	47
1962–1968	2,334	33	124
1968–1972	684	25	51
1972–1978	3,837	3	5

make diagnoses and effectively treat diseases, even though this will be formally against the law. Still, an increase of one [*sic!*] traditional doctor a year for the whole country is far from sufficient to keep the tradition alive. What is actually happening is that the link between plants (pharmacy) and diseases (medicine) is being severed. The result will be that the tradition will gradually degenerate into one in which practitioners are "pill-makers," with no experience in actual curing.

As for the recruitment to the various schools, we have only come across the following limited survey from the School of Traditional Medicine in Chiangmai, reproduced in table 16.

These figures show that there should be a sufficient number of students to keep traditional pharmacy alive in the North, provided that most of them actually pass their examinations and thereafter go into practice. We note that women are entering the tradition, even if at a slow rate.

6.3. THE ATTITUDE OF THE PATIENTS: THE MORE THE BETTER?

There have been various attempts to quantify the popularity of traditional medicine among the Thais, using statistics covering the actual use of the various curing alternatives. The statistics we have come across are all taken from surveys of limited areas, and they are therefore of limited value. Still, the similar trends in these sta-

TABLE 16

Candidates in Traditional Pharmacy, Chiangmai, 1964–1972[5]

	All candidates	Women	Monks/novices
1964–1965	10	0	0
1965–1966	20	3	0
1966–1967	20	0	1
1967–1968	22	2	3
1968–1969	40	8	4
1969–1970	70	5	10
1970–1971	60	5	8
1971–1972	45	1	2
Totals	287	24 (8%)	28 (10%)

tistics give us a fair indication of the popularity of traditional medicine.

The results of a survey in 1977 of some two thousand households in Suphanburi, Central Thailand, are shown in table 17.

Figures from two communes in Com Thong District, Chiangmai Province in Northern Thailand surveyed in 1976–1977 give the results shown in table 18.

A survey covering the period 1962–1965 is summarized as follows in table 19.

The Lampang Health Development Project reports the following figures for 1978 (see table 20).

We will not attempt to analyze these statistics in any detail. Suffice it to point out here that the traditional doctors have a very low score in all of them. Only 1 to 5 percent of the patients consult them. Our own experience in Northern Thailand during 1978 and 1979 points in the same direction, so to us the figures look quite reliable.

We consider the Chom Thong statistics in table 18 to be the most interesting because they contain preferences over time. The

5. Summaries from *nǎŋsýy ʔànúsɔ̌ɔn* . . . 1974:73–86.

TABLE 17

USE OF VARIOUS CURING ALTERNATIVES, SUPHANBURI, 1977

A. Percentage of respondents having ever used:[6]		
Western medicine		
Tambon (subdistrict) doctor	40	
Government health worker	58	
Medical doctor	61	
Amphoe (district) hospital	20	
Cangwat (province) hospital	62	
Private clinic	51	
Private hospital	14	
Injection doctor	38	
Traditional medicine		
Traditional doctor	40	
Spirit doctor (mawpi)	7	
Granny midwife	67	
Drugstores	98	
B. Where people prefer to go when they are sick (%):[7]		
Government hospitals, health stations	60.5	
Private hospitals, clinics	14.0	
Injection doctors	9.6	
Subtotal: Western medicine		84.1
Practitioner (maw)	2.6	
Traditional doctor	1.2	
Buddhist monk doctor	0.2	
Subtotal: Traditional medicine		4.0
Drugstore		11.4

C. Health provider gone to for most recent medical problems (%):[8]

	Minor illness	Serious medical problem
Government hospitals, health stations	21.5	65.6
Private hospitals, clinics	10.3	19.3
Injection doctors	5.2	3.7

6. Day et al. 1977:80 and 107 (figures have been rounded off).
7. Day et al. 1977:58 (condensed and rearranged).
8. Day et al. 1977:60 (condensed and rearranged).

TABLE 17 (*continued*)

USE OF VARIOUS CURING ALTERNATIVES, SUPHANBURI, 1977

Subtotal: Western medicine		37.0		88.6
Practitioner (maw)	1.6		2.3	
Traditional doctor (maw boran)	1.2		1.9	
Subtotal: Traditional medicine		2.8		4.2
Drugstores		58.0		4.5
Other		3.1		2.7

TABLE 18

USE OF VARIOUS CURING ALTERNATIVES, CHOM THONG, CHIANGMAI, 1976–1977[9] (percentages)

	First visit	Second visit	Third visit
Tambon doctor	1.0	8.9	5.5
Amphoe hospital	8.0	25.7	11.3
First-grade clinic	1.4	2.4	11.3
Midwife clinic	0.3	1.1	0.0
Private clinics	4.1	14.2	27.5
Injection doctors	2.4	17.9	11.3
Subtotal: Western medicine	17.2	70.2	66.9
Traditional doctors	1.0	1.1	5.5
Drugstore	69.4	10.9	0.0
Others	14.4	17.8	27.5

overall trend in the figures indicates that the first place to seek help is the drugstore. For the second visit, the patients prefer government hospitals, private clinics, or injection doctors. The figures for the third visit show that the majority still sticks to Western medicine, with private clinics now getting the highest score. At the same time, there is an increase in the score of traditional doctors, and particularly "others."

9. kaansỳgsǎa 1977:6 (figures have been rearranged).

TABLE 19

USE OF VARIOUS CURING ALTERNATIVES, CHIANGMAI, 1962–1965 (percent of personal visits)[10]

Modern health-care	50
Injection doctors	47
Ancient doctors	3

The statistics from Chom Thong thus show that patients often switch from one type of curer to another. Our experience indicates furthermore that none of the alternative curing methods is normally regarded as exclusive, which means that treatments commonly run in parallel. During the course of a disease a patient may very well simultanously use both various Western and traditional drugs, consult an unlicensed injection doctor, get magical treatment, and pay visits to various hospitals and clinics. This simultaneous use of several curing methods makes it extremely difficult to keep track of the sinuous curing path of the patients and, at the same time, makes it almost impossible to find out what actually cured them. Statements such as "My disease x was cured by medicine y" should therefore be taken with all possible caution and skepticism. Patients will normally not indicate (or remember) all the explanations possible but will choose the one that fits best with their worldview or

TABLE 20

USE OF VARIOUS CURING ALTERNATIVES, LAMPANG, 1978[11]

Of villagers who become ill:

50%	visit drug sellers or pharmacists
35%	go to private or state-run hospitals and clinics
15%	seek help from injectionists, herbalists, and magical healers

10. Condensed from C. E. Cunningham, ed. 1970:6–8 (precise survey area not indicated).

11. Lampang 1978:12.

prejudices, or they may answer according to the situation; that is, the answer they expect will make the investigator happy.

But beyond this "the-more-the-better" attitude to medicine, there are of course other conditions that influence the choice of curers. Certain diseases may, in the eyes of the local people, qualify for one type of curer, while other diseases qualify for other curers. In the Chom Tong statistics the patients who went directly to the herbalist on the first visit (1%) are likely to have had one of those diseases which typically require traditional treatment. One Western-trained physician said that patients with backache, nĩw, bàhòog, lídsaduaŋ, cancer, certain skin diseases, cut wounds, and mental diseases will normally seek traditional treatment.[12]

The increase to 5.5 percent for herbalists on a patient's third try for a cure is probably due to another set of factors. We have noted that many patients who turn to the traditional doctor will say that they have already been to the hospital, where the doctors recommended operation, amputation, expensive medicines, or just said that there was nothing they could do. Thus for reasons such as fear of an operation, the high cost of the treatment, or because they have nowhere else to go, people turn to the "way of nature" of the herbalists. Nowadays a sizable number of the herbalists' patients will therefore be serious cases that are difficult to cure, like cancer, or chronic diseases for which successful treatment is unlikely.

Another possible explanation for this increase is that the traditional treatment is actually more effective than the modern one, or that Western drugs have more side effects than traditional ones. People therefore prefer the traditional.

6.4. THE ATTITUDE OF THE GOVERNMENT: THE LESS THE BETTER?

The following news item clearly shows the attitude of the Ministry of Public Health toward recruitment to traditional medicine:

---

12. Dr. Somsong Raksapa, Deputy Chief, Provincial Medical Office, Lamphun. Personal communication, August 1978.

> NO GOVT NOD FOR HERBAL MEDICINE
>
> THE Public Health Ministry yesterday announced that it has never supported any schools or associations which give training in ancient medicine.
>
> Several private bodies, schools and associations have advertised that they can provide training for interested persons who will later receive special certificates for opening pharmacies or for practicing medicine.
>
> The ministry said it knew nothing about the advertisements and that a special division of the ministry was the only body allowed to issue the certificates.[13]

Furthermore, attitudes frequently met with in bureaucratic circles and among Western-trained physicians could be summarized as follows: Traditional drugs are harmless nonsense, although they make a valuable psychological supplement to Western treatment (or the unavailability of such), and at the same time give some people the means of earning a living. As traditional pharmacy poses no real competition to Western medicine and does not harm the patient, it is allowed to live, and is even encouraged. Traditional midwives and general traditional practitioners might on the other hand both harm the patient and become competitors of the Western practitioners.[14]

In section 6.2, where we discussed the recruitment to the tradition (tables 14 and 15), we noted the tremendous disparity between licenses in traditional pharmacy on one hand, and traditional medicine and midwifery on the other. One explanation for this trend is that there is money in being a traditional pharmacist, but not in practicing midwifery[15] or in being a general practitioner. Fol-

13. Bangkok Post, September 16, 1974.

14. We have the impression that at the military medical schools and in their courses there has been a relatively relaxed attitude toward traditional medicine, and we have met some doctors who have passed these medical courses and who today practice the most mixed combination of the two traditions we have encountered. In passing, it could also be mentioned that there is a heavy demand for protective measures—especially against bullet and knife wounds—among the military and the police and that there has developed an extensive magical tradition to satisfy these needs.

15. In fact, there seem to be no courses in traditional midwifery at Wat Pho anymore, but there are classes in Thai massage, although this branch of study is not registered with the Ministry of Public Health (Mulholland July 1979*a*:85).

lowing demand, the students therefore choose pharmacy. The attitude of the government, however, and the medical establishment mentioned above, together with the dwindling number of licenses in traditional medicine issued by the Ministry of Public Health, could well be interpreted to show that the ministry actively follows a policy aimed at limiting the number of general practitioners of the traditional school by making the examinations so difficult that students simply cannot pass them. We cannot confirm that this is a conscious policy of the ministry, but the facts point in that direction.

6.5. THE ATTITUDE OF WESTERN MEDICINE: SWALLOW OR INTEGRATE?

This negative—or at best indifferent—official policy toward traditional medicine is to some extent counteracted by certain tendencies on both a national and an international level.

In Thailand a growing nationalism among the elite has made traditional medicine *en vogue* in certain academic, bureaucratic, and business quarters. Some regard traditional medicine as a national heritage which is their duty to preserve, others want to use the traditional doctors to ensure better health services for the majority of the people, while others still see the possibility of using the experiences of traditional medicine to find new drugs and to start producing them to reduce the now enormous imports of Western drugs. Unfortunately these people do not seem to be interested in the tradition as a whole, but only in the pharmaceutical side of it.

These tendencies are strengthened by a worldwide trend that springs from the realization that, in the last two decades, development projects do not seem to have had the desired impact in the rural areas of the Third World. This fact, coupled with the industrialized nations' fears regarding the population explosion and economic instability, has led to an increasing interest being taken in the peasants and poor people of these areas. In the health sector, the World Health Organization (WHO) is focusing its attention on the already existing curers in the rural areas, having realized that Western medical treatment, as it is organized in most developing countries, does not reach the majority of the population. WHO and other development agencies thus favor some kind of integration of the traditional and modern health-care systems, along the Chinese model.

Even if we welcome this trend, which we hope will bring better health care to more people, we also notice a good deal of hypocrisy involved in these efforts. We believe that what basically is happening is that traditional curers are being used to serve the spread of the Western medical tradition, and that this exploitation will hasten the disintegration and destruction of the traditional medical systems.

The Lampang Health Development Project is a good example of how traditional midwives are being used to spread Western medicine. The project, which aims at expanding primary health care in Lampang province, is based on a strategy of employing local energy and talent. In respect to pre- and postnatal care and the birth itself, the project states that "cultural taboos, ignorance and lack of knowledge on the part of the parents and traditional practitioners often result in needless death."[16] Therefore traditional midwives are invited to participate in two-week courses at the Lampang Midwifery School, from which they will emerge as Traditional Birth Attendants (TBAs). The course is devoted to "aseptic techniques and modern methods of normal birth delivery, recognition of abnormal pregnancies for referral, personal hygiene, good child care practices, and nutrition for mother and child." The idea is clearly not to integrate traditional midwives with Western practices, but to make the traditional midwives into carriers of Western practices.

There are two prerequisites for any real integration in the true sense of the word. First, the parties to be integrated must be somehow equally strong, and, second, there must exist a mutual respect. None of these conditions is present. Western medicine is young, strong, and self-confident (to the point of being arrogant), endowed with official backing and the advantages derived from being part of

16. Lampang 1978:24.

an economically and culturally expanding force, while traditional medicine is old, weak, and internally rather disorganized, having no backing. And despite all lip service to, and verbalized claptrap about the tradition, Western medicine does not have any real respect for traditional medicine.

The "integration" taking place under these circumstances is bound to be on the conditions of the stronger. What is actually happening is that traditional medicine is being swallowed by the modern—the unpalatable parts being spit out or remaining undigested.

We do not want to be sentimental about the tradition, or overly sensitive about this development, but we do feel that Western culture may miss a lot, always rushing for "the juicy parts" without respect for the context and the whole. Traditional medicine is not just an overripe orange to be sucked for valuable pharmaceutical components for the immediate benefit of the Western pharmaceutical industry. It is a system belonging to a cultural tradition, and should be studied, appreciated, and used as such.

6.6. WILL HERBALISM SURVIVE?

The factors mentioned above—the recruitment to the tradition, the attitude of the government and the patients, as well as the competition from cosmopolitan medicine—are all interrelated and important for the survival of the tradition. We believe, though, that the fundamental precondition for its survival is that the practitioners of the tradition clean up their own house first. During this process, the herbalists will have to do away with secrecy and discard a lot of dogmatism and, instead, take their own practice and experience as a point of departure. It is essential for practitioners to strengthen their study of the traditional disease concepts, the relationship between the plants and the diseases, and to make the theoretical framework of the tradition more explicit. Nonherbalists can of course also do this—as we have tried to do it in this book—but to have any effect this soul-searching process must start from within. Only then can it have any impact on the tradition itself. Only then can the tradition regain its vitality.

Appendix

Compilation of Ethnobotanical Data

by
Terje Bjørnland and
Trond Schumacher

List of Medicinal Plants Collected in Chiangmai and Lamphun Provinces, Northern Thailand

The identification of the botanical material is a result of joint efforts by T. Bjørnland and T. Schumacher; critical taxa of various families have been revised by botanical colleagues as follows:

B. Hansen—Botanical Museum, University of Copenhagen - Acanthaceae
K. Larsen—Botanical Institute, University of Aarhus - Caesalpiniaceae and Zingiberaceae
I. Nielsen—Botanical Institute, University of Aarhus - Mimosaceae
R. Geesink—Rijksherbarium, Leiden - Fabaceae

Plant taxon	Vernacular[1]	Locality[2] (collection number)	Medical use(s)	Part(s) of plant used	Physical[3] quality	Preparation and administration
LICHENS:						
Usnea baileyi (Stirt.) Zahlbr.	fɔ̌ɔj lom	IIIc (341)	kɛ̃ɛ lom beŋ, kɛ̃ɛ lom phíd dyan	whole plant	indifferent	decoction per os, or decoction as vaporous bath
Usnea sp.	fɔ̌ɔj lom	XXIIId (281)	*as above*	" "	"	" " " "
PTERIDOPHYTA						
PSILOPHYTATAE						
PSILOTACEAE:						
Psilotum nudum (L.) Griseb.	wǎaj tànɔ̃ɔj	XVIc (202)	khǎaŋ, saaŋ	whole plant	indifferent	decoction as bath or vaporous bath
LYCOPODIATAE						
SELAGINELLACEAE:						
Selaginella sp.	kud fɔ̌ɔj ñãa laŋ kàj	XXIa (714)	saaŋ	whole plant	indifferent	decoction as bath or vaporous bath

EQUISETATAE						
EQUISETACEAE:						
Equisetum debile Roxb.	ñãa thɔ̀ɔd pɔ̂ŋ	Ia (405) XVIc (201) XXa (601)	nĩw, ñîaw khad	whole plant	indifferent	decoction per os
POLYPODIATAE						
MARATTIACEAE:						
Angiopteris erecta Hoffm.	kìib máa lom	IIIb (311)	lídsaduan twaan, bàhòog kõn pûud	root	indifferent	decoction per os
SCHIZACEAE:						
Lygodium flexuosum (L.) Sw.	kùud kɔ̀ɔŋ	IIId (552)	saaŋ	whole plant	indifferent	fresh, soaked in water, as bath or per os
SALVINIACEAE:						
Salvinia sp.	kǎa kɔ̀ɔg hǔu nǔu	XVIe (430)	luˀ tɔ́ɔŋ	whole plant	cool	fresh, soaked in water, per os, or decoction per os
SPERMATOPHYTA PINOPHYTINA						
CYCADATAE						
CYCADACEAE:						
Cycas sp.	bàpáaw tàw dɔɔj	XVIa (196)	jaa kɛ̃ɛ kǐn phid	root	indifferent	dried, ground, per os
PINATAE						
CUPRESSACEAE:						
Cupressus sempervirens L.	sǒn ciin	XXa (456)	kɛ̃ɛ ˀaj	cone	indifferent	decoction per os
PINACEAE:						
Pinus kesiya Gord.	sǒn kíaˀ	XXIIa (442)	kɛ̃ɛ ˀaj, fǐi	cone resin of bark	indifferent	decoction per os fresh, applied topically
PODOCARPACEAE:						
Podocarpus neriifolius D. Don	máj sílâa sɛ̀ɛ	XIXa (633)	khǎaŋ pɔ̀ɔŋ	whole plant	indifferent	decoction per os or as vaporous bath

LIST OF MEDICINAL PLANTS COLLECTED IN CHIANGMAI AND LAMPHUN PROVINCES, NORTHERN THAILAND (*continued*)

The identification of the botanical material is a result of joint efforts by T. Bjørnland and T. Schumacher; critical taxa of various families have been revised by botanical colleagues as follows:

B. Hansen—Botanical Museum, University of Copenhagen - Acanthaceae
K. Larsen—Botanical Institute, University of Aarhus - Caesalpiniaceae and Zingiberaceae
I. Nielsen—Botanical Institute, University of Aarhus - Mimosaceae
R. Geesink—Rijksherbarium, Leiden - Fabaceae

Plant taxon	Vernacular[1]	Locality[2] (collection number)	Medical use(s)	Part(s) of plant used	Physical[3] quality	Preparation and administration
MAGNOLIOPHYTINA						
ACANTHACEAE:						
Adhatoda vasica (L.) Nees	bua laa khǎaw	VIa (2) VIh (518) VIj (587)	khǎaŋ khañyy, nedsaa	leaves whole plant	warm	dried, crushed, per os dried, crushed, applied topically
Chroestes lanceolata (T. And.) B. Hansen	hɔ̂ɔm cáaŋ	XVIIc (725)	nedsaa, nedsỹŋ, kìaw, ceb tɔ́ɔŋ	whole plant whole plant	warm	dried, crushed, applied topically decoction per os
Crossandra infundibuliformis (L.) Nees	sǒŋ kɔɔlánii	VIIIj (423)	kǐn phid, maw hǔa	root	indifferent	dried, ground, per os
Eranthemum tetragonum Nees	hɔ̂ɔm cáaŋ	IIId (541)	nedsaa, nedsỹŋ, kìaw, ceb tɔ́ɔŋ	whole plant whole plant	warm	dried, crushed, applied topically decoction per os
Gendarussa vulgaris Nees	bua laa dam	XIIIa (190) IXb (225) VIIIf (302)	nedsaa, nedsỹŋ, jaa salǐimuun, láduu bà maa, khwaam dan	whole plant leaves, stem whole plant	warm	dried, crushed, soaked in water, applied topically dried, crushed, per os decoction per os

Pseuderanthemum andersonii (Mast.) Lindau	phájáb mêeg	XVIIa (481)	?	?	?	?
Rhinacanthus nasutus (L.) Kurz	ñãa man kàj	Xa (175) XVIe (432)	khwaam dan, kẽɛ nɔɔn bà lab	leaves, stem	indifferent	decoction per os
Ruellia tuberosa L.	ñãa lɔ́b lɛ̂ɛb	VId (125)	khãj	root	indifferent	decoction per os
Tetraglochidium cf. maingayi (Cl.) Brem.	hɔ̂ɔm cáaŋ dam	XXa (590)	kìaw, ceb tɔ́ɔŋ	whole plant	warm	decoction per os
	hɔ̂ɔm cáaŋ khǎaw	XXa (591)				
Thunbergia hossei C. B. Clarke	nǎam nɛ̂ɛ, laŋ cỳyd	XVIIa (488)	khãj, hɔ́ɔn naj,	bark, wood	indifferent	decoction per os
Thunbergia laurifolia Lindl.	nǎam nɛ̂ɛ, laŋ cỳyd	VIIIb (68) VIIIc (109) Xa (160) XXIVa (459)	ŋuu khob, kẽɛ cám	leaves	indifferent	chew fresh leaves, swallow the juice, apply the leaves topically
ALZOACEAE:						
Mollugo pentaphylla L.	ñãa tĩin nóg	VIIIc (95)	khãj, hɔ́ɔn naj	whole plant	indifferent khom	decoction per os
AMARANTHACEAE:						
Achyranthes aspera L.	ñãa khuaj ŋuu	XIIIa (183)	khãj, nĩw, ñîaw khad	whole plant root	indifferent	decoction per os decoction per os
Achyranthes bidentata Bl.	ñãa khuaj ŋuu	VIIIk (477)	khãj, nĩw, ñîaw khad	whole plant root	indifferent	decoction per os decoction per os
Aerva sanguinolenta (L.) Bl.	ñãa hǔa ped	XVIIa (496)	jaa tâad	flowers	indifferent	dried, crushed, per os
Alternanthera sessilis (L.) DC.	hɔ̂ɔm kìaw ŋən	VIIIg (353)	kìaw, tɔ́ɔŋ tẽn	whole plant	warm	decoction per os
Alternanthera sp.	phag pìaw	VIIIb (77)	jaa tâad	root	cool	decoction per os
Amaranthus spinosus L.	phag hǒm nǎam	IXc (383)	khĩi hâag	root	cool	fresh, soaked in water, solution per os
Celosia argentea L.	dãaj nám	VIj (585)	lom sǎan	whole plant	cool	dried, crushed, per os
Celosia cristata L.	dãaj ŋɔ̃ɔn kàj	VIIIf (289)	khĩi hâag	root	indifferent	fresh, soaked in water, solution per os

The identification of the botanical material is a result of joint efforts by T. Bjørnland and T. Schumacher; critical taxa of various families have been revised by botanical colleagues as follows:

B. Hansen—Botanical Museum, University of Copenhagen - Acanthaceae
K. Larsen—Botanical Institute, University of Aarhus - Caesalpiniaceae and Zingiberaceae
I. Nielsen—Botanical Institute, University of Aarhus - Mimosaceae
R. Geesink—Rijksherbarium, Leiden - Fabaceae

Plant taxon	Vernacular[1]	Locality[2] (collection number)	Medical use(s)	Part(s) of plant used	Physical[3] quality	Preparation and administration
Cyathula prostrata (L.) Bl.	ñãa khuaj ŋuu nɔ́ɔj	VIa (19)	khāj,	whole plant	indifferent	decoction per os
		VIi (529)	nīw, ñîaw khad	root		decoction per os
Gomphrena globosa L.	tàlɔ̄ɔm, dɔ̀ɔg dāaj tàlɔ̄ɔm	IXb (212)	khāj	root	indifferent	decoction, or dried, ground, per os
AMARYLLIDACEAE:						
Allium sativum L.	hɔ̌ɔm tiam	VIIIc (92)	lom phid dyan, piʔ, kìaw, sǎan, fɔ̂ɔg lŷad	bulb	warm	decoction per os
Crinum asiaticum L.	bua bog, lii lua	VIa (9)	nedsaa, nedsŷŋ	stem	warm	cut into pieces, warmed up, applied topically
ANACARDIACEAE:						
Anacardium occidentale L.	mámûaŋ hìmáphaan	VIIIm (661)	khāj, khǎaŋ	bark	indifferent	dried, ground, or decoction per os
Bouea oppositifolia (Roxb.) Meissn.	bàphǎaŋ	VIIIf (298)	khǎaŋ	bark	indifferent	dried, ground, per os
Melanorrhoea usitata Wall.	máj hág khīi mǔu	XXIVa (468)	kǐn phid,	bark	indifferent	dried, ground, per os
	máj hág lǔaŋ	VIIa (653)	khǎaŋ	bark	indifferent	dried, ground, per os

Semecarpus cf. curtisii King	mámûaŋ pàa, mámûaŋ nóg	XXIa (712)	lom phid dyan	bark, wood	indifferent	dried, ground, per os
Semecarpus sp.	máj hág lŭaŋ	IIIa (316)	khăaŋ	bark	indifferent	dried, ground, per os
Spondias pinnata (L. f.) Kurz	bàkɔ̀ɔg myaŋ, bàkɔ̀ɔg	XIIa (515)	kε̃ε lom, kĭn phid, khāj, maw hŭa	bark	cool	dried, ground, per os
ANNONACEAE:						
Anomianthus dulcis (Dunal) J. Sincl.	nom ŋua	VIIIa (41)	lídsaduaŋ naj lam sāj,	wood, root	indifferent	decoction per os
		IIa (267)	kīw, bàhòog lŷad			
Artabotrys uncinatus (Lam.) Merr.	sàbanŋaa tāj	VIIIg (365)	bàhòog,	root	indifferent	decoction per os
			kε̃ε lom	wood, bark		dried, ground, per os
Cananga odorata (Lam.) Hook. f. et Thoms.	sàbanŋaa	VIe (206)	kε̃ε lom	" "	"	" " " "
Ellipeiopsis cherrevensis (Finet et Gagnep.) R. E. Fries	nom mεεw	XXIVa (463)	bàhòog lŷad	root	indifferent	decoction per os
Fissistigma polyanthoides (DC.) Merr.	sàbanŋaa khya	IIIe (691)	bàhòog, kε̃ε lom	wood, bark	indifferent	decoction per os
Miliusa velutina Hook. f. et Thoms.	khăaŋ hŭa mŭu	IXb (220)	khăaŋ	wood, bark	indifferent	dried, ground, per os, or applied topically as powder
Polyalthia debilis Finet et Gagnep.	tàb tàw nɔ̆ɔj	IIa (250)	khăaŋ,	root	indifferent	dried, ground, per os
			tɔ́ɔŋ tēn, jaa tâad	root		decoction per os
APIACEAE:						
Centella asiatica (L.) Urban	phag nɔ̀ɔg	VIIIc (118)	khāj, hɔ́ɔn naj	whole plant	indifferent	dried, crushed, per os
Eryngium foetidum L.	phag chii kàlìaŋ	VIIIc (114)	satog, jaa tâad	whole plant	indifferent	dried, crushed, per os
APOCYNACEAE:						
Amalocalyx microlobus Pierre in Spire	khya ceen lŭaŋ	VIIIc (117)	bàhòog, ñîaw khad, ceb lăŋ cebˀεw	whole plant	indifferent	decoction per os

The identification of the botanical material is a result of joint efforts by T. Bjørnland and T. Schumacher; critical taxa of various families have been revised by botanical colleagues as follows:

B. Hansen—Botanical Museum, University of Copenhagen - Acanthaceae
K. Larsen—Botanical Institute, University of Aarhus - Caesalpiniaceae and Zingiberaceae
I. Nielsen—Botanical Institute, University of Aarhus - Mimosaceae
R. Geesink—Rijksherbarium, Leiden - Fabaceae

Plant taxon	Vernacular[1]	Locality[2] (collection number)	Medical use(s)	Part(s) of plant used	Physical[3] quality	Preparation and administration
Ervatamia divaricata (L.) Burk.	málíʔdin	IIId (536)	kǐn phid, lom phid dyan (emeticum)	whole plant	indifferent	dried, crushed, per os
Holarrhena antidysenterica DC.	mûug man lǔaŋ	VIIIa (39) IXb (234)	khǎaŋ, bàhòog	bark, wood	indifferent	dried, ground, per os
Plumeria sp.	cǎmpǎa laaw	XVIa (34)	fǐi	latex	warm	fresh latex applied topically
Rauwolfia serpentina Kurz	jɔ̂m tǐin mǎa, cáaŋ jâm pə̂ə	VIIIa (56) VIIIc (111)	jaa kɛ̃ɛ, lom piʔ, bamluŋ hǔa cǎj	root	indifferent	decoction per os
Thevetia peruviana. (Pers.) K. Schum.	sɛ̀ɛ sǎalaa	XVa (197)	fǐi	latex	warm	fresh latex applied topically
			nīw	root		decoction per os
Wrightia tomentosa Roem. et Schult.	máj mûug man nɔ́ɔj	XIIa (505)	bàhòog, bàhòog lŷad	bark, wood, root	indifferent	decoction per os
Wrightia cf. viridiflora Kerr	máj mûug man lǔaŋ	XIIa (507)	bàhòog lŷad,	bark	indifferent	decoction per os
			bàhòog, khǎaŋ	bark, wood, root		dried, ground, per os
ARACEAE:						
Acorus gramineus W. Ait.	haŋ khaaw	VIa (15)	khāj, hɔ́ɔn naj	whole plant	cool	dried, ground, per os or applied topically on throat
		VIIIe (271)	sǎan	whole plant		dried, crushed, per os

Aglaonema sp.	puu cáaŋ nɔ́ɔj	XVIIa (499)	fĭi	stem	indifferent	chopped into pieces, applied topically
Alocasia cf. alba Schott	kàdàad	XIXa (625)	khăaŋ	root	cool	dried, ground, per os
Amorphophallus sp. 1.	hŭa bug, bug wăan	IXa (133)	?	?	?	?
Amorphophallus sp. 2.	bug mŭu	IXa (157)	?	?	?	?
Arisaema sp. 1.	hŭa khâw khâa	XXIIIc (374)	jaa tâad, khab lŷad	root	warm	dried, ground, per os
Arisaema sp. 2	hŭa khâw khâa	XXIIa (444)	khāj, jaa tâad, khab lŷad	root	warm	dried, ground, per os
Colocasia esculenta (L.) Schott var. antiquorum (Schott) Hubb & Rehder	kàdàad	VIe (207)	khăaŋ	root	cool	dried, ground, per os
Lasia spinosa (L.) Thw.	phag năam	Ia (403)	khāj, ceb hŭa, maw hŭa, fĭi	root root	indifferent	dried, ground, per os dried, crushed, applied topically
Pistia stratiotes L.	kăa kɔ̀ɔg	XIVb (438)	luʔ tɔ́ɔŋ	leaves	cool	fresh, soaked in water, per os
Pothos cathcarti Schott	tuŋ wáʔ	IIIe (704)	saaŋ	whole plant	indifferent	decoction as vaporous bath
Pothos sp.	cag kheb	XVIIa (502)	sad khob, mɛɛŋ khob	whole plant	warm	fresh, applied topically
Scindapsus officinalis Schott	puu cáaŋ	XVIIa (487)	fĭi	root	cool	dried, ground, applied topically
Typhonium trilobatum (L.) Schott	bɔɔn bɛ̀ɛw	VIa (17)	fĭi	root	indifferent	chopped into pieces, applied topically
ARALIACEAE:						
Macropanax sp. 1.	ʔɔ̄ɔj cáaŋ	XIXa (615)	bàhòog phanládii	bark, wood	indifferent sweet	dried, ground, or decoction, per os
Macropanax sp. 2.	mákhùaŋ doŋ	XXVIIc (721)	ceb tɔ́ɔŋ	fruit	indifferent	dried, crushed, per os
Polyscias fruticosa (L.) Harms.	léb khúd, bàkhúd	VIa (8) VIj (586)	lom bàheŋkhúd	leaves, root	indifferent	dried, crushed, per os, or fresh, soaked in water to wash the face
Trevesia palmata (Roxb. ex Lindl.) Vis.	táaŋ pàa	XVIIb (567) XVIIc (726)	sàníbàad cág lom phid dyan	root bark, wood	indifferent	dried, ground, per os dried, ground, per os

The identification of the botanical material is a result of joint efforts by T. Bjørnland and T. Schumacher; critical taxa of various families have been revised by botanical colleagues as follows:

B. Hansen—Botanical Museum, University of Copenhagen - Acanthaceae
K. Larsen—Botanical Institute, University of Aarhus - Caesalpiniaceae and Zingiberaceae
I. Nielsen—Botanical Institute, University of Aarhus - Mimosaceae
R. Geesink—Rijksherbarium, Leiden - Fabaceae

Plant taxon	Vernacular[1]	Locality[2] (collection number)	Medical use(s)	Part(s) of plant used	Physical[3] quality	Preparation and administration
ARECACEAE:						
Borassus flabellifer L.	taan tànòod	XIIIa (199)	lom phid dyan	fruit	indifferent	dried, crushed, per os
Caryota mitis Lour.	kǐaŋ	XIIIa (195)	tùm khan	wood (marrow)	indifferent	fresh, applied topically
Phoenix acaulis Roxb.	pùm pêŋ	XVIIIa (603)	ceb tɔ́ɔŋ, luʔ tɔ́ɔŋ	root	indifferent	dried, ground, per os
ASCLEPIADACEAE:						
Calotropis gigantea (Willd.) W. T. Ait.	pàn thŷan	VIh (526)	khǎaŋ khañyy, fii	root latex	warm	decoction per os fresh, applied topically
Dischidia rafflesiana Wall.	kòod phuŋ plaa, kũaj máj	IXa (154)	saaŋ	leaves	indifferent	roasted leaves, per os
Myriopteron paniculatum Griff.	ʔɔ̃ɔj sǎam sǔan, ʔɔ̃ɔj sɛ̌ɛn sǔan	IXb (224) VIf (280)	khǎaŋ, khĩi hâag, kɛ̃ɛ lom, kɛ̃ɛ lom sàníbàad, jaa tâad	stem root stem stem	indifferent	dried, crushed, per os dried, ground, per os dried, crushed, by os decoction per os

Streptocaulon griffithii Hook. f.	khya ceen nɔ́ɔj	IIa (243)	cebˀɛw, ñîaw khad	whole plant	indifferent	decoction per os
Toxocarpus sp. 1.	khya ceen nɔ́ɔj	VIIIb (84)	ñîaw khad	" "	"	" " "
Toxocarpus sp. 2.	khya ceen lǔaŋ	VIIa (648)	cebˀɛw, bàhòog, ñîaw khad	whole plant	indifferent	decoction per os
Wattakaka volubilis (L.) Stapf.	phag húan mǔu	IXb (213)	khãj, sad khob, mɛɛŋ khob	leaves stem	indifferent	dried, crushed, per os dried, crushed, applied topically
Zygostelma benthamii Baill.	khya ceen nɔ́ɔj khǎaw	VIIIh (391)	ceb hǔa, cebˀɛw	stem	indifferent	decoction per os
ASTERACEAE:						
Ageratum conyzoides L.	sàab kǎa	XXIIa (455)	khãj jaa tâad	root whole plant	indifferent	decoction per os dried, crushed, per os
Anaphalis adnata DC.	nàad ŋən	XXIIa (446)	jaa tâad	whole plant	indifferent	dried, crushed, per os
Bidens pilosa L.	phag phed kuulaa	IIIa (308)	jaa tâad	whole plant	warm	dried, crushed, per os
Blumea cf. balsamifera DC.	nàad lǔaŋ	XVIb (59)	jaa tâad	whole plant	indifferent	dried, crushed, per os
Blumea clarkei Hook. f.	pàa hêw mɔ̌ɔŋ	XVIIb (581)	jaa tâad, phɔ̌ɔm hɛ̌ɛŋ lɛɛŋ nɔ́ɔj, khãj	leaves root	indifferent	dried, crushed, per os decoction per os
Blumea lanceolaria (Roxb.) Druce	lǔa sǎam kwian	XVIIc (723)	bàhòog, ceb laŋ cebˀɛw, jaa bamluŋ kǎmlaŋ	root	indifferent	decoction per os
Elephanthopus scaber L.	ñãa sǎam sib sɔ̌ɔŋ hâag	IIId (540)	jaa bamluŋ kǎmlaŋ	root	indifferent	decoction per os
Eupatorium odoratum L.	ñãa myaŋ waaj	XVIIa (486)	khwaam dan, samǎan phɛ̌ɛ	root leaves	indifferent	decoction per os fresh, applied topically
Inula cappa (D. Don.) DC.	nàad kham	IXa (145) XXIIa (452)	jaa tâad	leaves, root	indifferent	dried, crushed, per os
	nàad ŋən	IXc (380)	jaa tâad	whole plant	indifferent	dried, crushed, per os
Inula cf. polygonata DC.	nàad ŋən	Ia (402)	jaa tâad	whole plant	indifferent	dried, crushed, per os
Microglossa pyrifolia (Lam.) O. Ktze.	phakaa kɔɔŋ pàa	IIIe (688)	khǎaŋ lammánâad	bark, wood	indifferent	decoction per os

The identification of the botanical material is a result of joint efforts by T. Bjørnland and T. Schumacher; critical taxa of various families have been revised by botanical colleagues as follows:

B. Hansen—Botanical Museum, University of Copenhagen - Acanthaceae
K. Larsen—Botanical Institute, University of Aarhus - Caesalpiniaceae and Zingiberaceae
I. Nielsen—Botanical Institute, University of Aarhus - Mimosaceae
R. Geesink—Rijksherbarium, Leiden - Fabaceae

Plant taxon	Vernacular[1]	Locality[2] (collection number)	Medical use(s)	Part(s) of plant used	Physical[3] quality	Preparation and administration
Saussurea sp.	phag pāŋ	XXa (597)	khǎaŋ luˀ tɔ́ɔŋ	root	indifferent	decoction per os
Senecio cf. nagensium C. B. Clarke	nàad phaa	XXIIIa (369)	jaa tâad, jaa bamluŋ kǎmlaŋ	root	indifferent	decoction per os
Sonchus sp.	phag phed pàa	XXa (595)	jaa ˀaajúˀ wádthánáˀ	flowers	indifferent	dried, crushed, per os
Vernonia cinerea (L.) Less.	ñāa sǎam wan ñāa láˀɔ̄ɔŋ fáa	VIk (669)	khǎj pāaŋ	whole plant	indifferent	decoction per os
Vernonia elaeagnifolia DC.	láan phǐi pāaj sɛ̌ɛn phǐi klua	VIa (643)	kǐn phid	bark, wood, root	indifferent	dried, ground, per os
Vernonia cf. kingii C. B. Clarke	lǔa sǎam kwian	XXIIb (677)	bàhòog, ceb laŋ cebˀɛw jaa bamluŋ kǎmlaŋ	bark, wood, root	indifferent	decoction per os dried, crushed, per os
Vernonia parishii Hook. f.	nàad kham	IIIc (338)	jaa bamluŋ kǎmlaŋ, jaa ˀaajúˀ wádthána, jaa tâad	leaves, root	indifferent	dried, crushed, per os
Vernonia cf. sutepensis Kerr	lǔa sǎam kwian	XVIIa (495)	bàhòog, ceb laŋ cebˀɛw, jaa bamluŋ kǎmlaŋ	bark, wood, root	indifferent	decoction per os
Vernonia volkameriaefolia DC.	máj sāan	XIXa (611)	khǎaŋ	bark, wood	indifferent	dried, ground, per os

Vernonia sp.	jaa kɛ̃ɛ tõn diaw	XIXa (612)	jaa bamluŋ kămlaŋ, lom phid dyan	whole plant stem	indifferent	decoction per os dried, crushed, per os
Vicoa indica (L.) DC.	khwaaj săam ŋăan	XXIVa (462)	jaa bamluŋ kămlaŋ	whole plant	indifferent	decoction per os
Asteraceae *indeterm.*	phag kàad kòb	VIIIc (100)	fíi, ŋuu khob	whole plant	indifferent	crushed, applied topically, chewed, juice swallowed, remnants applied topically
BALSAMINACEAE:						
Impatiens cf. psittacina Hook. f.	lɔb lɛb dɛɛŋ	IIIa (319)	năŋ mãj	leaves	indifferent	fresh, applied topically
BERBERIDACEAE:						
Mahonia siamensis Takeda	ŋîaŋ păa dug	XXIIb (675)	kĭn phid	bark, wood	indifferent	dried, ground, per os
BETULACEAE:						
Betula alnoides Buch.-Ham. in D. Don	kămlaŋ sўa khôoŋ, lɛ̃ɛn hàj	IIId (544)	jaa bamluŋ kămlaŋ, jaa tâad	bark	indifferent	decoction per os
Betula sp.	padcamaw	XXa (598)	lom săan	bark, wood	indifferent	dried, crushed, per os
BIGNONIACEAE:						
Millingtonia hortensis L. f.	kăa sàlɔɔŋ	Xa (161)	kĭn phid (emeticum)	bark, root	indifferent	dried, ground, per os
Oroxylum indicum (L.) Vent.	máléd máj	XVIa (35)	jaa tâad, jaa ˀaajúˀ wádtháná?	bark	warm	dried, crushed, per os
BIXACEAE:						
Bixa orellana L.	bàkaaj ñŭm	VIIIa (53)	thàaj pháñâad	fruit	indifferent	dried, crushed, per os
BOMBACACEAE:						
Bombax ceiba L.	tĭin ped	VIIIm (660)	khăaŋ	bark, wood	indifferent	dried, ground, per os

LIST OF MEDICINAL PLANTS COLLECTED IN CHIANGMAI AND LAMPHUN PROVINCES, NORTHERN THAILAND (*continued*)

The identification of the botanical material is a result of joint efforts by T. Bjørnland and T. Schumacher; critical taxa of various families have been revised by botanical colleagues as follows:

B. Hansen—Botanical Museum, University of Copenhagen - Acanthaceae
K. Larsen—Botanical Institute, University of Aarhus - Caesalpiniaceae and Zingiberaceae
I. Nielsen—Botanical Institute, University of Aarhus - Mimosaceae
R. Geesink—Rijksherbarium, Leiden - Fabaceae

Plant taxon	Vernacular[1]	Locality[2] (collection number)	Medical use(s)	Part(s) of plant used	Physical[3] quality	Preparation and administration
BRASSICACEAE:						
Brassica sp.	máléd phag kòod	VIIIg (361)	bamluŋ hŭa căj	seeds	indifferent	dried, crushed, per os
BROMELIACEAE:						
Ananas comosus (L.) Merr.	bàkhànád	VIIIf (286)	nīw, măa wɔ̄ɔ khob	root leaves	indifferent	decoction per os fresh, applied topically
BUDDLEJACEAE:						
Buddleja asiatica Lour.	pùag nám	XXa (593)	nīw	root	indifferent	decoction per os
CAESALPINIACEAE:						
Afzelia xylocarpa Craib	mákhâa hŭa kham	XVId (406)	jaa thìib khāj, jaa thìib píd	seeds	indifferent	dried, ground, per os
Bauhinia purpurea L.	sôm sīaw	VIIIh (385)	jaa tâad, khăaŋ	bark "	indifferent	decoction per os dried, ground, per os
Bauhinia variegata L.	máj sīaw	IIIe (700)	khăaŋ	bark	indifferent	dried, ground, per os
Bauhinia viridescens Desv.	sôm sīaw naa	IXa (150)	jaa tâad	bark	indifferent	decoction per os

Caesalpinia digyna Rottler	năam căaj, mákhĭi hɛ̆ɛd	VIIIc (96)	săan, fĭi săan naj tɔ́ɔŋ,	root	indifferent	dried, ground, or decoction per os
		IIa (241) VIIIm (658)	khăaŋ	wood		fresh, chewed, applied topically in mouth
	năam pùu ñâa	IXc (382)	tăa dɛɛŋ	whole plant	indifferent	infusion as eye bath
Caesalpinia pulcherrima (L.) Sw.	sɔɔmphɔɔ lÿaŋ	VIIIf (292)	lídsaduaŋ naj lam sāj, bàhòog lŷad	root	indifferent	decoction per os
Caesalpinia sappan L.	máj fāaŋ	Xa (164)	bàhòog lŷad	wood	indifferent	decoction per os
Caesalpinia sp.	khĭi leg pàa	IXa (130)	săan	root	indifferent	decoction per os
Cassia alata L.	léb myyn lŭaŋ	VIi (528)	jaa thàaj,	leaves	indifferent	decoction per os
			hýan nám, phaj nám, khĭi khàag	leaves		fresh, applied topically
Cassia fistula L.	lom lɛ́ɛŋ	IIa (249)	khăaŋ khañyy,	leaves	indifferent	dried, crushed, per os
		VIh (520)	khăaŋ lammánâad	bark		fresh, chewed, applied topically in mouth
Cassia javanica L.	kăaláphýg	VIIIg (362)	fĭi	bark, wood	indifferent	dried, ground, applied topically
		XVIe (433)	khāj	〃 〃		dried, ground, per os
Cassia occidentalis L.	léb myyn lŭaŋ	VIIIf (300)	khāj	root	indifferent	decoction per os
Cassia siamea Lam.	khĭi leg	VIIId (237)	jaa thàaj	seeds	indifferent	decoction per os
Cassia tora L.	léb myyn nɔ́ɔj	VIIIb (72)	khāj	root	indifferent	decoction per os
	léb myyn	VIIIg (364)	〃	〃		〃 〃 〃
Delonix regia (Hook. f.) Rafin.	somphɔɔ tāj	VIIIf (288)	lídsaduaŋ, bàhòog lŷad	root	indifferent	decoction per os
Peltophorum dasyrhachis Baker in Hook. f.	săan kham	VIIIg (367)	fĭi săan naj tɔ́ɔŋ, lom săan	bark, wood	indifferent	decoction per os
Saraca bijuga Prain	kàsôm chûn, sōm cŷn	VIIIc (120)	jaa bamluŋ hŭa cǎj,	bark	indifferent	dried, crushed, per os
			lom	flowers		dried, crushed, powder as inhalant
Tamarindus indica L.	bàkhăam	XVIIa (482)	piʔ	pericarp (of fruit)		dried, crushed, per os
Caesalpiniaceae *indeterm.*	săan ŋən	VIIIg (368)	phaj, tùm,	bark	indifferent	dried, ground, per os
			lom săan, fĭi săan naj tɔ́ɔŋ	bark, wood		decoction per os

The identification of the botanical material is a result of joint efforts by T. Bjørnland and T. Schumacher; critical taxa of various families have been revised by botanical colleagues as follows:

B. Hansen—Botanical Museum, University of Copenhagen - Acanthaceae
K. Larsen—Botanical Institute, University of Aarhus - Caesalpiniaceae and Zingiberaceae
I. Nielsen—Botanical Institute, University of Aarhus - Mimosaceae
R. Geesink—Rijksherbarium, Leiden - Fabaceae

Plant taxon	Vernacular[1]	Locality[2] (collection number)	Medical use(s)	Part(s) of plant used	Physical[3] quality	Preparation and administration
CANNABACEAE:						
Cannabis sativa L. var. indica (Lam.) C. B. Clarke	kanchaa	VIIIg (356) VIIIh (395)	*stimulant*	leaves	indifferent	dried, smoked as inhalant
CANNACEAE:						
Canna glauca L.	bua láwoŋ dɔ́ɔg lỹaŋ	VIIa (646)	lom khȳn	root	indifferent	dried, ground, per os
CAPPARACEAE:						
Capparis sepiaria L.	nǎam léb mɛɛw	VIIIb (67) IXb (223)	kĭn phid	root	indifferent	dried, ground, per os
Capparis cf. zeylanica L.	léb mɛɛw nɔ́ɔj	IXb (221)	kĭn phid	root	indifferent	dried, ground, per os
CAPRIFOLIACEAE:						
Sambucus javanica Bl.	dɔ̀ɔg ʔuun	VIIIb (64)	kĭn phid	root	indifferent	dried, ground, per os
Viburnum inopinatum Craib	dɔ̀ɔg ʔuun pàa	IIId (555)	khǎaŋ lammánâad	bark, wood	indifferent	fresh, chewed, applied topically

CELASTRACEAE:						
Celastrus cf. paniculatus Willd.	bàtὲεg	IXb (228)	bàhòog, lídsaduaŋ	root	indifferent	decoction per os
Euonymus cf. colonoides Craib	máj nóg khɔ̀ɔ	XVIIc (717)	khăaŋ	bark	indifferent	dried, ground, per os
Lophopetalum wallichii Kurz	kămlaŋ ŋua thə̌əŋ	XVIa (51) XVId (407)	jaa bamluŋ kămlaŋ jaa tâad	bark	indifferent	decoction per os
	cáaŋ phỳag	VIIa (650)	luˀ tɔ́ɔŋ, thàaj pháñâad	bark	indifferent	decoction per os
CLEOMACEAE:						
Cleome gynandra L.	phag sīan bāan	VIIIb (78)	*edible*	whole plant	indifferent	
Cleome viscosa L.	sōm sīan phĭi	VIIIb (79)	khăaŋ, khăaŋ khañyy, khĭi khûu	root	indifferent	dried, ground, per os
CLUSIACEAE:						
Garcinia cf. delpyana Pierre	bàdan	VIIIg (366)	khàad wídtamin sii, khāj	fruit	indifferent	dried, crushed, per os
Mesua ferrea L.	bun nâag	Xa (159)	bamluŋ hŭa căj	flowers	indifferent	dried, crushed, per os or as inhalant
COMBRETACEAE:						
Calycopteris floribunda Lam.	tĭin tàŋ	IVa (638)	bàhòog	bark, wood	indifferent	decoction per os
Combretum latifolium Bl.	hε̌εn khya	XIIIa (187) XXIa (710)	khăan, khăaŋ hɔ́ɔn khɔɔ	bark, wood " "	indifferent	dried, ground, per os decoction per os or dried, ground, applied topically in mouth
Combretum quadrangulare Kurz	sàkεε, phε̂εŋ	VId (126)	khăaŋ, kĭn phid, fĭi	bark, wood bark	indifferent	dried, ground, per os dried, crushed, applied topically
		VIIIf (301)	luˀ tɔ́ɔŋ	bark	indifferent	dried, ground, or decoction per os
		IVa (635)	nĩw	bark, wood		decoction per os

The identification of the botanical material is a result of joint efforts by T. Bjørnland and T. Schumacher; critical taxa of various families have been revised by botanical colleagues as follows:

B. Hansen—Botanical Museum, University of Copenhagen - Acanthaceae
K. Larsen—Botanical Institute, University of Aarhus - Caesalpiniaceae and Zingiberaceae
I. Nielsen—Botanical Institute, University of Aarhus - Mimosaceae
R. Geesink—Rijksherbarium, Leiden - Fabaceae

Plant taxon	Vernacular[1]	Locality[2] (collection number)	Medical use(s)	Part(s) of plant used	Physical[3] quality	Preparation and administration
Combretum cf. sundaicum Miq.	khāw mīn khya	XIXa (629)	tǎa lŷaŋ	bark, wood	indifferent	decoction per os
Terminalia bellerica (Gaertn.) Roxb.	hɛ̌ɛn tōn	IXa (136)	khǎaŋ	bark	indifferent	dried, ground, or decoction per os
			khǎaŋ pàag pỳaj	fruit		applied topically (lips)
Terminalia chebula Retz	bàná?	VIIIa (42)	sǎan, jaa thàaj	fruit	indifferent	dried, ground, per os
CONNARACEAE:						
Connarus semidecandrus Jack.	khǎaŋ dɛɛŋ	IIId (556)	khǎaŋ	bark, wood	indifferent	dried, ground, per os
Ellipanthus tomentosus Kurz	máj mûug man nɔ́ɔj	VIIa (652)	bàhòog	bark, root	indifferent	decoction per os
CONVOLVULACEAE:						
Argyreia mollis (Burm. f.) Choisy	cǐi cɔ̄ɔ lǔaŋ	Ia (400)	khāj, lu? tɔ́ɔŋ	root whole plant	indifferent	decoction per os " " "

Argyreia cf. osyrensis (Roth) Choisy in DC.	mǔu pɔ̀j	IIa (261)	jaa tâad, jaa ʔaajúʔ wádtháná?	stem, leaves	indifferent	dried, crushed, per os
Argyreia sp. 1.	cǐi cɔ̃ɔ lǔaŋ	IIIc (342)	khãj, luʔ tɔ́ɔŋ	root whole plant	indifferent	decoction per os " " "
	mǔu pɔ̀j	XXIVa (467)	jaa tâad, jaa ʔaajúʔ wádtháná?	stem, leaves	indifferent	dried, crushed, per os
Argyreia sp. 2.	cǐi cɔ̃ɔ lǔaŋ	Ia (408)	khãj luʔ tɔ́ɔŋ	root whole plant	indifferent	decoction per os " " "
Ipomoea obscura (L.) Ker-Gawl.	ñaa tooŋ wáʔ	VIIIi (392)	tǎa dɛɛŋ	whole plant	indifferent	soaked in water, solution applied topically (eyes)
Ipomoea cf. trilobata L.	cǐi cɔ̃ɔ bãan	VIIIk (474)	tɔ́ɔŋ sǐa	whole plant	indifferent	decoction per os
Porana racemosa Roxb.	khya nám myg	IIId (558)	mỹn	whole plant	indifferent	soaked in water, solution as bath (topically)
CUCURBITACEAE:						
Gymnopetalum cochinchinense (Lour.) Kurz	bànɔɔj caa	IIa (239)	hɔ́ɔn naj	fruit	indifferent	fresh, per os
Luffa cylindrica (L.) Roem.	bùab khǒm	IXc (384)	khĩi haŋkɛɛ	fruit	indifferent	fresh, soaked in water, solution applied topically
Solena cf. heterophylla Lour.	tɛ̌ɛŋ thỳan	IIa (264)	jaa tâad, jaa ʔaajúʔ wádtháná?	whole plant	indifferent	dried, crushed, per os
Trichosanthes rubriflos Cayla	thǎw wan prîaw	IIIa (303)	khãj	whole plant fruit	indifferent	dried, crushed, per os decoction per os
Trichosanthes tricuspidata Lour.	phag sàab	IIIa (305)	hɔ́ɔn naj	fruit	cool	fresh, mashed, applied topically on head
		IIId (530)	khĩi khòog khĩi haŋkɛɛ	"		fresh, soaked in water, solution applied topically
cf. Trichosanthes sp.	bàhàm pàw	Xa˙ (172)	sad khob (mǎa wɔ́ɔ, ŋuu), phaj	whole plant	indifferent	dried, crushed, applied topically

LIST OF MEDICINAL PLANTS COLLECTED IN CHIANGMAI AND LAMPHUN PROVINCES, NORTHERN THAILAND (*continued*)

The identification of the botanical material is a result of joint efforts by T. Bjørnland and T. Schumacher; critical taxa of various families have been revised by botanical colleagues as follows:

B. Hansen—Botanical Museum, University of Copenhagen - Acanthaceae
K. Larsen—Botanical Institute, University of Aarhus - Caesalpiniaceae and Zingiberaceae
I. Nielsen—Botanical Institute, University of Aarhus - Mimosaceae
R. Geesink—Rijksherbarium, Leiden - Fabaceae

Plant taxon	Vernacular[1]	Locality[2] (collection number)	Medical use(s)	Part(s) of plant used	Physical[3] quality	Preparation and administration
CUSCUTACEAE:						
Cuscuta sp.	khya khǎw kham	XVIe (431)	bamluŋ hǔa cǎj, jaa ˀaajúˀ wádthánáˀ	whole plant	warm	dried, crushed, per os
CYPERACEAE:						
Carex baccans Nees	fɛ̀ɛg hɔ̌ɔm	XVIIIa (596)	kǐn phid	root	warm	dried, ground, per os
Cyperus corymbosus Rottb.	kog ˀii jib	VIIIf (293)	khāj	root	indifferent	dried, crushed, applied topically on head
Cyperus rotundus L.	ñāa bàníw mǔu	Xa (168)	jaa ˀaajúˀ wádthánáˀ,	root	indifferent	dried, crushed, per os
			jaa bamluŋ kǎmlaŋ			decoction per os
DIOSCOREACEAE:						
Dioscorea bulbifera L.	bàhàm pàw, hǔa lɔ́ɔj luu	XVIIa (484) IIId (546)	phaj, sad khob (mǎa wɔ́ɔ, ŋuu)	bulbs on stem	indifferent	dried, crushed, applied topically
Dioscorea hispida Dennst.	kɔ̌ɔj	IIa (252)	mɛɛŋ khian	root	indifferent	fresh, chopped into pieces, applied topically

EBENACEAE:						
Diospyros ehretioides A. DC.	tab tàw tõn	XVIIb (584)	jaa bamluŋ kămlaŋ	bark	indifferent	decoction per os
Diospyros malabarica (Desv.) Kost.	máj thàan faj phĭi	XVa (203)	khăaŋ, jaa thìib, thàaj pháñâad	bark	indifferent	dried, ground, per os
Diospyros mollis Griff.	máklya	VIc (22)	jaa thàaj, thàaj pháñâad	fruits	indifferent	dried, crushed, per os
Diospyros cf. pilosula (A. DC.) Hiern.	doŋ dam	Xa (173)	kĭn phid	bark, wood, root	indifferent	dried, crushed, per os
			khăaŋ	bark, wood		dried, ground, per os
Diospyros rhodocalyx Kurz	mákŏo	VIIa (649)	jaa thàaj, jaa bamluŋ kămlaŋ	fruits bark	indifferent	dried, crushed, per os decoction per os
Diospyros cf. variegata Kurz	doŋ dam	XIIa (509)	kĭn phid	bark, wood, root	indifferent	dried, crushed, per os
			khăaŋ	bark, wood		dried, ground, per os
Diospyros sp.	mákŏo	XVIa (37)	jaa thàaj, jaa bamluŋ kămlaŋ	fruits bark	indifferent	dried, crushed, per os decoction per os
ELAEAGNACEAE:						
Elaeagnus latifolia L.	málɔ̀ɔd	IIId (531)	kĭn phid	bark, wood	indifferent	dried, ground, per os
ERICACEAE:						
Lyonia ovalifolia (Wall.) Drude	mỳad tob	XXIIa (454)	khăaŋ,	bark, wood	indifferent	fresh, chewed, applied topically
			jaa thàaj	bark		dried, ground, per os
Vaccinium sprengelii (Don) Sleumer	máj mỳad	XXIIb (683)	khăaŋ lŭaŋ	bark, wood	indifferent	dried, ground, per os
ERYTHROXYLACEAE:						
Erythroxylum cuneatum (Miq.) Kurz	tăan, tăan khàmoj	IXa (137)	saaŋ	whole plant root	indifferent	dried, ground, or decoction per os

The identification of the botanical material is a result of joint efforts by T. Bjørnland and T. Schumacher; critical taxa of various families have been revised by botanical colleagues as follows:

B. Hansen—Botanical Museum, University of Copenhagen - Acanthaceae
K. Larsen—Botanical Institute, University of Aarhus - Caesalpiniaceae and Zingiberaceae
I. Nielsen—Botanical Institute, University of Aarhus - Mimosaceae
R. Geesink—Rijksherbarium, Leiden - Fabaceae

Plant taxon	Vernacular[1]	Locality[2] (collection number)	Medical use(s)	Part(s) of plant used	Physical[3] quality	Preparation and administration
EUPHORBIACEAE:						
Antidesma brunneum Hook f.	bàmāw, māw lyysii, māw sǎaj	IIa (256)	phɛ̌ɛ píd	bark, wood, leaves	indifferent	dried, crushed, applied topically
			ŋuu khob	leaves		fresh, chewed, saliva swallowed, remnants applied topically
			kɛ̃ɛ lom, fïi sǎan	bark, wood		dried, ground, per os
Aporosa dioica Muell. Arg. in DC.	mỳad tob	XXIa (713)	jaa thàaj	bark	indifferent	dried, ground, per os
Aporosa villosa Baill.	mỳad tob	VIIIa (43)	khǎaŋ	bark, wood	"	fresh, chewed, applied topically
Baccaurea sapida Muell. Arg. in DC.	bàfaj bàfaj pàa, bàfaj dyan hāa	VIIIf (295) XXIa (709) XVIIc (719)	nīw, cebˀɛw khǎaŋ hɔ́ɔn khɔɔ	bark, root	indifferent	decoction per os
				bark, wood		dried, ground, per os
Baliospermum axillare Bl.	pāw tɔ̌ŋ tɛ̀ɛg	XIIIa (185)	khǎaŋ, jaa thàaj	latex root	warm	dried, applied topically dried, crushed, per os
Baliospermum cf. montanum Muell. Arg. in DC.	pāw tɔ̌ŋ tɛ̀ɛg	VIIIl (607)	khǎaŋ, jaa thàaj	latex root	warm	dried, applied topically dried, crushed, per os
Bischofia cf. javanica Bl.	kùm bog	XXIa (706)	nedsaa, nedsy̌ŋ	bark	warm	dried, crushed, applied topically (legs)

Breynia glauca Craib	phía faan, dab píd	VIa (13) VId (124) VIIIg (355)	fĭi	leaves	indifferent khom	fresh, mashed, applied topically
Breynia sp.	máj kâan pǎa dɛɛŋ	VIIIa (31)	khǎaŋ,	bark, wood, root	indifferent	dried, ground, per os
			bàheŋ, khǎj pàa	root		fresh, crushed, applied topically
Cleidion spiciflorum (Burm. f.) Merr.	dii mĭi	VIIIf (297)	tǎa dɛɛŋ	leaves	indifferent khom	fresh, soaked in water, solution applied topically
	mǎw lŷad	IIIc (336)	fɔ̂ɔg lŷad, khaaw pǎa lăŋ kə̀əd	bark, wood, leaves	warm	dried, crushed, per os, or soaked in water, solution as bath
	máj mádùug	IIIe (702)	bàhòog	bark, wood, root	indifferent	decoction per os
Croton birmanicus Muell. Arg.	hàdsàkhyyn	VIa (6) VIf (276) VIh (519)	kìaw, nedsaa	leaves	indifferent	dried, crushed, applied topically
Croton cf. calococcus Kurz	baj lăŋ khǎaw	IIa (265)	jaa kɛ̃ɛ, luˀ tɔ́ɔŋ	root	indifferent	dried, ground, per os
Croton cf. joufra Roxb.	pāw nɔ́ɔj	VIb (21)	kìaw, nedsaa,	leaves	warm	dried, crushed, per os
		VIh (521)	khab lŷad khab nám, khaaw pǎa lăŋ kə̀əd	leaves		dried, crushed, or decoction per os or as bath
Croton oblongus Burm. f.	pāw lŭaŋ	IVa (639)	khab lŷad khab nám, khaaw pǎa lăŋ kə̀əd	leaves	indifferent	dried, crushed, or decoction per os or as bath
Croton tiglium L.	bàkhàŋ, màag khàŋ	VIa (5) VIIIc (116) VIf (274)	jaa thàaj	fruits	indifferent	dried, crushed, per os
Drypetes roxburghii (Wall.) A. Shaw	paˀoŋ nóg	XIIIa (192)	kĭn phid, jaa kɛ̃ɛ	bark	indifferent	dried, ground, or decoction per os
Euphorbia hirta L.	ñāa nám myg	IXb (211)	khǎj	whole plant root	indifferent	decoction per os
Euphorbia tirucalli L.	kíaˀtian	IVa (637)	fĭi	latex	warm	fresh, applied topically
Gelonium multiflorum Juss.	mádùug, mádùug lŷam	IXa (134) VIIIm (664)	bàhòog	bark, wood, root	indifferent	decoction per os

The identification of the botanical material is a result of joint efforts by T. Bjørnland and T. Schumacher; critical taxa of various families have been revised by botanical colleagues as follows:

B. Hansen—Botanical Museum, University of Copenhagen - Acanthaceae
K. Larsen—Botanical Institute, University of Aarhus - Caesalpiniaceae and Zingiberaceae
I. Nielsen—Botanical Institute, University of Aarhus - Mimosaceae
R. Geesink—Rijksherbarium, Leiden - Fabaceae

Plant taxon	Vernacular[1]	Locality[2] (collection number)	Medical use(s)	Part(s) of plant used	Physical[3] quality	Preparation and administration
Glochidion lanceolarium Dalz.	khĩi mɔ̂ɔd, khàj mɔ̂ɔd	VIa (4) VId (123)	máam too, khɔɔ fɔ̂ɔg	bark	indifferent	dried, chopped into pieces, heated, applied as skin paints over the affected spots
		IXb (236)	lom phid dyan, nĩw	bark, wood bark, wood		dried, crushed, per os decoction per os
Glochidion sphaerogynum Kurz	" "	IIId (554)	máam too, khɔɔ fɔ̂ɔg, lom phid dyan	bark bark, wood	indifferent	*as above* (4, 123, 236)
Jatropha curcas L.	bàhùŋ, bàhùŋ húa	VIIIc (93) VIIIg (360)	nĩw, luʔtɔ́ɔŋ	bark, wood root	indifferent	decoction per os
			phaj	"		dried, crushed, applied topically
Jatropha gossypifolia L.	bàhùŋ dɛɛŋ	VIIIc (115)	jaa thàaj	seeds, fruits	indifferent	fresh, mashed, juice (oil) per os
Mallotus philippinensis (Lam.) Muell. Arg.	bàkaaj khàd, bàkaaj ñũm	IIIc (348) IIId (534)	jaa thàaj, thàaj sãj dyan	fruits, bark	indifferent	dried, crushed, per os
Mallotus sp.	bàkaaj khad	VIa (18)	jaa thàaj, thàaj sãj dyan	fruits, bark	indifferent	dried, crushed, per os
Megistostigma burmanicum (Kurz) A. Shaw	hɔ̃ɔ sàpaaj khwaaj	XVIIa (501)	jaa bamluŋ kămlaŋ	stem	indifferent	decoction per os

Phyllanthus emblica L.	mákhǎam pɔ̃m	IXa (140) IIIc (343)	jaa tâad, jaa thàaj, khǎaŋ	fruits bark	indifferent	fresh, per os dried, ground, per os
Phyllanthus pulcher (Baill.) Muell. Arg.	thɔɔlánii sǎan, bàkhǎam pɔ̃m din	XIIIa (182) VIf (277) VIh (525)	sǎan, lom sǎan, fïi sǎan, lom sàníbàad	whole plant whole plant	indifferent	decoction per os dried, crushed, per os
Phyllanthus roseus (Craib & Hutch.) Beille	bàdii kàj	XVIIa (500)	khãj	bark, wood	indifferent	dried, ground, per os
Phyllanthus urinaria L.	faj dyan hãa	VIIIc (119)	bawwǎan, khãj	whole plant	indifferent	decoction per os
Ricinus communis L.	bàhùŋ heb	VIIIc (104)	jaa thàaj	seeds	indifferent	fresh, mashed, juice (oil) per os
Sauropus cf. amoebiflorus A. Shaw	phag wǎan tõn	VIIIc (106)	lom bàheŋkhúd	root	indifferent	dried, crushed, per os
Sauropus androgynus Merr.	phag wǎan bãan	IIc (473)	lom bàheŋkhúd	root	cold	dried, crushed, per os
FABACEAE:						
Abrus sp.	mákàm tǎa kàj	VIIIc (102)	khǎaŋ, jaa thàaj	bark	indifferent	dried, crushed, per os
Atylosia sp.	tĩin nóg nɔ́ɔj	XXa (604)	bàhòog	root	indifferent	decoction per os
Crotalaria alata D. Don	ñãa khɔɔ tuŋ, ñãa tuŋ húŋ	IXc (378) Ia (397)	khǎaŋ, saaŋ	whole plant	indifferent	decoction per os or used topically as bath
Crotalaria albida Roth.	tɛ̀ɛd cɛ́ʔ	XVIIa (492)	jaa bamluŋ kǎmlaŋ	whole plant	indifferent	decoction per os
Dalbergia sp. 1.	sàbãa	IXa (135)	khǎaŋ, jaa thàaj	seeds "	indifferent	fresh, chewed, used topically in mouth crushed, per os
Dalbergia sp. 2.	pĩi khya	XVIIb (570)	khǎaŋ	bark, wood	indifferent	fresh, chewed, used topically in mouth, or per os
Derris elliptica (Roxb.) Benth.	lǎj	XVIIa (494)	bỳa pǎa	whole plant	indifferent	crushed, dissolved in a pond (fish poison)
Derris thyrsiflora Benth.	pǎn khɛ̌ɛ	VIIIa (55)	hɔ́ɔn nàj , khĩi hâag	bark, root	indifferent	dried, crushed, per os
Derris sp.	tỳŋ khya ŋən	XVIIb (576)	lom sàníbàad	bark, wood	indifferent	fresh, ground, per os
cf. Derris sp.	máj ked jùag	XIIa (513)	khãj sàn	seeds	indifferent	decoction per os
Desmodium polycarpum DC.	khǎaŋ khan ñãa	IIa (245) IIb (425)	khǎaŋ	root	indifferent	decoction per os
	ked pǎa lə̌əm	IIId (539)	hɔ́ɔn nàj, jaa bamluŋ kǎmlaŋ	root, whole plant	warm	decoction per os

The identification of the botanical material is a result of joint efforts by T. Bjørnland and T. Schumacher; critical taxa of various families have been revised by botanical colleagues as follows:

B. Hansen—Botanical Museum, University of Copenhagen - Acanthaceae
K. Larsen—Botanical Institute, University of Aarhus - Caesalpiniaceae and Zingiberaceae
I. Nielsen—Botanical Institute, University of Aarhus - Mimosaceae
R. Geesink—Rijksherbarium, Leiden - Fabaceae

Plant taxon	Vernacular[1]	Locality[2] (collection number)	Medical use(s)	Part(s) of plant used	Physical[3] quality	Preparation and administration
Desmodium motorium (Houtt.) Merr.	khǎaŋ khɛ̂ŋ khɛ́ʔ	Ia (396)	khǎaŋ	whole plant	indifferent	decoction per os
Desmodium pulchellum Benth.	ñāa lûug lîib	Ia (401)	kǐn phid	root	indifferent	dried, ground, per os
Desmodium renifolium (L.) Schindl.	ked pǎa lǝ̌ǝm	IIIb (322)	hɔ́ɔn naj, jaa bamluŋ kǎmlaŋ	root whole plant	warm	decoction per os " " "
	ñāa lŷad nàaj	IIId (538)	khab lŷad khab nám, khaaw pǎa lǎŋ kə̀əd, láduu bà maa	root	"	decoction per os
Desmodium styracifolium (Osb.) Merr.	khǎaŋ pɔɔj khǎaw	IIb (426)	khǎaŋ pàag pyàj	bark, wood	indifferent	dried, ground, per os
Desmodium triflorum DC.	ñāa tǎan saaj	VIIIh (386)	khāj	whole plant	indifferent	decoction per os
Desmodium velutinum (Willd.) DC.	ñāa tyg mɛɛw lûug lîib tōn	XVIIa (489) IIId (557)	khāj kə̀əd ŋâaj	whole plant " "	indifferent "	decoction per os fresh, soaked in water, used as bath or vaporous bath
Desmodium sp.	ñāa lŷad nàaj	IIIb (326)	khab lŷad khab nám, khaaw pǎa lǎŋ kə̀əd, láduu bà maa	root	warm	decoction per os

Dolichos lablab L.	thùa máp̀ɛɛb	VIIIm (656)	khāj, khāj khȳn	root	indifferent	dried, crushed, applied topically on head
Eriosema sp.	máa mɛ̂ɛ kàm	Ia (399)	jaa bamluŋ kămlaŋ, jaa tâad	whole plant	indifferent	decoction per os
Erythrina sp.	thɔɔŋ lăaŋ	IXb (210)	khăaŋ hɔ́ɔn khɔɔ,	bark	indifferent	dried, ground, per os
		IVa (636)	khāj, hɔ́ɔn naj	"		crushed, applied topically on head
			kɛ̃ɛ lom	bark, wood		dried, ground, per os
Flemingia lineata W. Ait.	kăa săam pìig	XXIIIa (375)	jaa bamluŋ kămlaŋ	root	indifferent	decoction per os
	khamīn mádtrii	XVIIb (579)	khāj, lom săan	root	indifferent	decoction per os
Flemingia macrophylla (Willd.) O. Ktze.	bàhĭŋ mēn	IIId (542)	nīw, bàhòog	root	indifferent	decoction per os
Flemingia sp.	bàhĭŋ mēn	XVIIa (490)	nīw, bàhòog	root	indifferent	decoction per os
Gliricidia sepium (Jacq.) Steud.	kɛɛ fàlàŋ	VIIa (645)	khăaŋ	bark, wood	indifferent	dried, ground, or decoction per os
Indigofera hirsuta L.	léb myyn dɔ̀ɔg dɛɛŋ	VIIIf (299)	khāj	root	indifferent	decoction per os
Lespedeza sp.	kăa săam pìig	XXIIb (681)	jaa bamluŋ kămlaŋ, jaa tâad, ceb ˀɛw	root	indifferent	fresh, in alcoholic tincture or decoction per os
Milletia aff. pachylola Drake	khya lăj dɛɛŋ	IIIc (344)	bỳa păa	bark, wood, leaves	indifferent	crushed, dissolved in a pond
Milletia cf. piscidia Wight	khăaŋ khăaw	IIIc (331)	khăaŋ pàag pỳaj	bark, wood	indifferent	crushed, or decoction per os
Mucuna pruriens DC.	măa ñ̆yaŋ	VIIIk (458)	bàhòog kōn pûud	root	indifferent	decoction per os
Psophocarpus tetragonolobus DC.	thùa puu	VIIIg (352) VIIIj (411) VIIIj (420)	khāj, khāj khȳn	root	indifferent	crushed, applied topically on head
Pueraria collettii Prain	kwăaw khya	IIId (553)	jaa ˀaajúˀ wádthánáˀ	whole plant	indifferent	dried, crushed, per os
Pueraria mirifica A. Shaw et Suvat.	kwăaw khya dɛɛŋ	IXb (217) VIIIm (667)	jaa ˀaajuˀ wádthánáˀ, jaa tâad, jaa bamluŋ kămlaŋ	root	indifferent	dried, crushed, per os

The identification of the botanical material is a result of joint efforts by T. Bjørnland and T. Schumacher; critical taxa of various families have been revised by botanical colleagues as follows:

B. Hansen—Botanical Museum, University of Copenhagen - Acanthaceae
K. Larsen—Botanical Institute, University of Aarhus - Caesalpiniaceae and Zingiberaceae
I. Nielsen—Botanical Institute, University of Aarhus - Mimosaceae
R. Geesink—Rijksherbarium, Leiden - Fabaceae

Plant taxon	Vernacular[1]	Locality[2] (collection number)	Medical use(s)	Part(s) of plant used	Physical[3] quality	Preparation and administration
Pueraria sp.	kwǎaw dam	XIXa (623)	jaa ˀaajúˀ wádthánáˀ	root	indifferent	dried, crushed, per os
Sesbania grandiflora (L.) Pers.	kɛɛ khǎaw	IIc (471)	khĩaw phúˀ	bark	indifferent	fresh, chewed, applied topically in mouth
Tephrosia purpurea Pers.	léb myyn nɔ́ɔj dɔ́ɔg khǎaw	VIIIh (393)	khãj	root	indifferent	decoction per os
Urariopsis cordifolia (Wall.) Schindl.	lûug lîib tõn	IXb (227)	kə̀əd ŋâaj	whole plant	indifferent	fresh, soaked in water, used as bath or vaporous bath
Fabaceae 1. *indeterm.*	jaa kɛ̃ɛ hâag lỹaŋ	IIIc (337) IIIc (339)	jaa tâad	root	indifferent	decoction per os
Fabaceae 2. *indeterm.*	mɛ̂ɛ nám nɔɔŋ	XVIIb (565)	hɔ́ɔn naj	bark, wood	cool	fresh, ground, per os
FAGACEAE:						
Castanopsis argentea (Bl.) A. DC.	máj kɔ̀ɔ	XVIe (428)	khĩaw phúˀ	bark	indifferent	fresh, chewed, applied topically
Lithocarpus craibianus Barnett	kɔ̀ɔ mòn	XXIIb (682)	khǎaŋ ŋỳag buam	bark	indifferent	fresh, chewed, applied topically

FLACOURTIACEAE:						
Casearia glomerata Roxb.	phĭi sȳa lŭaŋ sĭi sȳa lŭaŋ	XVIIb (578)	jaa thàaj, jaa salĭimuun	bark	indifferent	dried, crushed, per os
Casearia grewiaefolia Vent. var. cinerea (Turcz.) Sleum.	phĭi sȳa lŭaŋ sĭi sȳa lŭaŋ	VIa (3) VId (121) IXb (216)	jaa thàaj, jaa salĭimuun	bark	indifferent	dried, crushed, per os
ICACINACEAE:						
Apodytes dimidiata Arn.	máj nâw naj	IIIc (345)	jaa tâad	bark	indifferent	decoction per os
Gomphandra quadrifida (Bl.) Sleum.	mádam phĭi pɛ̆ɛŋ	XIXa (632)	lom sàníbàad	fruit	indifferent	dried, crushed, per os
IRIDACEAE:						
Belamcanda chinensis (L.) DC.	wâan mîid ñáb	Xa (165)	hɔ́ɔn naj, fĭi, năŋ mā̆j	root leaves	cool	dried, crushed, per os fresh, mashed, applied topically
JUGLANDACEAE:						
Engelhardtia serrata Bl. var. cambodica Manning	khâa hod	IIIb (323)	lom phid dyan	bark, wood, leaves	warm	decoction per os
Engelhardtia spicata Bl. var. colebrookeana K. & V.	máhăŋ kàan	XXIIb (678) XXIIb (687)	jaa salĭimuun, khăaŋ lammánâad, khăaŋ ŋỳag buam	bark "	indifferent	dried, crushed, per os dried, crushed, applied topically
LAMIACEAE:						
Ajuga cf. macrosperma Wall.	hɔ̂ɔm cáaŋ doŋ, hɔ̂ɔm dɔɔj	XXIa (707)	kìaw, ceb tɔ́ɔŋ	whole plant	warm	decoction per os
Elsholtzia cf. blanda Benth.	tamjɛɛ pàa	XXIIb (670)	bàhòog	root	indifferent	decoction per os
Mentha arvensis L.	ñāa hɔ̆ɔm dùan	VIIIj (416)	ceb tɔ́ɔŋ, khīi khàag nám nom, khīi sīan	whole plant leaves	indifferent	fresh, per os fresh, crushed, per os
Ocimum sanctum L.	kɔɔm kɔ̂ɔ dam	VIIIc (85)	ceb tɔ́ɔŋ, kĭn phid, jaa ʔaajuʔ wádthánáʔ, jaa tâad	whole plant	warm	dried, crushed, per os

List of Medicinal Plants Collected in Chiangmai and Lamphun Provinces, Northern Thailand (*continued*)

The identification of the botanical material is a result of joint efforts by T. Bjørnland and T. Schumacher; critical taxa of various families have been revised by botanical colleagues as follows:

B. Hansen—Botanical Museum, University of Copenhagen - Acanthaceae
K. Larsen—Botanical Institute, University of Aarhus - Caesalpiniaceae and Zingiberaceae
I. Nielsen—Botanical Institute, University of Aarhus - Mimosaceae
R. Geesink—Rijksherbarium, Leiden - Fabaceae

Plant taxon	Vernacular[1]	Locality[2] (collection number)	Medical use(s)	Part(s) of plant used	Physical[3] quality	Preparation and administration
Orthosiphon aristatus (Bl.) Miq.	ñãa nùad mɛɛw	VIa (10) VIIIc (88) VIh (524)	ceb ˀɛw, ñîaw khad, bàhòog	whole plant or root	indifferent	decoction per os
Salvia plebeia R. Br.	kɔɔm kɔ̂ɔ khǎaw	IIa (254)	jaa ˀaajúˀ wádthánáˀ	whole plant	warm	decoction per os
LAURACEAE:						
Cinnamomum cf. iners Bl.	haaŋ kɛɛŋ laaŋ kɛɛŋ	XXIIIa (372)	bamluŋ hǔa cǎj	bark	indifferent	dried, crushed, per os
Cinnamomum sp.	haaŋ khái laaŋ khái	XVIIb (572)	jaa tâad	bark	indifferent	dried, crushed, per os
Lindera thomsonii Allen	puu tõn	XXa (589)	jaa ˀaajúˀ wádthánáˀ	leaves	indifferent	dried, crushed, per os
Litsea cubeba (Lour.) Pers.	càkhaj tõn	IIIb (310)	tɔ́ɔŋ tẽn, tɔ́ɔŋ fə́ə	fruits	indifferent	dried, crushed, per os
Litsea glutinosa (Lour.) C. B. Rob.	máj mìi, phag mìi	VIIIa (40)	kǐn phid, khâab	root leaves	indifferent	dried, ground, per os decoction, applied topically
Neolitsea cuipala (D. Don) Kost.	paˀ cãw pɛ̀ɛd paˀoŋ	XIXa (614)	kɛ̃ɛ lom	bark, wood	indifferent	dried, ground, per os

Phoebe grandis (Nees) Merr.	máj pig tɔ̌ɔŋ	IIIe (695)	kɛ̃ɛ lom	bark	indifferent	dried, ground, per os
Phoebe lanceolata (Roxb.) Nees	sùláphíd kham	IIIe (333)	kǐn phid, jaa kɛ̃ɛ	bark, wood	indifferent	dried, ground, per os
LECYTHIDACEAE:						
Careya arborea Roxb.	puj, kàdoon sɔɔj	XIIa (508)	khǎaŋ	bark	indifferent	dried, crushed, per os
LILIACEAE:						
Asparagus filicinus D. Don	máa khɔ̂ɔg tɛ̀ɛg	IIIc (340)	jaa tâad, jaa bamluŋ kǎmlaŋ, jaa ʔaajúʔ wádthánáʔ	fruits, roots	indifferent	decoction per os
Aspidistra sutepensis K. Larsen	thâw nâŋ hûŋ	XIXa (613)	jaa bamluŋ kǎmlaŋ	root	indifferent	decoction per os
Cordyline terminalis Kunth.	màag púu	VIf (275)	ceb hǔa, maw hǔa	root, leaves	indifferent	dried, ground, per os fresh, soaked in water, solution to wash the head
Dianella ensifolia (L.) Red.	wâan mîid ñáb	XXIIIa (351)	hɔ́ɔn naj, fĭi, nǎŋ mãj	root leaves	cool	dried, ground, per os fresh, mashed, applied topically
Disporopsis longifolia Craib	wâan khãaw cìi	XVIIc (724)	jaa bamluŋ kǎmlaŋ	root	indifferent	decoction per os
Dracaena angustifolia Roxb.	cǎn pàa	XVIIa (498)	kǐn phid, hǔa cǎj tẽn, khǎaŋ, jaa tâad	wood ″	indifferent	dried, crushed, per os decoction per os
	pháaw pan lam	XVIIb (575)	kɛ̃ɛ píd (jaa thìib)	bark, wood	indifferent	fresh, crushed, per os
Dracaena sp.	cǎn pàa mǎa	XVa (194)	kǐn phid, hǔa cǎj tẽn, khǎaŋ, jaa tâad	wood ″	indifferent	dried, crushed, per os decoction per os
Gloriosa superba L.	dɔɔŋ dyŋ	XIIIa (188)	pooŋ, ʔammapâad, nedsaa	root	warm	dried, crushed, or decoction both per os and applied topically

The identification of the botanical material is a result of joint efforts by T. Bjørnland and T. Schumacher; critical taxa of various families have been revised by botanical colleagues as follows:

B. Hansen—Botanical Museum, University of Copenhagen - Acanthaceae
K. Larsen—Botanical Institute, University of Aarhus - Caesalpiniaceae and Zingiberaceae
I. Nielsen—Botanical Institute, University of Aarhus - Mimosaceae
R. Geesink—Rijksherbarium, Leiden - Fabaceae

Plant taxon	Vernacular[1]	Locality[2] (collection number)	Medical use(s)	Part(s) of plant used	Physical[3] quality	Preparation and administration
Ophiopogon reptans Hook. f.	khɔ́ɔn saden	XIXa (617)	khāj	root	warm	dried, ground, per os
LOBELIACEAE:						
Lobelia nicotianaefolia R. & S.	dɔ̀ɔg dāaj pàa	XXa (592) XXa (600)	lom bàheŋkhúd	root	indifferènt	dried, ground, per os
Pratia begonifolia Lindl.	phag hâag kūaj	XXIIIa (370)	hɔ́ɔn naj, jaa tâad	whole plant	cool	decoction per os
LOGANIACEAE:						
Strychnos nux-blanda A. W. Hill	mátə̂ŋ, máj tûm	XVIa (38) IXb (235)	khǎaŋ, ŋuu khob	bark, wood bark	indifferent	dried, ground, per os fresh, crushed, applied topically
LORANTHACEAE:						
Dendrophtoe pentandra (L.) Miq.	kǎa fàag kǎa fàag saa	XXIIa (441) IIId (545)	kǐn phid, lom khȳn " " " "	bark, wood " "	indifferent	dried, ground, per os " " " "
Viscum ovalifolium DC.	kǎa fàag léb káw	IVa (642)	lom phid dyan	bark, wood	indifferent	dried, ground, per os

LYTHRACEAE:						
Lagerstroemia balansae Koehne	máj pǔaj	IIa (263)	kǐn phid (emeticum)	bark, leaves	indifferent	fresh, chewed, then swallowed
Lagerstroemia calyculata Kurz	máj hēw	XIIa (516)	khāj	fruits	indifferent	dried, crushed, per os
Lagerstroemia macrocarpa Voigt	cɔ̀ɔ lɔ̂ɔ	XVIa (32)	khǎaŋ pàag pỳaj, tùm, phɛ̌ɛ phúaʔ	fruits	indifferent	dried, ground, per os
MAGNOLIACEAE:						
Michelia champaca L.	cǎmpǎa	XVa (205)	jaa kɛ̄ɛ, luʔ tɔ́ɔŋ, khǎaŋ	bark " "	indifferent	dried, crushed, per os decoction per os boiled, bark chewed, used topically (mouth)
Paramichelia baillonii (Pierre) Hu	cǎmpǐi	VIIIc (110)	jaa kɛ̄ɛ, luʔ tɔ́ɔŋ, khǎaŋ	bark " "	indifferent	dried, crushed, per os decoction per os boiled, bark chewed, used topically (mouth)
MALVACEAE:						
Abelmoschus moschatus Medic. ssp. moschatus	pɔ̌ɔ fāaj	IIId (543)	khǎaŋ, saaŋ	root	cool	decoction per os
Abutilon hirtum (Lam.) Sweet	bàkɔ̀ŋ khāaw	Xa (179)	khāj	root	indifferent	decoction per os
Abutilon indicum (L.) Sweet ssp. indicum	bàkɔ̀ŋ khāaw	VIIIh (394)	khāj	root	indifferent	decoction per os
Gossypium barbadense L.	fāaj	Xa (166)	jaa thàaj	seeds	indifferent	dried, crushed, per os
Hibiscus sabdariffa L.	bàtěŋ kheŋ	VIIIf (291) VIIIj (418)	khāj	fruits	indifferent	decoction per os
Thespesia lampas (Cav.) Dalz. et Gibs.	fāaj pàa	XVIIa (497)	kɛ̄ɛ hâag	fruits	indifferent	mashed, soaked in water, solution per os
Urena lobata L.	ñāa phǒm ñūŋ	XXIIa (449) XVIIb (582)	khāj	root	indifferent	decoction per os

The identification of the botanical material is a result of joint efforts by T. Bjørnland and T. Schumacher; critical taxa of various families have been revised by botanical colleagues as follows:

B. Hansen—Botanical Museum, University of Copenhagen - Acanthaceae
K. Larsen—Botanical Institute, University of Aarhus - Caesalpiniaceae and Zingiberaceae
I. Nielsen—Botanical Institute, University of Aarhus - Mimosaceae
R. Geesink—Rijksherbarium, Leiden - Fabaceae

Plant taxon	Vernacular[1]	Locality[2] (collection number)	Medical use(s)	Part(s) of plant used	Physical[3] quality	Preparation and administration
Wissadula periplocifolia (L.) Presl.	bàhɛ̃n nóg	VIIIk (478)	ceb ʔɛw, khãj	whole plant root	indifferent	decoction per os " " "
MARANTACEAE:						
Schumannianthus sp.	jɛ̀ŋ	XIIIa (184)	khãj, khăaŋ khãj sàníbàad	root root	indifferent	dried, crushed, per os dried, ground, per os
MELASTOMATACEAE:						
Memecylon scutellatum Triana	mỳad fɔɔŋ	XVIIIa (602)	khăaŋ	bark, wood	indifferent	dried, ground, per os
MELIACEAE:						
Azadirachta indica Juss.	sàdaw, sàliam	VIIIa (52)	khãj, khãj càb sàn	bark or whole plant	indifferent	decoction per os

MENISPERMACEAE:						
Cissampelos pareira L. var. hirsuta (DC.) Forman	khǒŋ khàmǎw ñāa mǔu nɔ́ɔj	VIIIa (47) IIIa (306)	phɛ̌ɛ phúaˀ " "	leaves "	indifferent	dried, crushed, applied topically
Tiliacora triandra Diels	cɔɔj naaŋ	VIIIg (358)	fĭi sǎan, kǐn phid kɛ̃ɛ cám	root leaves	indifferent	dried, ground, or decoction per os fresh, mashed, per os
Tinospora cf. crispa (L.) Hook. f. et Thoms.	cûŋcaliŋ	IIa (255)	kɛ̃ɛ lom, khāj pāaŋ	leaves, stem stem	indifferent	dried, crushed, per os decoction per os
MIMOSACEAE:						
Acacia catechu (L.) Willd. f. catechu	sĭi sìad	Xa (180)	phɛ̌ɛ nâw pỳaj	bark	indifferent	decoction, used topically
Acacia megaladena Desv. var. indo-chinensis Niels.	sōm pɔ̀ɔj	VIIIc (94)	khàad wídtámin sii	root	warm	dried, ground, per os
Acacia megaladena Desv. var. megaladena	nǎam hǎn	IIId (549)	lom sāan	bark, wood	warm	dried, ground, per os
Acacia rugata (Lam.) Merr.	sōm pɔ̀ɔj	IIId (532)	khàad wídtámin sii	root	warm	dried, ground, per os
Adenanthera pavonina L. var. microsperma (T. & B.) Niels.	mákàm tǎa	IIId (535)	khǎaŋ, jaa thàaj	bark	indifferent	dried, ground, per os
Albizia chinensis (Osb.) Merr.	máj sǎan	XXIa (715)	lom sǎan, fĭi sǎan naj tɔ́ɔŋ	bark	indifferent	dried, ground, per os decoction per os
Albizia lucidior (Steud.) Niels.	pǎn khɛ̌ɛ	XIIa (510)	hɔ́ɔn naj, ˀaahǎan sĭa, kǐn phid	bark, root	cool	dried, ground, per os
Archidendron clypearia (Jack.) Niels.	máj pìig nỳaŋ	IIIe (690)	khǎaŋ	bark, wood	indifferent	dried, ground, per os
Archidendron glomeriflorum (Kurz) Niels.	bàkhīi kǎa khɛɛ fɔ̌ɔj	XXIIa (445) XXIIb (679)	bàhòog khǎaŋ, khǎaŋ lammánâad	root bark, wood " "	indifferent indifferent	decoction per os dried, ground, per os fresh, chewed, used topically in mouth
Mimosa pudica L. var. hispida Brenan	ñāa ciˀ ñɔ̂ɔb	IIb (427)	ñîaw khad, jaa tâad, jaa bamluŋ kǎmlaŋ	root	indifferent	decoction per os

The identification of the botanical material is a result of joint efforts by T. Bjørnland and T. Schumacher; critical taxa of various families have been revised by botanical colleagues as follows:

B. Hansen—Botanical Museum, University of Copenhagen - Acanthaceae
K. Larsen—Botanical Institute, University of Aarhus - Caesalpiniaceae and Zingiberaceae
I. Nielsen—Botanical Institute, University of Aarhus - Mimosaceae
R. Geesink—Rijksherbarium, Leiden - Fabaceae

Plant taxon	Vernacular[1]	Locality[2] (collection number)	Medical use(s)	Part(s) of plant used	Physical[3] quality	Preparation and administration
Pithecellobium dulce (Roxb.) Benth.	bàkhǎam thêed	VIIIj (424) VIh (527)	lom, khwaam dan	bark root	indifferent	dried, ground, per os fresh, crushed, per os
Xylia xylocarpa (Roxb.) Taub. var. kerrii (Craib et Hutch.) Niels.	pŷag máj dɛɛŋ	IXb (218)	phɛ̌ɛ, tùm	bark	indifferent	dried, ground, or decoction, used topically
Mimosaceae *indeterm.*	kaaŋ khĩi mɔ̂ɔd	VIII1 (606)	khǎaŋ, bàhòog	bark bark, wood	indifferent	dried, ground, per os decoction per os
MORACEAE:						
Artocarpus heterophylla Lam.	bànǔn	VIIIe (269) VIIIk (475)	luʔ tɔ́ɔŋ	bark, latex	indifferent	decoction per os
Artocarpus lakoocha Roxb.	pùag hàad	IIIb (312)	jaa thàaj, thàaj sǎj dyan	latex	indifferent	dried, per os
Broussonetia papyrifera Vent.	pàan sǎa	XIIa (511)	ceb hǔa, maw hǔa	root	indifferent	dried, ground, or decoction per os
Ficus cf. altissima Bl.	phag hŷad	VIIIj (414)	kǐn phid luʔ tɔ́ɔŋ	bark, wood, root bark	indifferent	decoction per os " " "

Ficus cf. ampelas Burm.f.	máj haj nóg kog	XVIIb (564)	luˀ tɔ́ɔŋ	latex	indifferent	dried, per os
Ficus glomerata Roxb.	dỳa kīaŋ	XIIa (517)	luˀ tɔ́ɔŋ, khǎaŋ	bark, wood	indifferent	dried, crushed, per os
Ficus hispida L. f.	mádỳa	XIIIa (200)	luˀ tɔ́ɔŋ	latex	indifferent	dried, per os
Ficus rumphii Bl.	máj salǐi	XXIVa (469)	luˀ tɔ́ɔŋ	latex	indifferent	dried, per os
Ficus subincisa J. E. Smith	máj khɔ̀ɔj pàa	IIId (561)	luˀ tɔ́ɔŋ	latex	indifferent	dried, per os
Ficus tinctoria (L. f.) Forst. f. ssp. gibbosa (Bl.) Corner	máj haj	Xa (169)	luˀ tɔ́ɔŋ	latex	indifferent	dried, per os
Ficus sp.	dỳa lɔ̆ɔŋ lɛ̆ɛŋ	XXIa (708)	luˀ tɔ́ɔŋ	latex	indifferent	dried, per os
Streblus asper Lour.	khɔ̀j	VIIIb (75) IVa (641)	luˀ tɔ́ɔŋ	bark, latex	indifferent	decoction per os
MORINGACEAE:						
Moringa oleifera Lam.	phag ˀìi hym bàkhɔ́n kɔ̃m	IXa (147) VIIIf (285)	jaa tâad " "	bark "	warm "	decoction per os " " "
MYRISTICACEAE:						
Myristica cf. tenuivenia J. Sincl.	muaŋ lŷad	XVIIb (566)	bàhòog lŷad, khab nám khaaw pǎa	root	indifferent	decoction per os
MYRSINACEAE:						
Ardisia sp. 1.	cîi pug dɔɔj	XIXa (609)	jaa kɛ̃ɛ	bark, wood	indifferent	dried, ground, per os
Ardisia sp. 2.	càm khǎaw	XIXa (628)	jaa kɛ̃ɛ lom, maw hǔa	bark, wood	indifferent	dried, ground, per os
Embelia parviflora Mez.	mátǎaj waaj	XIXa (618)	bỳa maw mǎa	fruits	indifferent	crushed, mixed with food
Maesa montana A. DC.	bàmāw, māw lyysǐi	IIIc (332)	jaa kɛ̃ɛ lom phɛ̌ɛ píd	bark, wood	indifferent	dried, ground, per os
	sàtàban	XIXa (619)	ŋuu khob	bark, wood, leaves		chewed, juice swallowed, remnants applied topically
	bàmāw khwaaj	XXIIb (671)	khǎaŋ	bark, wood	indifferent	dried, ground, per os
Maesa sp.	bàhòog tōn dìaw	IIIe (692)	bàhòog	root	indifferent	decoction per os
Myrsine semiserrata Wall. in Roxb.	bàhāa doŋ	XVIIIa (588)	khǎaŋ, luˀ tɔ́ɔŋ	bark	indifferent	dried, crushed, per os

The identification of the botanical material is a result of joint efforts by T. Bjørnland and T. Schumacher; critical taxa of various families have been revised by botanical colleagues as follows:

B. Hansen—Botanical Museum, University of Copenhagen - Acanthaceae
K. Larsen—Botanical Institute, University of Aarhus - Caesalpiniaceae and Zingiberaceae
I. Nielsen—Botanical Institute, University of Aarhus - Mimosaceae
R. Geesink—Rijksherbarium, Leiden - Fabaceae

Plant taxon	Vernacular[1]	Locality[2] (collection number)	Medical use(s)	Part(s) of plant used	Physical[3] quality	Preparation and administration
MYRTACEAE:						
Psidium guajava L.	ñɔ̂ɔd bàkũaj	VIIIj (410)	luʔ tɔ́ɔŋ	bark, wood, leaves	indifferent, bitter	decoction per os
Syzygium cf. balsameum (Wight) A. M. et J. M. Cowan	máhãa doŋ	XXIIb (673)	luʔ tɔ́ɔŋ, khăaŋ	bark	indifferent	dried, crushed, per os
Syzygium cf. javanicum Miq.	bàcum puu, chumphûu khăaw	VIIIm (665)	khăaŋ	bark, wood	indifferent	dried, ground, per os
Syzygium cf. pseudoformosum (King) Merr. & Perry	bàcum puu, chumphûu pàa	XVIIc (720)	khăaŋ, khăaŋ lŭaŋ	bark, wood	indifferent	dried, ground, per os
Syzygium sp.	bàkĭaŋ	VIIIc (112)	luʔ tɔ́ɔŋ, khàad wídtámin sii,	fruit	indifferent	dried, per os
			khãj	root		decoction per os
Tristania rufescens Hance	máj màmûn	XXIIb (686)	khãj	bark, wood	indifferent	dried, ground, per os
Myrtaceae *indeterm.*	sõm pɔ̃ɔŋ	XVIIa (483)	bàhòog	root	indifferent	decoction per os

NELUMBONACEAE:						
Nelumbo nucifera Gaertn.	bua lǔaŋ	VIg (439)	jaa bamluŋ hǔa cǎj " " " "	flowers root	indifferent	dried, crushed, per os dried, ground, or decoction, per os
NYMPHAEACEAE:						
Nymphaea pubescens Willd.	bua sǎaj	XVIe (429)	jaa bamluŋ hǔa cǎj	flowers	indifferent	dried, crushed, sniffed (inhalant)
	dɔ̀ɔg páan dɛɛŋ	XIVb (437)	jaa bamluŋ kǎmlaŋ	"		decoction per os
OCHNACEAE:						
Ochna integerrima (Lour.) Merr.	máj tǎan lÿaŋ	IXb (229)	saaŋ	whole plant, root	indifferent	decoction per os
OLEACEAE:						
Jasminum anastomosans DC.	málíʔ din	IIIe (694)	kǐn phid	bark, wood, root	indifferent	dried, ground, per os
Jasminum sambac (L.) W. Ait.	málíʔ	IXa (151)	kǐn phid,	bark, wood, root	indifferent	dried, ground, per os
			lom phid dyan	whole plant		dried, crushed, per os
Jasminum cf. sambac (L.) W. Ait.	málíʔ	IXa (152)	*as above*	" "	"	" " " "
OPILIACEAE:						
Opilia cf. amentacea Roxb.	phag naaŋ jɛ́ɛm	XVIIIa (605)	jaa tâad, jaa bǎmluŋ kǎmlaŋ	bark, wood	indifferent	decoction per os
ORCHIDACEAE:						
Arundina graminifolia (D. Don) Hochr.	ŋúan tàag ŋǎaj	IXc (381)	khǎj, jaa tâad kǐn phid	whole plant root	indifferent	dried, crushed, per os dried, ground, per os

The identification of the botanical material is a result of joint efforts by T. Bjørnland and T. Schumacher; critical taxa of various families have been revised by botanical colleagues as follows:

B. Hansen—Botanical Museum, University of Copenhagen - Acanthaceae
K. Larsen—Botanical Institute, University of Aarhus - Caesalpiniaceae and Zingiberaceae
I. Nielsen—Botanical Institute, University of Aarhus - Mimosaceae
R. Geesink—Rijksherbarium, Leiden - Fabaceae

Plant taxon	Vernacular[1]	Locality[2] (collection number)	Medical use(s)	Part(s) of plant used	Physical[3] quality	Preparation and administration
OXALIDACEAE:						
Averrhoa carambola L.	bàfyaŋ	Xa (170)	nĩw	root, fruits	indifferent	decoction per os
Biophytum petersianum Klotzsch	kàthŷyb ñɔ̂ɔd	IXa (144)	khãj	whole plant	indifferent	decoction per os
Oxalis corniculata L.	sõm sǎŋkǎa	XVIa (27) XVIIIa (599)	jaa tâad, jaa ʔaajúʔ wádtháńáʔ	whole plant	indifferent	dried, crushed, per os
PANDANACEAE:						
Pandanus sp.	tə̌əj	IIId (548)	khǎaŋ	root	indifferent	dried, ground, per os
PAPAVERACEAE:						
Papaver somniferum L.	dɔ̀ɔg fìn	IIId (562)	luʔ tɔ́ɔŋ, rôog thɔ́ɔ cǎj	latex	indifferent bitter	dried, per os
PASSIFLORACEAE:						
Passiflora foetida L.	phag khɛ̂ɛb cég	IXb (215)	jaa tâad, jaa ʔaajúʔ wádtháńáʔ	whole plant	indifferent	dried, crushed, or decoction, per os

PIPERACEAE:						
Peperomia pellucida (L.) Kunth.	phag sǎŋ	IXb (208)	hɔ́ɔn naj, khĭi hâag	whole plant	cool	fresh, soaked in water, solution per os
Piper boehmeriaefolium DC.	puu din púu	XVIIb (573)	jaa tâad	stem, leaves	indifferent	dried, crushed, per os
Piper aff. boehmeriaefolium DC.	sàkháan	Xa (162)	jaa tâad	stem, leaves	warm	dried, crushed, per os
Piper leptostachyum A. Rich.	diipǐi	VIIIe (270)	jaa tâad, sǎan, lom phid dyan	fruit	warm	dried, crushed, per os
Piper cf. longum L.	puu liŋ nóg	VIa (20) IXa (146)	jaa tâad, khǎaŋ, khǎaŋ lammánâad	whole plant	warm	dried, crushed, per os
Piper sarmentosum Roxb.	phag puu liŋ, phag khɛ̃ɛ	VIIIb (69) VIII1 (608)	jaa tâad	whole plant	warm	dried, crushed, per os
Piper sp. 1.	puu kɛɛŋ	XXIIIa (376) XXIIa (448)	jaa tâad	stem, leaves	warm	dried, crushed, per os
Piper sp. 2.	puu din	XVIIb (563)	jaa tâad	leaves	indifferent	dried, crushed, per os
PLANTAGINACEAE:						
Plantago cf. asiatica L.	ñãa ˀen jŷyd	VId (122)	cám naj	whole plant	indifferent	dried, crushed, mixed with alcohol, applied topically
Plantago erosa Wall. in Roxb.	ñãa ˀen jŷyd	XXIIa (440)	*as above*	" "	"	" " "
PLUMBAGINACEAE:						
Plumbago rosea L.	pid piw dɛɛŋ	VIIIc (108) Xa (176)	jaa tâad, khab lŷad, lom phid dyan	whole plant root whole plant	warm	dried, crushed, per os decoction per os dried, crushed, per os
Plumbago zeylanica L.	pid piw khǎaw	Xa (177)	fǐi	root		dried, crushed, applied topically
POACEAE:						
Arundo donax L.	ñãa ˀɔɔ nɔ́ɔj	VIIIg (354)	khwaam cǎm dii	stem	indifferent	fresh, chewed together with honey

The identification of the botanical material is a result of joint efforts by T. Bjørnland and T. Schumacher; critical taxa of various families have been revised by botanical colleagues as follows:

B. Hansen—Botanical Museum, University of Copenhagen - Acanthaceae
K. Larsen—Botanical Institute, University of Aarhus - Caesalpiniaceae and Zingiberaceae
I. Nielsen—Botanical Institute, University of Aarhus - Mimosaceae
R. Geesink—Rijksherbarium, Leiden - Fabaceae

Plant taxon	Vernacular[1]	Locality[2] (collection number)	Medical use(s)	Part(s) of plant used	Physical[3] quality	Preparation and administration
Bambusa cf. blumeana Schult.	máj phàj cɛ̃ɛ	VIIIh (388)	nĩw	root	indifferent	decoction per os
Coix lacryma-jobi L.	bàdəəj hǐn	Xa (167) VIIIf (296) VIIIj (421) VIh (522)	nĩw	root	indifferent	decoction per os
Dactyloctenium aegyptiacum (L.) P. Beauv.	ñãa phàag khwaaj	XIVa (25)	nĩw	whole plant	indifferent	decoction per os
Eleusine indica (L.) Gaertn.	ñãa phàag khwaaj	XIVa (24)	nĩw	whole plant	indifferent	decoction per os
Imperata cylindrica (L.) Raeusch	ñãa khaa	IIa (251)	khǎaŋ, thàaj sãj dyan	root	indifferent	decoction per os
Saccharum officinarum L.	ʔɔ̃ɔj dam	IIb (435)	jaa tâad	stem	indifferent	decoction per os
Thyrsostachys siamensis Gamble	máj hûag	VIIIh (387)	nĩw	root	indifferent	decoction per os
Thysanolaena maxima (Roxb.) O. Ktze	ñãa tɔ̀ɔŋ kǒŋ	IIId (537)	bàhòog lŷad	root	indifferent	decoction per os
Poaceae *indeterm.*	hǔa ñãa khom baaŋ	IXc (379)	kǐn phid	root	indifferent	dried, crushed, per os

POLYGALACEAE:						
Polygala arillata D. Don	chaaŋ sàtan	XIXa (621)	jaa ˀaajúˀ wádthánáˀ	whole plant	indifferent	dried, crushed, per os
Xanthophyllum siamense Craib	dỳa kiaŋ	IIIc (349)	khǎaŋ	bark, wood	indifferent	dried, ground, per os or chewed (topical)
	máj mádaˀ	IIIe (703)	bàhòog	bark, wood	indifferent	decoction per os
PONTEDERIACEAE:						
Eichhornia crassipes (Mart.) Solms	phag tob	XIVb (436)	bamluŋ hǔa cǎj	flowers	indifferent	dried, crushed, per os
PORTULACACEAE:						
Portulaca oleracea L.	phag bīa	IXb (226)	jaa tâad, saaŋ	root whole plant	cool	dried, ground, per os soaked in water, solution used as bath
PRIMULACEAE:						
Lysimachia laxa Baudo	ñāa khāaw sǎan	XXIIIa (371)	fĭi	leaves	indifferent	fresh, mashed, applied topically
			kɛ̃ɛ lom, khāj	root		dried, ground, per os
PROTEACEAE:						
Helicia cf. nilagirica Bedd.	mádii khwaaj	XXIIb (680)	khǎaŋ	bark, wood	indifferent	dried, ground, per os
PUNICACEAE:						
Punica granatum L.	bàkɔ́ɔ	VIa (1)	jaa kɛ̃ɛ	pericarp (of fruit)	indifferent	dried, crushed, per os
		XVIb (65) VIIIJ (415)	luˀ tɔ́ɔŋ	leaves		decoction per os
RANUNCULACEAE:						
Clematis sp.	cǔaŋ khya	XXIIb (672)	sàníbàad	whole plant	indifferent	dried, crushed, per os

The identification of the botanical material is a result of joint efforts by T. Bjørnland and T. Schumacher; critical taxa of various families have been revised by botanical colleagues as follows:

B. Hansen—Botanical Museum, University of Copenhagen - Acanthaceae
K. Larsen—Botanical Institute, University of Aarhus - Caesalpiniaceae and Zingiberaceae
I. Nielsen—Botanical Institute, University of Aarhus - Mimosaceae
R. Geesink—Rijksherbarium, Leiden - Fabaceae

Plant taxon	Vernacular[1]	Locality[2] (collection number)	Medical use(s)	Part(s) of plant used	Physical[3] quality	Preparation and administration
RHAMNACEAE:						
Ventilago calyculata Tul.	kɔ̂ŋ kὲεb	VIIIa (29) IIa (260)	bàhòog, ceb lăŋ ceb ʔεw	bark, wood	indifferent	decoction per os
Ziziphus mauritiana Lam.	bàtan tõn	VIIIj (422)	khăaŋ naj pàag, khăaŋ hɔ́ɔn khɔɔ	bark, wood	indifferent	dried, crushed, per os
Ziziphus oenoplia (L.) Mill.	tan khɔ̌ɔ	VIIIh (390)	khăaŋ, ceb lăŋ ceb ʔεw	bark, wood " "	indifferent	dried, ground, per os decoction per os
Ziziphus rugosa Lam.	máj bàkhwâad	VIIIm (662)	bàhòog, ceb lăŋ ceb ʔεw	bark, wood	indifferent	decoction per os
Ziziphus sp.	năam kõoŋ dam	XIXa (626)	săan, lom săan	bark, wood	indifferent	dried, ground, per os
ROSACEAE:						
Parinarium anamensis (Hance) J. E. Vid.	mámyy	VIIa (651)	khăaŋ	bark, wood	indifferent	dried, ground, per os
Prunus persica (L.) Batsch	bàmòŋ, fũuŋ khɔ̂ɔb	IIIb (313) VIIIk (479)	tùm sug, tùm săj hɔ́ɔn naj	bark, wood	indifferent	dried, ground, per os
Rubus alceifolius Poir.	bàhúu, bàhúu kham	IIIc (330)	ceb lăŋ ceb ʔεw	root	indifferent	decoction per os

ROXBURGHIACEAE:						
Stemona cf. burkillii Prain	nɔ̌ɔn taaj jàag	IXa (155)	khāa mɛɛŋ	root	indifferent	ground, used as insecticide
Stemona cf. collinsae Craib	nɔ̌ɔn taaj jàag	IXa (46) IXa (156)	*as above*	"		" " " "
RUBIACEAE:						
Canthium sp.	nǎam léb lɔ̀ɔg	XIXa (624)	kǐn phid	bark, wood, root	indifferent	dried, ground, per os
Catunaregam spinosa (Thunb.) Tirveng.	dig diam	IIId (550)	sànîbàad	bark, wood	indifferent	dried, ground, per os
Catunaregam aff. spinosa (Thunb.) Tirveng.	dig diam	XXIVa (461)	*as above*	" "		" " " "
Catunaregam tomentosa (DC.) Tirveng.	máj tɛ́ɛŋ	IIa (262)	khǎaŋ	bark, wood	indifferent	dried, ground, used topically (mouth)
		XXIVa (464)	baw wǎan	bark, wood		decoction per os
Ixora finlaysoniana Wall.	khěm khǎaw	VIIIm (655)	jaa thìib	root	indifferent	dried, ground, per os
Ixora sp. 1.	sōm sug	XIXa (634) XXIa (716A)	sànîbàad, kǐn phid, khīi hâag sɔ̌ɔŋ kɔɔŋ	bark, wood, root	indifferent	dried, ground, per os
Lasianthus sp.	kɔ́ɔŋ din	XVIIc (722)	lom sǎan	root	indifferent	dried, ground, per os
Meyna sp.	máj mákhéd	IXb (233)	bỳa pǎa	fruit	indifferent	squashed, dissolved into a pond (fish poison)
Mitragyna parvifolia Korth.	sàpáan kǎa, máj sɛ?	IVa (644)	khǎaŋ lammánâad	bark	indifferent	decoction per os or chewed
Morinda citrifolia L.	jɔɔ	IIa (240)	jaa tâad	fruit	indifferent	fresh, per os
Oxyceras horrida Lour.	nǎam léb káw, nǎam líd káw	VIIIb (71) IXb (222) IVa (640)	kǐn phid	bark, wood, root	indifferent	dried, ground, per os
Paederia sp. 1.	ñāa tod mǎa	XVIc (83)	ceb lǎŋ ceb ʔɛw, bàhòog	leaves, stem	indifferent	decoction per os
Paederia sp. 2.	cáa ñāa tod mǎa	IXc (377)	ceb lǎŋ ceb ʔɛw, bàhòog	leaves, stem	indifferent	decoction per os
Wendlandia cf. tinctoria A. DC.	sɔ̃ɔj hɔ̌ɔm kǎj	XXIIb (685)	khǎaŋ	bark, wood	indifferent	dried, ground, per os
Wendlandia sp.	máj máhóg fáa	XXIIb (676)	khǎaŋ	bark, wood	indifferent	dried, ground, per os

The identification of the botanical material is a result of joint efforts by T. Bjørnland and T. Schumacher; critical taxa of various families have been revised by botanical colleagues as follows:

B. Hansen—Botanical Museum, University of Copenhagen - Acanthaceae
K. Larsen—Botanical Institute, University of Aarhus - Caesalpiniaceae and Zingiberaceae
I. Nielsen—Botanical Institute, University of Aarhus - Mimosaceae
R. Geesink—Rijksherbarium, Leiden - Fabaceae

Plant taxon	Vernacular[1]	Locality[2] (collection number)	Medical use(s)	Part(s) of plant used	Physical[3] quality	Preparation and administration
RUTACEAE:						
Aegle marmelos (L.) Corr.	bàpin	VIIIc (89) Xa (163)	jaa tâad	fruit	indifferent	decoction per os
Citrus grandis (L.) Osb.	sōm ˀoo	IIIe (693)	khīi hâag sɔ̌ɔŋ kɔɔŋ	pericarp (of fruit)	indifferent	heated, soaked in water, solution per os
			mɛɛŋ khian	juice of pericarp		used topically (head)
			kǐn phid	bark, wood		dried, ground, per os
Citrus hystrix DC.	bàkhùud	XVIb (62)	lom piˀ	pericarp	indifferent	dried, crushed, per os
Euodia lepta (Spreng.) Merr.	saliam doŋ	XIXa (610)	khāj sàn	bark, wood	indifferent khom	decoction per os
Hesperethusa crenulata (Roxb.) Roem.	máj khaˀ cɛˀ	VIIIc (107)	sīw	bark	indifferent	dried, ground, used topically
Micromelum minutum (Forst. f.) Wight et Arn.	cáa phag wǎan cīi jɔ́ɔj	IIIe (689) XVIIc (718)	lom bàheŋkhúd khāj pāaŋ	root bark, wood	indifferent indifferent	dried, ground, per os dried, ground, or decoction, per os
Toddalia asiatica (L.) Lam.	phag pɛɛm pàa	IIId (560)	lom bàheŋkhúd, jaa tâad	whole plant	cool	dried, crushed, per os
		XXIa (711)	tǎa dɛɛŋ	leaves		fresh, soaked in water, solution applied topically (eyes)

Zanthoxylum avicennae (Lam.) DC.	bàkhwɛ̃n, bàkhɛn kɛ̀ɛn nɔ̃ɔj	IIIc (347)	luʔ tɔ́ɔŋ, kad tɔ́ɔŋ	fruit	warm	dried, crushed, or decoction, per os
Zanthoxylum myriacanthum Hook. f.	bàhàad nɔ̃ɔj, bàhàad náam	IIIc (346)	luʔ tɔ́ɔŋ	bark	indifferent	decoction per os
SALICACEAE:						
Salix tetrasperma Roxb.	kháj nûn	VIIIh (389) XIIa (512)	khɔɔ fɔ̂ɔg	bark	indifferent	dried, crushed, per os and used topically as throat paints
SALVADORACEAE:						
Azima tetracantha Lam.	pid tɔ́ʔ	IIc (472)	khāj hâag sàag, jaa thìib	bark, wood	indifferent	dried, ground, per os
SANTALACEAE:						
Henslowia sessilis Craib	kăa fàag, máj tĩin nóg	XXIIa (443)	kĭn phid, lom khȳn	bark, wood	indifferent	dried, ground, per os
SAPINDACEAE:						
Allophylus cobbe (L.) Raeusch	saliam pàa	XVIIb (568)	khāj cab sàn	whole plant	indifferent	decoction per os
Arfeuillea arborescens Pierre	khīi nɔ̆ɔn	VIIa (647)	bàhòog	bark	indifferent	decoction per os
Lepisanthes tetraphylla (Vahl) Radlk.	mŏŋ khaa cyʔ, phag jîaw wua	IXb (232)	bàhòog,	bark, wood	indifferent	decoction per os
			ceb lăŋ ceb ʔɛw, lídsaduaŋ, khāj	" "		dried, ground, per os

The identification of the botanical material is a result of joint efforts by T. Bjørnland and T. Schumacher; critical taxa of various families have been revised by botanical colleagues as follows:

B. Hansen—Botanical Museum, University of Copenhagen - Acanthaceae
K. Larsen—Botanical Institute, University of Aarhus - Caesalpiniaceae and Zingiberaceae
I. Nielsen—Botanical Institute, University of Aarhus - Mimosaceae
R. Geesink—Rijksherbarium, Leiden - Fabaceae

Plant taxon	Vernacular[1]	Locality[2] (collection number)	Medical use(s)	Part(s) of plant used	Physical[3] quality	Preparation and administration
SAPOTACEAE:						
Mimusops elengi L.	kɛ̃ɛw	VIIIc (113)	jaa bamluŋ kǎmlaŋ, khīaw phúʔ	flowers bark	indifferent	dried, crushed, per os chewed (topical)
SAURURACEAE:						
Houttuynia cordata Thunb.	phag khãaw tɔɔŋ	VIIIj (409)	lom piʔ	whole plant	indifferent	dried, crushed, per os
SAXIFRAGACEAE:						
Saxifraga sp.	hɔ̌ɔm dùan nám	VIIIg (359)	bamluŋ hǔa cǎj	whole plant	indifferent	dried, crushed, used as inhalant
SCROPHULARIACEAE:						
Scoparia dulcis L.	ñāa khad nɔ́ɔj	VIIIc (101)	khāj	whole plant	indifferent	decoction, per os or as bath

SIMAROUBACEAE:						
Brucea javanica (L.) Merr.	hadsàkhyn	IXa (143) IIa (246) IIa (257)	khāj	bark, wood	indifferent	decoction per os
Eurycoma longifolia Jack.	hɛɛpancan	XXIVa (460)	khăaŋ, saaŋ	bark, wood	indifferent	dried, ground, per os
Harrisonia perforata (Blanco) Merr.	máj cîi	IIa (268)	phɛ̆ɛ	fruit	indifferent	decoction, solution applied topically
		IIId (547)	kìaw	fruit		heated, chopped in pieces, applied topically
		VIIIm (659)	khăaŋ, khăaŋ lammánâad	bark, wood		dried, ground, per os
Irvingia malayana A. Benn.	mámŷyn	XXIVa (465)	khāj tăa lўaŋ	pericarp (of fruit)	indifferent	dried, crushed, per os
Picrasma javanica Bl.	bàkɔɔm khŏm	XVIIb (577)	kĭn phid (*laxative*)	bark	indifferent	dried, crushed, per os
SMILACACEAE:						
Smilax biumbellata T. Koyama	khāw jen tāj, daw nɔ́ɔj	IXb (230)	lídsaduaŋ, lom săan	root	indifferent	decoction per os
Smilax lanceifolia Roxb.	daw, khāw jen tāj, daw nɔ́ɔj	IIIa (325) XIXa (630) IIId (551)	lídsaduaŋ, lom săan	root	indifferent	decoction per os
Smilax ovalifolia Roxb.	daw lŭaŋ	XVIa (28) IXb (231) VIIIf (290)	lídsaduaŋ, lom săan	root	indifferent	decoction per os
SOLANACEAE:						
Datura metel L. var. alba (Nees) C. B. Clarke	bàkhўa bāa khăaw	Xa (178)	sàníbàad bāa	root	indifferent	dried, ground, per os
Datura metel L. var. metel	bàkhўa bāa dam	VId (127) VIf (273)	sàníbàad bāa	root	indifferent	dried, ground, per os
Nicotiana tabacum L.	ñāa múan khỳn	XVIIa (503)	khāa mɛɛŋ	leaves	indifferent	fermented leaves soaked in water, solution used topically

The identification of the botanical material is a result of joint efforts by T. Bjørnland and T. Schumacher; critical taxa of various families have been revised by botanical colleagues as follows:

B. Hansen—Botanical Museum, University of Copenhagen - Acanthaceae
K. Larsen—Botanical Institute, University of Aarhus - Caesalpiniaceae and Zingiberaceae
I. Nielsen—Botanical Institute, University of Aarhus - Mimosaceae
R. Geesink—Rijksherbarium, Leiden - Fabaceae

Plant taxon	Vernacular[1]	Locality[2] (collection number)	Medical use(s)	Part(s) of plant used	Physical[3] quality	Preparation and administration
Solanum ferox L.	bàkhŷa pùu	VIIIk (476)	phɛ̌ɛ phúaʔ, khǎaŋ, kǐn phid	leaves stem	indifferent	*used as above* dried, crushed, per os
Solanum indicum L.	bàkhwɛ́ŋ khǒm	VIa (16) XVIa (44) VIIIj (413) VIIIn (668)	khǎaŋ hɔ̌ɔn khɔɔ, lom sǎan, khāj, kǐn phid, jaa tâad	root fruit	indifferent	dried, ground, per os dried, crushed, per os
Solanum seaforthianum Andr.	bàkhwɛ́ŋ khya	Xa (174)	khīi hâag sɔ̌ɔŋ kɔɔŋ	whole plant	indifferent	decoction per os
Solanum torvum Sw.	bàkhwɛ́ŋ kulaa	VIIIm (657)	khāj	bark, wood	indifferent	dried, ground, or decoction, per os
Solanum verbascifolium L.	máj fàa pɛ̃ɛŋ	XVIIa (485)	khāj hâag sàad	root	indifferent	dried, ground, or decoction, per os
Solanum sp.	bàkhŷa khỳn bàkhŷa cɛ̃ɛ	VIIIb (76)	jaa tâad	root	indifferent	dried, crushed, per os
SONNERATIACEAE:						
Duabanga sonneratioides Buch.-Ham.	máj sàbāa	XIIa (504)	phɛ̌ɛ phúaʔ	bark	indifferent	dried, crushed, used topically

STAPHYLEACEAE:						
Turpinia pomifera DC.	máj mûaŋ kɔ̃ɔm	IIIe (697)	bàhòog	bark, wood, root	indifferent	decoction per os
Turpinia sphaerocarpa Hassk.	máj khám, máj wid doŋ	XIXa (620)	kɛ̃ɛ lom	bark	indifferent	dried, ground, per os
STERCULIACEAE:						
Pterospermum semisagittatum Roxb.	máj hăm hɔ̂ɔg	IIa (248)	khĩaw phúʔ	bark	indifferent	fresh, chewed (topical)
Sterculia foetida L.	pỳag pɔ̃ɔ	VIIIj (417)	khĩi sĩan	bark	indifferent	dried, crushed, soaked in water, solution applied topically
Waltheria indica L.	pàa hêw mɔ̆ɔŋ	IIa (266)	nàaj ʔɔ̀ɔn phia, jaa tâad	leaves	indifferent	dried, crushed, per os
			khãj, phɔ̆ɔm hɛ̃ɛŋ lɛɛŋ nɔ́ɔj	root		decoction per os
SYMPLOCACEAE:						
Symplocos hookeri C. B. Clarke in Hook. f.	mádii kàj	XXIa (716)	khãj,	bark, wood	indifferent	decoction per os
			tăa dɛɛŋ	fruit		mashed, soaked in water, solution applied topically
TACCACEAE:						
Tacca integrifolia Ker-Gawl.	dii ŋuu wãa	XVIc (189) IIIa (309) IIIe (705)	bamluŋ hŭa căj, jaa tâad	whole plant	indifferent	dried, crushed, per os
			khăaŋ, kĭn phid, pɔɔŋ, jaa bamluŋ kămlaŋ	root		dried, ground, per os
THEACEAE:						
Anneslea fragrans Wall.	níw myy phácãw	XXIIa (453)	khăaŋ	bark, wood	indifferent	dried, ground, per os
	hãa pháʔoŋ	XXIIb (684)	khăaŋ khañyy, khĩi khûu	" "		decoction per os

The identification of the botanical material is a result of joint efforts by T. Bjørnland and T. Schumacher; critical taxa of various families have been revised by botanical colleagues as follows:

B. Hansen—Botanical Museum, University of Copenhagen - Acanthaceae
K. Larsen—Botanical Institute, University of Aarhus - Caesalpiniaceae and Zingiberaceae
I. Nielsen—Botanical Institute, University of Aarhus - Mimosaceae
R. Geesink—Rijksherbarium, Leiden - Fabaceae

Plant taxon	Vernacular[1]	Locality[2] (collection number)	Medical use(s)	Part(s) of plant used	Physical[3] quality	Preparation and administration
Camellia caudata Wall.	săalápii pàa	XXIIa (447)	khăaŋ, kɛ̃ɛ lom, bamluŋ hŭa căj	bark flowers	indifferent	dried, crushed, per os dried, crushed, inhaled
Camellia sinensis (L.) O. Ktze	mīaŋ	IIId (533)	luʔ tɔ́ɔŋ	leaves	indifferent	decoction per os
Eurya acuminata DC.	māw săaj	IIId (559)	phɛ̆ɛ píd ŋuu khob	bark, wood, leaves leaves	indifferent	dried, crushed, used topically fresh, chewed, juice swallowed, remnants applied topically
THYMELAEACEAE:						
Daphne involucrata Wall.	khĕm khăaw pàa	XIXa (631)	kɛ̃ɛ lom, fĭi săan naj tɔ́ɔŋ jaa thìib (lom, tùm, khāj) fĭi săan naj tɔ́ɔŋ	bark, wood root bark, wood	indifferent	dried, ground, per os dried, ground, per os decoction per os

TILIACEAE:						
Colona floribunda (Kurr) Craib	pɔ̆ɔ tɛ̆ɛŋ	IIIe (701)	lom bàheŋkhúd	bark, wood	indifferent	dried, ground, per os
Grewia lacei Drum. et Craib	pɔ̆ɔ mŷyn	XXIVa (466)	khīi haŋkɛɛ	bark	indifferent	decoction, solution applied topically
Grewia microcos L.	bàkɔɔm	Xa (181)	tùm khan	leaves	indifferent	fresh, mashed, used topically
Triumfetta bartramia L.	ñāa phŏm ñūŋ	XVIIb (583)	khāj	root	indifferent	decoction per os
ULMACEAE:						
Celtis philippinensis Blanco	máj kêŋ khīi phácāw	IIIb (327)	kɛ̃ɛ lom	bark, wood	indifferent	dried, ground, per os
Celtis tetrandra Roxb.	máj had	XIIa (514)	bàhòog	bark, wood	indifferent	decoction per os
Celtis cf. timorensis Spanoghe	máj had	IIIe (696)	*as above*	" "		" " "
Trema orientalis (L.) Bl.	máj ñâab	IIIe (698)	jaa kɛ̃ɛ	bark, wood	indifferent	dried, ground, per os
URTICACEAE:						
Boehmeria nivea (L.) Gaud.	pàan săa	XVIIa (480)	lom bàheŋkhúd, kĭn phid	bark, wood, root "	indifferent	dried, ground, or decoction, per os decoction per os
Debregaesia velutina Gaud.	phag mŭu	XXIIIb (373)	khāj	root	indifferent	dried, ground, per os
VERBENACEAE:						
Callicarpa candicans (Burm. f.) Hochr.	sàpháan kón	IXa (139)	kĭn phid, kĭn sàlɛ̆ɛŋ (*laxative*)	root	indifferent	dried, crushed, per os
Clerodendrum fragrans (Vent.) R. Br.	pîŋ sɔ́ɔn, ñāa liŋ cɔ̂ɔn khăaw	VIIIb (73) IIIa (304)	bàhòog, lídsaduaŋ twaan, tùm	root "	indifferent	decoction per os dried, ground, used topically
Clerodendrum serratum (L.) Moon	pîŋ dɛɛŋ, ñāa liŋ cɔ̂ɔn dɛɛŋ	IIIa (307)	bàhòog, lídsaduaŋ twaan, tùm	root "	indifferent	decoction per os dried, ground, used topically

The identification of the botanical material is a result of joint efforts by T. Bjørnland and T. Schumacher; critical taxa of various families have been revised by botanical colleagues as follows:

B. Hansen—Botanical Museum, University of Copenhagen - Acanthaceae
K. Larsen—Botanical Institute, University of Aarhus - Caesalpiniaceae and Zingiberaceae
I. Nielsen—Botanical Institute, University of Aarhus - Mimosaceae
R. Geesink—Rijksherbarium, Leiden - Fabaceae

Plant taxon	Vernacular[1]	Locality[2] (collection number)	Medical use(s)	Part(s) of plant used	Physical[3] quality	Preparation and administration
Clerodendrum squamatum Vahl	pîŋ dɛɛŋ, ñāa líŋ cɔ̂ɔn dɛɛŋ	IXa (142)	bàhòog, lídsaduaŋ twaan,	root	indifferent	decoction per os
			tùm	″		dried, ground, used topically
Clerodendrum sp. 1.	léb myy naaŋ	IIIb (328)	khǎaŋ	whole plant	indifferent	dried, crushed, per os
Clerodendrum sp. 2.	pîŋ khǎaw	IIIe (699)	jaa ʔaajúʔ wádthánáʔ, jaa tâad	root	indifferent	decoction per os
Congea tomentosa Roxb.	khyaʔɔ̀ɔn dɛɛŋ	IIa (259) VIIIm (654)	bàhòog	bark, wood	indifferent	decoction per os
Duranta repens L.	thian khāaw tɔ̀ɔg	IIa (242)	maw hǔa	bark, wood	indifferent	fresh, crushed, per os
Gmelina arborea Roxb.	máj phǎa sǐan, tɔɔŋ sǎa	VIIIm (663)	jaa kɛ̃ɛ	bark, wood	indifferent	dried, ground, per os
Lantana camara L.	ñāa khīi tûud	IXb (214) VIIIm (666)	khǎaŋ, khīi tûud	bark, wood	indifferent	decoction per os
Nyctanthes arbor-tristis L.	sàpáan kǎa, máj sɛɛ	XIVa (26)	lom kìaw, nedsaa	bark, wood, leaves	indifferent	dried, ground, per os
		XIa (457)	khǎaŋ lammánâad	bark		decoction as rinse water and per os

Tectona grandis L. f.	sàg	VIIIf (294)	kĭn phid, lom bàheŋkhúd	fruit bark	indifferent	decoction per os dried, crushed, per os
Vitex peduncularis Schauer	tĭin ped khya	VIIIa (48)	khăaŋ	bark, wood, root	indifferent	dried, ground, per os
Vitex trifolia L.	phĭi sȳa nɔ́ɔj, sĭi sȳa nɔ́ɔj	VIIIb (74)	ja tâad jaa salĭimuun	whole plant	warm	dried, crushed, per os
VIOLACEAE:						
Rinorea virgata (Thw.) O. Ktze	hɔˀ sáthɔ́ɔn	IIe (470)	khāj hâag sàad, hɔ́ɔn naj	bark, wood	indifferent	dried, crushed, per os
VITACEAE:						
Cayratia pedata (Lour.) Juss.	sōm máˀɔ̀ɔb	XIIIa (191)	khăaŋ, saaŋ	whole plant	indifferent	soaked in water, solution as bath and per os
Cayratia tenuifolia Gagnep. in Lecomte	ñāa pog tɔ̆ɔ	XXIIb (674)	lom piˀ, piˀ fáa mɛ̂ɛb, khāj jaa tâad	whole plant " "	indifferent	decoction per os dried, crushed, per os
Cayratia trifolia (L.) Domin	ñāa pog tɔ̆ɔ	IIa (253) VIIIg (350)	lom piˀ, piˀ fáa mɛ̂ɛb, khāj jaa tâad	whole plant " "	indifferent	decoction per os dried, crushed, per os
Cissus cf. discolor Bl.	cĭi cɔ̄ɔ lŭaŋ	Ia (398)	khāj	root	indifferent	decoction per os
Cissus cf. siamica Planch. in DC.	khya khăw mûag khăaw	VIIIb (80) VIIIe (272)	maw hŭa	stem	indifferent	dried, crushed, per os
cf. Cissus sp.	bàdỳa thăw, bàdỳa khya	XIIIa (186)	lúˀ tɔ́ɔŋ	whole plant	indifferent	decoction per os
Leea acuminata C. B. Clarke	khĭaŋ khêŋ máa dɛɛŋ	VIIIa (50) IXa (129)	bàhòog	root	indifferent	decoction per os
Leea crispa L.	khĭaŋ khêŋ máa khăaw	VIIIa (49) IXa (128)	bàhòog	root	indifferent	decoction per os
ZINGIBERACEAE:						
Alpinia sp.	khàa	VIIIb (60) VIIIf (283)	ceb tɔ́ɔŋ, kad tɔ́ɔŋ ceb tɔ́ɔŋ	root "	warm	boiled and eaten " " "

List of Medicinal Plants Collected in Chiangmai and Lamphun Provinces, Northern Thailand (*continued*)

The identification of the botanical material is a result of joint efforts by T. Bjørnland and T. Schumacher; critical taxa of various families have been revised by botanical colleagues as follows:

B. Hansen—Botanical Museum, University of Copenhagen - Acanthaceae
K. Larsen—Botanical Institute, University of Aarhus - Caesalpiniaceae and Zingiberaceae
I. Nielsen—Botanical Institute, University of Aarhus - Mimosaceae
R. Geesink—Rijksherbarium, Leiden - Fabaceae

Plant taxon	Vernacular[1]	Locality[2] (collection number)	Medical use(s)	Part(s) of plant used	Physical[3] quality	Preparation and administration
Amomum sp. 1.	máʔīi	IXa (138) IIIb (321)	jaa tâad	root	warm	dried, powdered, per os
Amomum sp. 2.	hǔa bahaŋ ŋâŋ	XVIIa (491)	ceb tɔ́ɔŋ, jaa tâad	root	warm	dried, powdered, per os
Boesenbergia sp. 1.	hǔa láʔɛɛn	VIIIc (86)	bamluŋ hǔa cǎj, fǐi sǎan naj tɔ́ɔŋ	root	warm	dried powdered, per os
Boesenbergia sp. 2.	khǐŋ tàw	VIIIc (90)	jaa tâad, ceb tɔ́ɔŋ	root	warm	dried, powdered, per os
Boesenbergia sp. 3.	wāan màhǎa nin	VIIIc (97)	kad tɔ́ɔŋ, luʔ tɔ́ɔŋ fǐi, phɛ̌ɛ píd, ŋuu khob	whole plant " "	warm	dried, crushed, per os dried, crushed, used topically
Boesenbergia sp. 4.	hɛɛw dam	IXa (131)	ceb tɔ́ɔŋ, jaa tâad	root	warm	dried, powdered, per os
Boesenbergia sp. 5.	hǔa kǎmbid	IXa (132)	ceb tɔ́ɔŋ, jaa tâad	root	warm	dried, powdered, per os
Curcuma sp.	khāw mīn, khāw mīn jùag	VIIIf (282)	fǐi, tùm khan, sǎan, fǐi sǎan	root	warm	dried, powdered, used topically dried, powdered, per os
Hedychium stenopetalum Lodd.	ćii kúg	VIIIf (284) IIIb (320)	bamluŋ kǎmlaŋ lǎŋ kə̀əd	root, stem	indifferent	decoction both per os and as steam bath
Kaempferia galanga L.	wāan phɛ̀n din jen	VIIIc (87)	jaa tâad	root	indifferent	dried, powdered, per os or as inhalant

Zingiber sp. 1.	puuləəj lŭaŋ	VIa (14)	ceb tɔ́ɔŋ, kad tɔ́ɔŋ, lu? tɔ́ɔŋ	root	warm	boiled and eaten
Zingiber sp. 2.	puuləəj	VIIIb (66)	*as above*	"	"	" " "
Zingiber officinale (L.) Roscoe	khĭŋ	XVIc (204)	jaa tâad	root	warm	dried, powdered, per os
Zingiber sp. 3.	hŭa kămbid	VIf (278)	ceb tɔ́ɔŋ, jaa tâad	root	warm	dried, powdered, per os
Zingiber sp. 4.	khăw mīn khy̆n	VIf (279)	khāj, jaa tâad	root	warm	dried, powdered, per os
Zingiber sp. 5.	khĭŋ pàa	IIIa (324)	khāj hɔ́ɔn naj, ceb tɔ́ɔŋ, kad tɔ́ɔŋ	root	warm	dried, powdered or decoction per os
INDETERMINATA:						
	dii ŋuu tōn	XVIIb (571)	kĭn phid, kĭn sàlɛ̆ɛŋ (*laxative*)	root	indifferent	fresh, ground, per os
	hàdsàkhŭn thêed	VIIIa (58) IIa (258)	kɛ̃ɛ ?aj	bark, wood	indifferent	fresh, soaked in water, solution mixed with sugar, per os
	hɔ̃ɔ sàpaaj khwaaj	IIIc (335)	jaa bamluŋ kămlaŋ	bark, wood	indifferent	decoction per os
	kaaŋ khĭi mɔ̂ɔd	IIIc (349)	khăaŋ, bàhòog	bark bark, wood	indifferent	dried, ground, per os decoction per os
	kămlaŋ cáaŋ phy̆ag	VIIIc (98)	jaa bamluŋ kămlaŋ, jaa tâad	bark, wood, root bark	indifferent	decoction per os dried, crushed, per os
	kămlaŋ cáaŋ săan	IXb (209)	jaa bamluŋ kămlaŋ, jaa tâad	bark, wood, root bark	indifferent	decoction per os dried, crushed, per os
	kampɔɔŋ	XXIIa (451)	khāj	root	indifferent	decoction per os
	khăw wua	IIIb (315)	bàhòog, ceb lăŋ ceb ?ɛw	root	indifferent	decoction per os
	kĭaŋ phaa bāan	VIIIj (419)	tăa dɛɛŋ, lom kìaw	leaves whole plant	indifferent	mashed, water added, solution applied topically decoction per os
	máj bàkhwád	XIIa (506)	bàhòog, bàhòog lŷad		indifferent	decoction per os

The identification of the botanical material is a result of joint efforts by T. Bjørnland and T. Schumacher; critical taxa of various families have been revised by botanical colleagues as follows:

B. Hansen—Botanical Museum, University of Copenhagen - Acanthaceae
K. Larsen—Botanical Institute, University of Aarhus - Caesalpiniaceae and Zingiberaceae
I. Nielsen—Botanical Institute, University of Aarhus - Mimosaceae
R. Geesink—Rijksherbarium, Leiden - Fabaceae

Plant taxon	Vernacular[1]	Locality[2] (collection number)	Medical use(s)	Part(s) of plant used	Physical[3] quality	Preparation and administration
	máj kǎj	XVIIb (580)	khǎaŋ pàag pỳaj	bark	indifferent	fresh, crushed, applied topically
	máj máda	XVIIIa (594)	bàhòog	bark, wood	indifferent	decoction per os
	máj ʔii hὲεg	XIXa (627)	khǎaŋ, pɔɔŋ	bark, wood	indifferent	decoction per os
	mŷad khɔ̀n	IXa (141)	khǎaŋ, bàhòog	bark	indifferent	dried, ground, per os decoction per os
	ñãa khêŋ kàj	XIIIa (193)	sad khob, ŋuu khob	leaves	indifferent	chewed, juice swallowed, remnants applied topically
	ñãa sãj cáaŋ, khya sãj cáaŋ	IXa (148)	lom phid dyan, sàníbàad,	stems, leaves	indifferent	dried, crushed, per os or in aqueous solution as bath
			tùm dεεŋ	" "		soaked in water, solution as bath
	nǎam léb sy̌a	XIXa (622)	kε̃ε píd	bark, wood	indifferent	dried, ground per os
	phájáb mɔ̀ɔg	XVIe (434)	lom khy̌n	root	indifferent	fresh, ground, per os
	phag pεεm	VIIIf (287)	lom bàheŋkhúd, khwaam dǎn,	whole plant	cool	dried, crushed, per os decoction per os
			tǎa dεεŋ	leaves		soaked in water, solution applied topically

	saaŋ ciŋ	XIXa (616)	săan, lom săan	bark	cool	dried, ground, per os
	sămpan tỹŋ	Xa (171)	*local anaesthetic*	whole plant	warm	mashed, juice applied topically
		VIIIg (357)				
	sõm pɔ̃ɔŋ	XXIIa (450)	bàhòog	root	indifferent	decoction per os

1 The medicinal plants with entry on the local vernacular name is found in Index 3 on page xxx.
2 Localities and dates of collecting are found following this list.
3 For a summary of the physical qualities of the drugs, see section 3.8.6.

LOCALITIES (ALTITUDES), COLLECTING DATES, AND INFORMANTS

1. BAN HUAY CHANG KHIAN—DOI SUTHEP (350–800 m), Amphoe Muang, Cangwat Chiangmai: (a) 19 October 1978 (Pradit).
2. BAN HUAY SAI (350 m), Amphoe Muang, Cangwat Chiangmai: (a) 24 August 1978 (Pradit); (b) 26 October 1978 (Pradit); (c) 30 November 1978 (Pradit).
3. BAN KONG HAE (700–1,100 m), Amphoe Mae Rim, Cangwat Chiangmai: (a) 7 September 1978 (Pradit); (b) 7 September 1978 (Pradit and Bunchuaj Wajwongrob); (c) 14 September 1978 (Pradit and Bunchuaj Wajwongrob); (d) 21 December 1978 (Pradit and Inta Munpanind); (e) 15 February 1979 (Pradit and Inta Munpanind).
4. BAN LAN (300 m), Amphoe Muang, Cangwat Lamphun: (a) 1 February 1979 (Pradit).
5. BAN MAE MAE (550 m), Amphoe Mae Rim, Cangwat Chiangmai: (a) 14 September 1978 (Pradit).
6. BAN MUANG NGA (300 m), Amphoe Muang, Cangwat Lamphun: (a) 3 July 1978 (Po Liang Tan); (b) 12 July 1978 (Po Liang Tan); (c) 13 July 1978 (Mo Suphab); (d) 2 August 1978 (Po Liang Tan); (e) 14 August 1978 (Po Liang Tan); (f) 26 August 1978 (Po Liang Tan); (g) 27 October 1978 28 January 1979 (Pradit); (h) 17 December 1978 (Po Liang Tan); (i) 20 December 1978 (Po Liang Tan); (j) 10 January 1979 (Po Liang Tan); (k) 4 February 1979 (Pradit).
7. BAN NONG HUA (300 m), Amphoe Muang, Cangwate Lamphun: (a) 1 February 1979 (Pradit).
8. BAN PONG NOI (350 m), Amphoe Muang, Cangwat Chiangmai: (a) 19 July 1978 (Pradit); (b) 25 July 1978 (Pradit); (c) 27 July 1978 (Pradit); (d) 22 August 1978 24 February 1979 (Pradit); (e) 24 August 1978 (Pradit); (f) 29 August 1978

(Pradit); (g) 21 September 1978 (Pradit); (h) 12 October 1978 (Pradit); (i) 12 October 1978 (Khru Ded); (j) 26 October 1978 (Pradit); (k) 30 November 1978 (Pradit); (1) 14 January 1979 (Pradit); (m) 3 February 1979 (Pradit); (n) 4 February 1979 (Pradit).

9. BAN PONG NOI—DOI SUTHEP (350–700 m), Amphoe Muang, Cangwat Chiangmai: (a) 3 August 1978 (Pradit); (b) 17 August 1978 (Lung Peng); (c) 12 October 1978 (Pradit).

10. BAN RAM PERNG (350 m), Amphoe Muang, Cangwat Chiangmai: (a) 8 August 1978 (Pradit).

11. BAN SARAPHI CANG KHOENG (300 m), Amphoe Saraphi, Cangwat Chiangmai: (a) 29 November 1978 (Po Liang Tan).

12. BAN THAP DUA ARBORETUM (500 m), Amphoe Mae Taeng—Amphoe Chiang Dao, Cangwat Chiangmai: (a) 14 December 1978 (Pradit).

13. BAN UBOSOT (350 m), Amphoe Muang, Cangwat Chiangmai: (a) 10 August 1978 (Pradit).

14. CHIANGMAI (350 m), Amphoe Muang, Cangwat Chiangmai: (a) 16 July 1978 (Po Liang Tan); (b) 26 October 1978 (Pradit).

15. CHIANGMAI ARBORETUM (350 m), Amphoe Muang, Cangwat Chiangmai: (a) 10 August 1978 (Pradit).

16. CHIANGMAI UNIVERSITY (350 m), Amphoe Muang, Cangwat Chiangmai: (a) 19 July 1978 (Pradit); (b) 25 July 1978 (Pradit); (c) 10 August 1978 (Pradit); (d) 19 October 1978 (Pradit); (e) 26 October 1978 (Pradit).

17. DOI CHIANG DAO (500–700 m), Amphoe Chiang Dao, Cangwat Chiangmai: (a) 14 December 1978 (Pradit); (b) 4 January 1979 (Pradit and Lung Pom); (c) 22 February 1979 (Pradit and Lung Pom).

18. DOI INTHANON (500 m), Amphoe Chom Thong, Cangwat Chiangmai: (a) 11 January 1979 (Pradit).

19. DOI INTHANON (1,200 m), Ban Manad, Amphoe Mae Chaem, Cangwat Chiangmai: (a) 18 January 1979 (Pradit, Phua Nannoi, and Phua Muad).

20. DOI INTHANON (2,400–2,580 m), Amphoe Mae Chaem, Cangwat Chiangmai: (a) 11 January 1979 (Pradit).

21. DOI INTHANON (1,000 m), Nam Tok, Amphoe Mae Chaem, Cangwat Chiangmai: (a) 20 February 1979 (Pradit).

22. DOI PUI (1,600–1,685 m), Amphoe Muang, Cangwat Chiangmai: (a) 9 November 1978 (Pradit); (b) 8 February 1979 (Pradit).

23. DOI SUTHEP (1,400 m), Amphoe Muang, Cangwat Chiangmai: (a) 21 September 1978 (Pradit); (b) 21 September 1978 (local Meo); (c) 21 September 1978 (local Thai); (d) 27 August 1978 (Pradit).

24. WAT DOI KHEO (350 m), Amphoe Hang Dong, Cangwat Chiangmai: (a) 30 November 1978 (Pradit).

Bibliography

Thai authors, when writing in Thai, are alphabetized according to their first names.

A Barefoot Doctor's Manual
1977 Pennsylvania: Running Press.

Beyer, C.
1907 "About Siamese Medicine," *Journal of the Siam Society* 4:1–9.

Boesch, E. E.
1972 *Communication Between Doctors and Patients in Thailand.* Part 1: "Survey of the Problem and Analysis of the Consultations." Saarbrücken: Sozialpsychologische Forschungsstelle für Entwicklungsplanung, Universität des Saarlandes.

Bradley, D. B.
1865 *Siamese Practice of Medicine.* Bangkok Calendar 1865 (reprinted in *Social Science Review* [Bangkok] 5:103–119, 1967).

Breakey, G. F., and E. Voulgaropoulos
1976 *Laos Health Survey: Mekong Valley 1968–69.* Honolulu: University Press of Hawaii.

Brun, V.
1980 *The Relationship between Drugs and Diseases in Northern Thai Traditional Medicine.* Paper presented at ASOMPS IV, Bangkok.

Burling, R.
1964 "Cognition and Componential Analysis: God's Truth or Hocus-Pocus?" *American Anthropologist* 66:20–28.

Chan- Ok

1955 *Contribution à l'étude de la thérapeutique traditionelle en pays khmer.* Paris: Faculté Médecine, Université de Paris. Thesis.

Collins, D. C.

1906 *An English Laos Dictionary.* Chiangmai: Mission Press (reprinted 1972, England: Westmead, Gregg International Publishers Ltd.).

cɔɔ cɔɔ sɔ̌ɔ

1966 *phódcanaanúkrom phaasǎaphâagnɨ̌a* (A Northern Thai Dictionary). Bangkok: ʔàgsɔ̌ɔnsǎmphan.

Cullimore, D. H.

1875 *The Burmese, What Do They Know of Medicine?* Madras.

Cunningham, C. E.

1970 "Thai 'Injection Doctors': Antibiotic Meditors,' *Social Science and Medicine* 4:1–24.

Cunningham, C. E. (ed.)

1970 *Studies of Health Problems and Health Behavior in Saraphi District, North Thailand.* Chiangmai: Chiangmai University.

Damrong Khun Ying

1931 *Siamese Midwifery in the Old Days.* Bangkok.

Damrong Rajanuphab

1968 *níthaan booraankhádii* (*Tales from Ancient Times*). Bangkok: sǐnlápaabannaakhaan. (First printing, 1944.)

Davis, R.

1974 *Muang Metaphysics: A Study of Northern Thai Myth and Ritual.* Sidney: University of Sidney. Thesis.

Day, F. A., and B. Leoprapai

1977 *Patterns of Health Utilization in Upcountry Thailand.* Bangkok: Institute for Population and Social Research, Mahidol University.

Dhani Nivat

1933 "The Inscriptions of Wat Phra Jetubon," *Journal of the Siam Society* 26:143–170.

Dunn, F. L.

1976 "Traditional Asian Medicine and Cosmopolitan Medicine as Adaptive Systems," in *Asian Medical Systems: A Comparative Study,* ed.

C. Leslie. Berkeley, Los Angeles, London: University of California Press.

Feltus, G. H.
1924 *Samuel Reynolds. House of Siam, pioneer medical missionary, 1847–1876.* New York.

Filliozat, J.
1964 *The Classical Doctrine of Indian Medicine: Its Origins and Its Greek Parallels* (English version by Dev Raj Chanana). New Delhi: Munshiram Manoharlal.

Foster, G. M.
1976 "Disease Etiologies in Non-Western Medical Systems," *American Anthropologist* 78:773–782.

Foster, G. M., and B. G. Anderson
1978 *Medical Anthropology.* New York: John Wiley & Sons.

Frake, C. O.
1961 "The Diagnosis of Disease Among the Subanum of Mindanao," *American Anthropologist* 63:113–132.

Gilmette, J. D., and I. H. Burkhill
1930 "The Medical Book of Malayan Medicine," *Gardens' Bulletin* [Singapore] 6:323–474.

Gilmette, J. D., and H. W. Thomson
1939 *A Dictionary of Malayan Medicine* (reprinted 1971, London: Oxford University Press).

Goldschmidt, A. M. F., and B. Höfer
1972 *Communication Between Doctors and Patients in Thailand.* Part II: "Analysis of the Interviews with Doctors. Analysis of the Interviews with Patients." Saarbrücken: Sozialpsychologische Forschungsstelle für Entwicklungsplanung, Universität des Saarlandes.

Griswold, A. B.
1965 The Rishis of Wat Pó, in: *Felicitation volumes of Southeast-Asian studies presented to His Highness Prince Dhaninivat Kromamun Bidyalabh Bridhyakorn.* 2:319–328. Bangkok: The Siam Society.

Halpern, J. M.
1963 "Traditional Medicine and the Role of the Phi in Laos," *Eastern Anthropologist* 16:191–200.

Hanks, J. R.
1963 *Maternity and Its Rituals in Bang Chan.* Data Paper 51, Southeast Asia Program. New York: Cornell University.

Hart, D. V.
1970 *Bisayan Filipino and Malayan Humoral Pathologies: Folk Medicine and Ethnohistory in Southeast Asia.* Data Paper 76, Southeast Asia Program. New York: Cornell University.

Hauck, M. M.
1959 *Maternal and Child Health in a Siamese Rice Village: Nutritional Aspects. Studies in Bang Chan 1952–1954.* Data Paper 39, Southeast Asia Program. New York: Cornell University.

Hinderling, P.
1972 *Volkstümliche Medizin in Thailand. Interviews mit traditionellen Ärzten über Erklärungssysteme und Therapien. Aspekte der Interaktion zwischen Ärzten und Patienten.* Saarbrücken: Sozialpsychologische Forschungsstelle für Entwicklungsplanung, Universität des Saarlandes.

Hofbauer, R.
1943 "A Medical Retrospect of Thailand," *Journal of the Siam Society* 34:183–200.

Huard, P.
1963 "Le médicine cambodgienne traditionelle," *France-Asie* 19:676–686.

Ionescu-Tongyonk, J.
1981 "Explication of Wind Illness in Northern Thailand," *Transcultural Psychiatric Research Review* 18:42–45.

Irvine, W.
1982 *The Thai-Yuan 'Madman', and the Modernising, Developing Thai Nation as Bounded Entities under Threat: A Study in the Replication of a Single Image.* London: School of Oriental and African Studies. Thesis.

Jaspan, M. A.
1969 *Traditional Medical Theory in South-East Asia.* Hull: University of Hull publication.

júwadii tàpàniijaakɔɔn
1979 *wíwádthánaakaan khɔ̌ɔŋ kaanphɛ̂ɛdthaj tâŋtɛ̀ɛ sàmǎjrɔ̂əmtôn conthɤ̌ŋ cùlácɔɔmklâw.* (Evolution of Thai medicine from the earliest times to the Reign of King Chulalongkorn.) Bangkok; Chulalongkorn University. Thesis.

kaansỳgsǎa kaancèbkhâj khɔ̌ɔŋ pràchaakɔɔn naj tambon bâanlǔaŋ lɛ́ʔ tambon bâanpɛ̀ʔ, ʔamphəə cɔɔmthɔɔŋ, caŋwàd chiangmàj (A Study of Diseases of the Population in Ban Luang and Ban Pae Communes, Com Thong District, Chiangmai Province).
1977 Ciangmai: Chiangmai University (research paper by group of third-year medical students, 1976–1977). Mimeographed.

khɔ̂ɔsɔ̀ɔb lɛ́ʔ chàlɔ̌əj pheesàdchákamthaj phɛ̌ɛnbooraan (the correct answers to examination questions in traditional Thai pharmacy).
1973 Bangkok: sàmaakhom phɛ̂ɛdphɛ̌ɛnbooraan, wád máhǎathâad (Society of Traditional Doctors, Wat Mahathad).

khûumyy kaansỳgsǎa wíchaapheesàdchákɔɔnthaj (A Manual for Studies in Thai Pharmacy).
1969 Bangkok: sàmaakhom rooŋrian phɛ̂ɛdphɛ̌ɛnbooraan naj pràthêedthaj, wád phráchêedtùphon (Society of the School of Traditional Medicine in Thailand, Wat Pho).

khûumyy kaansỳgsǎa wíchaawêedchákam (A Manual for Medical Studies).
1970 Bangkok: sàmaakhom rooŋrian phɛ̂ɛdphɛ̌ɛnbooraan naj pràthêedthaj, wád phráchêedtùphon (Society of the School of Traditional Medicine in Thailand, Wat Pho).

Konoshima, M., M. Tabata, and D. Pecheraply
1973 "On a Thai native doctor and his folk medicine," *Tonan Ajia Kenkyu* (Southeast Asian Studies) 11:238–255 (in Japanese).

Kunstadter, P.
1978 "Do Cultural Differences Make Any Difference? Choice Points in Medical Systems Available in Northwestern Thailand," in *Culture and Healing in Asian Societies,* A. Kleinmann et al., eds. Cambridge, Mass.: Schenkman Publishing Co.

láddaawan bunrádtànákɔɔnkìd and thànɔ̌ɔmcìd sùphaawítaa
1975 *chɤ̂y phɤ̂ydsàmǔnphraj lɛ́ʔ pràjòod* (Names of Medicinal Plants and Their Use). Bangkok: Mimeographed.

ládthíthamniam tàaŋtàaŋ (Various Traditional Customs). 2 vols.
1961– 1963 Bangkok: hɔ̌ɔsamùd hɛ̀ɛŋ châad. (The National Library).

Lafont, P.-B.
1959 "Practiques médicales des Thai noirs du Laos de l'ouest," *Anthropos* 54:819–840.

Lampang Health Development Project: A Thai Primary Health Care Approach.
1978 Bangkok: Ministry of Public Health.

Leslie, C.
1973 "Toward the Comparative Study of Asian Medical Systems," *Current Anthropology* 14:508–510.

Leslie, C. (ed.)
1976 *Asian medical systems: A comparative study.* Berkeley, Los Angeles, London: University of California Press.

Lord, D. C.
1969 *Mo Bradley and Thailand.* Grand Rapids, Mich.: Wm. B. Ferdonans Publishing Co.

maaníd maanídcàrəən
1971 *phódcanaanúkromthaj* (A Thai Dictionary). Bangkok: ʔèegkàsǐnlápàkaanphim.

Macdonald, K. N.
1879 *The Practice of Medicine Among the Burmese.* Edinburg: Maclachlan and Stewart (reprinted by AMS Press, New York, 1979).

Macey, P.
1910 "L'art de guérir au Laos," *Revue indochinoise,* Janvier 1910.

McFarland, G. B.
1944 *Thai-English Dictionary.* California: Stanford University Press.

McFarland, B. B.
1958 *McFarland of Siam.* New York: Vantage Press.

McGilvary, D.
1919 *A Half Century among the Siamese and the Lao.* New York: Fleming H. Revell Co.

McKay, D. A.
1971 "Food, Illness, and Folk Medicine: Insights from Ulu Trengganu, West Malaysia," *Ecology and Food Nutrition* 1:67–72.

mêed rádtànáprasìd
1965 *phódcanaanúkrom thajjuan-thaj-ʔaŋkrìd* (A Northern Thai-Bangkok Thai-English Dictionary). Bangkok.

Muecke, M. A.
1979 "An Explication of 'Wind illness' in Northern Thailand," *Culture, Medicine and Psychiatry* 3:267–300.

Mulholland, J.
1977 *Thai Traditional Medicine: A Preliminary Investigation.* Canberra: Australian National University. Thesis.
1979*a* "Thai Traditional Medicine: Ancient Thought and Practice in a Thai Context," *Journal of the Siam Society* 67:80–115.
1979*b* *Thai Traditional Medicine: The Treatment of Diseases Caused by the Tridosa.* Paper presented at IASTAM I, Canberra.
1979*c* "Traditional Medicine in Thailand," *Hemisphere* 23:224–229.

năŋsỳy ʔànúsɔ̀ɔn khánáʔphɛ̂ɛdphɛ̌ɛnbooraan: sàthǎanphájaabaan banthawthúg booraan phâagnỳa khróbrɔ̂ɔb cèd pii (A Commemorative Volume for the Traditional Doctors: The 7th Anniversary of the Traditional Clinic in Northern Thailand).
1974 Chiangmai: sàmaakhom rooŋrian phɛ̂ɛdphɛ̌ɛnbooraan hɛ̀ɛŋ pràthɛ̂ɛdthaj sǎakhǎaphâagnỳa (The Northern Branch of the Association of Traditional Doctors in Thailand).

nídthêedsùgkìd (khǔn-)
1953 *ʔaajúráwêed sỳgsǎa: wíchaaphɛ̂ɛd phɛ̂ɛnbooraan* (Āyurvedic Studies: Traditional Medicine). Bangkok: phiisǐi phûmchuusǐi (2d ed.), 1973.

nítàjásǎan pheesàd-ʔaajúráwêed (Pharmaceutical and Āyurvedic Journal).
1964 Bangkok: sàmaakhom pheesàd lɛ́ʔ ʔaajúráwêedbooraan hɛ̀ɛŋ pràthêedthaj (The Āyurvedic Society of Thailand).

Opler, M. E.
1963 "The Cultural Definition of Illness in Village India," *Human Organization* 22:32–35.

pàrinjaa ʔùthídchálaanon
1974 *khambanjaaj wíchaaphɛ̂ɛd phɛ̌ɛnbooraan* (Explanations to Tra-

ditional Medicine). Bangkok: kɔɔŋwíchaakaan phɛ̂ɛdphɛ̌ɛnbooraan, wád máhǎathâad (Traditional Doctor Study Division, Wat Mahathad).

phɛ̂ɛdsàad sǒŋkhrɔ́ʔ (Medical Assistance). 3 vols.

1964–1976 Bangkok: sàmaakhom rooŋrian phɛ̂ɛdphɛ̌ɛnbooraan, wád phráchêedtùphon (Society of the School of Traditional Medicine, Wat Pho).

phíchaan phádthánaa

1966 *khwaampenmaa khɔ̌ɔŋ kaanphɛ̂ɛd myanthaj* (Accounts from the History of Medicine in Thailand). Bangkok: ʔoodian satoo (Odeon Store).

phídsànáprásàadwêed

1970 *wêedchásỳgsǎa: phɛ̂ɛdsàadsǎŋkhèeb* (Medical Studies: An Outline). Bangkok: rooŋrian wêedchásàmoosɔ̌ɔn.

phódcanaanúkrom phɛ̂ɛd pheesàd thaj (A Dictionary of Thai Medical and Pharmaceutical Terms).

1964 Bangkok: sàmaakhom pheesàd lɛ́ʔ ʔaajúráwêedbooraan hɛ̀ɛŋ pràthêedthaj (The Āyurvedic Society of Bangkok).

Piat, M.

1965 "Médecine populaire au Cambodge," *Bulletin de la Societé des Etudes Indochinoises* [Saigon] 40:301–315.

Poshakrishna, U.

1963 "Geschichte der Chirurgie in Thailand, 1828–1922," *Journal of the Siam Society* 51:59–78.

Pottier, R.

1971 "Le végétal dans la pharmacopée traditionelle lao," *Bulletin de la Societé botanique de France* 118:263–273.

1972 "Introduction á l'étude des pratiques therapeutiques Lao," *Asie du Sud-Est et Monde Insulindien* 3:173–193.

pràmuan sàbphákhun jaathaj wâadûaj phrýgsàchâad wádthùthâad lɛ́ʔ sàdwádthùʔ naanaachánid (A Compilation of the Properties of Various Thai Drugs from the Botanical, Mineral, and Animal Kingdoms). 3 vols.

1963–1969 Bangkok: sàmaakhom rooŋrian phɛ̂ɛdphɛ̌ɛnbooraan naj pràthêedthaj, wád phráchêedtùphon (The Society of the School of Traditional Medicine in Thailand, Wat Pho).

pràsə̀əd lÿaŋkeesɔ̌ɔn

1962 "pràwàd kaanphɛ̂ɛd naj samăjlăŋ khɔ̌ɔŋ rádchákaanthîihâa (B.E. 2432–2453)," (The Medical History of the Latter Part of the Fifth Reign [1889–1910]), *sǎansìrírâad* (Siriraj Journal) 1962: 562–567.

Riley, J. N., F. L. Mitchell, Jr., and D. Bensky

1979 *Thai Manipulative Medicine as represented in the Wat Pho Epigraphies.* Revised version of a paper presented at ICTAM 1, Canberra. Mimeographed.

Riley, J. N., and S. Sermsri

1974 *The variegated Thai medical system as a context for birth control services.* Working Paper no. 6. Bangkok: Institute for Population and Social Research, Mahidol University.

sàmăj canthâwímon

1954 "kaanphɛ̂ɛd khɔ̌ɔŋ pràthêedthaj: rádchákaan thîisăam - rádchákaan thîisìi" (Medicine in Thailand: The 3rd and the 4th Reigns), *Journal of the Medical Association of Thailand* 37:317–330.

sămraan woŋphâa

1952 "pràwàdkaanphɛ̂ɛdthaj: tamraajaa càag sìlaacaarÿg wád râadcháʔoorásăaraam (History of Thai Medicine: The Medical Treatise inscribed at Raja-orasaram temple)," *sǎansìrírâad* (Siriraj Journal) Jan. 1952.

sàmŭn phraj (Medicinal plants).

1978 Journal published by sàthăaban sòŋsə̌əm kaankhónkhwáa sàmŭnphraj ràwàaŋ pràthêed (International Institute of Pharmacological Research Extension). Nakorn Pathon.

sàŋàd plèeŋwaaníd

n.d. *pràwàdkaanphɛ̂ɛd khɔ̌ɔŋ pràthêedthaj* (A Medical History of Thailand). Pp. 117–129. (Publisher and locale unknown.)

Sassady, K.

1962 *Contribution à l'étude de la médecine laotienne.* Thèse No. 326. Paris: Faculté de Médecine, Université de Paris.

Scarpa, A.

1964 "La medicina tradizionale del Siam secondo un manoscritto su scorza d'albero," *Castalia* 20:3–8.

Schneider, J.

1975 *Communication Between Doctors and Patients in Thailand.* Part V, "The Doctor's Image as Rated by Himself and Others." Saarbrücken: Sozialpsychologische Forschungsstelle für Entwicklungsplanung, Universität des Saarlandes.

Schumacher, T.

1979 *Diagnostic and therapeutic practices in Northern Thai Traditional Medicine.* Paper presented at IASTAM I, Canberra.

1980 *Medico-botanical investigations in Northern Thai Traditional Medicine.* Paper presented at ASOMPS 4, Bangkok.

sèeg sɔ̆ɔnlam

n.d. *nɛɛwkhwaamrúu kaansỳgsǎa wêedchákam phɛ̌ɛnbooraan* (Insights in the Study of Traditional Medicine). Bangkok: sàmaakhom phɛ̂ɛdphɛ̌ɛnbooraan, wád máhǎathâad (Society of Traditional Doctors, Wat Mahathad).

sǐnthɔɔn chajchàkan

1977 *khûumyysỳgsǎa làgwíchaa pheesàdchákam phɛ̌ɛnbooraan* (A Study Manual in the Principles of Traditional Pharmacy). Chiangmai: rooŋphájaabaan banthawthúg booraan phâagnỳa (The traditional clinic in Northern Thailand).

Smith, M.

1947 *A Physician at the Court of Siam.* London: Country Life Ltd.

Spire, C.

1907 *Les Laotiens: Coutumes, Hygiène, Pratiques médicales.* Paris: Librairie Maritime et Coloniale.

Strange, H.

1973 "Illnesses and Treatments in a Malay Village," *Asian Journal of Medicine* 9:362–366.

sùd sɛ̌ɛŋwíchian

1978 "cùdcòb khɔ̆ɔŋ phɛ̂ɛdphɛ̌ɛnbooraan lɛ́ʔ kaanrə̂əmtôn khɔ̆ɔŋ kaanphɛ̂ɛdphɛ̌ɛnpàdcùban khɔ̆ɔŋthaj" (The End of Traditional Medicine and the Beginning of Modern Medicine in Thailand), *waarásǎan sǎŋkhomsàadkaanphɛ̂ɛd* 1:20–27.

tamraajaa caarýg wádrâadcháʔooród lɛ́ʔ phráʔoosòd phránaaraaj (Medical Manuals: Inscriptions at Raja-orot Temple and the Medicines of Naraj).

1979 Bangkok: khrooŋkaan phǝ̌ǝjphrɛ̂ɛʔèegkàlág khɔ̌ɔŋ thaj (Ministry of Education).

tamraa pheesàdchákamthaj phɛ̌ɛnbooraan (A textbook in Traditional Thai Pharmacy).
1973 Bangkok: sàmaakhom phɛ̂ɛdphɛ̌ɛnbooraan, wád máhǎathâad (Society of Traditional Doctors, Wat Mahathad).

tamraapheesàd phrábàadsǒmdèdphráʔnâŋklâwcâwjùuhǔa (Medical Texts Which His Majesty King Rama III Had Engraved at Phra Chetuphon Temple [Wat Pho] in B.E. 2375 [A.D. 1832]).
1977 Bangkok: Association of the Traditional Medical School.

tamraa pràmuan làg pheesàd (A Textbook in the Fundamentals of Pharmacy).
1978 Bangkok: rooŋrian phɛ̂ɛdphɛ̌ɛnbooraan, wád phráchêedtùphon (School of Traditional Medicine, Wat Pho).

tamraajaa sàmǔnphraj laannaa (Traditional Lanna Thai Medical Text).
1979 Compiled by Palm Leaf Text Studies Program. Chiangmai: Faculty of Social Sciences, University of Chiangmai.

Tantivatana, P., and D. Pongluk
1979 *Traditional and Folk Medicine in Thailand.* Paper presented at IASTAM I, Canberra.

Umemoto, D. L.
1980 "Medicine and Massage," *Sawaddi 1980* (Jan-Feb): 13–16 (+39).

Vidal, J.
1958 "La thérapeutique par les plantes au Laos," *Journal d'Agriculture tropicale et de botanique appliquée* 5:601–616.
1963 "Médecine populaire et plantes médecinales du Laos," *Communication à la Societé Française d'Homéopathie* 7:533–542.
1972 "Manuscrits de médecine populaire lao et leur intérêt ethnolinguistique. Langues et Techniques, Nature et Societé, "in *Approche ethnologique. Approche naturaliste.* J. M. C. Thomas and L. Bernot, eds. Paris: Klincksiek.

Vilaiporn Bharabhutanonda
1980 "The Medical Role of the 'Doctor Bhikku' in Bangkok and Rural Communities," *Journal of National Research Council of Thailand* 12:11–60.

waarásăan săŋkhomsàadkaanphɛ̂ɛd (Journal of Medical Sociology)
1978– 1980 Bangkok: Faculty of Social Sciences and Humanities, Mahidol University, *1* (2) (1978), *1* (3) (1978), *2* (4) (1980).

Wales, H. G. Q.
1933 "Siamese Theory and Ritual Connected with Pregnancy, Birth and Infancy," *Journal of the Royal Anthropological Institute of Great Britain and Ireland* 63:441–451.

WHO (World Health Organization)
1978 "The promotion and development of traditional medicine," *World Health Organization Technical Report Series* 622:1–40.

Yoddumnern, Benja
1974 *The Role of Thai Traditional Doctors.* Bangkok: Mahidol University, Institute for Population and Social Research.
1976 *khwaamchŷa lɛ́ʔ booríphôognísăj khɔ̆ɔŋ pràchaachon thaaŋphâagnŷa khɔ̆ɔŋ pràthêedthaj* (Beliefs and Nutritional Habits of the Inhabitants of Northern Thailand). Bangkok. Mimeographed.

Århem, P.
1977 "Traditional Medicine in Northern Thailand," *The Scandinavian Institute of Asian Studies, Special Publication no. 5:* 133–136.

Indexes

Note: The following index includes, besides relevant words from the text proper with normal page references, the medical terms occurring in the vocabularies (pp. 48–52, 54–59, 144, 151–155), as well as "medical use" in the List of Medicinal Plants in the Appendix. Instead of page references to the occurrences of these words, we have inserted their English translation. These translations serve as a dictionary for the words in the column "medical use"—which have been translated nowhere else in the book—and at the same time save readers the time to search for a word in the vocabularies inside the book, when the only information they would get there is a translation.

The special phonetic signs used to transcribe Northern Thai (underlined below) have been given the following position in the alphabet:

a, b, c, d, e, $\underline{\varepsilon}$, $\underline{\text{ə}}$, f, g, h, i, j, k, l, m, n, $\underline{\text{ŋ}}$, $\underline{\text{ñ}}$, o, $\underline{\text{ɔ}}$, p, r, s, t, u, w, y.

Index of Northern Thai Medical Terms

Index of Western Medical Terms and Related Terminology

Index of Botanical Vernacular Names

COMPARATIVE STUDIES OF HEALTH SYSTEMS AND MEDICAL CARE

John M. Janzen, *The Quest for Therapy in Lower Zaire*

Paul U. Unschuld, *Medical Ethics in Imperial China: A Study in Historical Anthropology*

Margaret M. Lock, *East Asian Medicine in Urban Japan: Varieties of Medical Experience*

Jeanie Schmit Kayser-Jones, *Old, Alone, and Neglected: Care of the Aged in Scotland and in the United States*

Arthur Kleinman, *Patients and Healers in the Context of Culture: An Exploration of the Borderland between Anthropology, Medicine, and Psychiatry*

Stephen J. Kunitz, *Disease Change and the Role of Medicine: The Navajo Experience*

Carol Laderman, *Wives and Midwives: Childbirth and Nutrition in Rural Malaysia*

Victor G. Rodwin, *The Health Planning Predicament: France, Québec, England, and the United States*

Michael W. Dols and Adil S. Gamal, *Medieval Islamic Medicine: Ibn Riḍwān's Treatise "On the Prevention of Bodily Ills in Egypt"*

Leith Mullings, *Therapy, Ideology, and Social Change: Mental Healing in Urban Ghana*

Jean de Kervasdoué, John R. Kimberly, and Victor G. Rodwin, editors, *The End of an Illusion: The Future of Health Policy in Western Industrialized Nations*

Arthur J. Rubel, Carl W. O'Nell, and Rolando Collado-Ardón, *Susto, a Folk Illness*

Paul U. Unschuld, *Medicine in China: A History of Ideas*

Paul U. Unschuld, *Medicine in China: A History of Pharmaceutics*

Glenn Gritzer and Arnold Arluke, *The Making of Rehabilitation: A Political Economy of Medical Specialization, 1890–1980*

Arthur Kleinman and Bryon Good, editors, *Culture and Depression: Studies in the Anthropology and Cross-Cultural Psychiatry of Affect and Disorder*

Judith Justice, *Policies, Plans, and People: Culture and Health Development in Nepal*

Paul U. Unschuld, *Nan-ching—The Classic of Difficult Issues*

Viggo Brun and Trond Schumacher, *Traditional Herbal Medicine in Northern Thailand*

Designer:	Marvin Warshaw
Compositor:	Publisher's Typography
Text:	10/12 Baskerville
Display:	Baskerville
Printer:	Edwards Bros., Inc.
Binder:	Edwards Bros., Inc.